Understanding CARE, WELFARE and COMMUNITY

Care, welfare and community are three key concepts in contemporary social policy. This reader covers a wide range of topics associated with them and which are relevant to the delivery of care and support to adults living in the community. It includes a wide-ranging collection of articles by leading writers and researchers, some previously published, some newly commissioned. It also has first-hand accounts by users and providers of care and welfare in the community. Groups covered include people with mental health problems, homeless people, older people, people with learning difficulties and people with impairments. The focus throughout is on how policies and practice can be developed appropriately and sensitively through an understanding of current issues.

The chapters are grouped into four sections, each with an introduction:

- Power and Inequality
- Difference and Identity
- Rights and Risk
- Territories and Boundaries.

Most of the material relates to a diverse turn-of-the-century Britain, but this is set in a wider context enabling the student to explore the alternative realities of other countries or other times.

Understanding Care, Welfare and Community provides an integrated, multidisciplinary overview of the many different aspects of community care. It is appropriate for students and professionals following a wide range of courses in social work, nursing, care, health, social policy, medicine, voluntary work and welfare services. It will also be a valuable resource for teachers and policy makers.

Bill Bytheway, Vivien Bacigalupo, Joanna Bornat, Julia Johnson, Susan Spurr, all work in the School of Health and Social Welfare at The Open University.

Open University Course:
Care, Welfare and Community (K202)

This Reader forms part of The Open University course *Care, Welfare and Community* (K202), a 60 points second level undergraduate course. It is an optional course for the BA/BSc (Open) and the BA/BSc in Health and Social Care, as well as being a core course for the Diploma in Health and Social Welfare. A shorter version of K202 is also a component of the National Open Learning Programme (NOLP), which leads to a Diploma in Social Work (DipSW) and a Diploma of Higher Education (DipHE SW) awarded by The Open University.

The chapters in this book have been designed as a source for students during their study of this course. The primary focus throughout is how policies and practice can be sensitively and appropriately developed through an understanding of current issues surrounding care, welfare and community. Opinions expressed in the Reader are not necessarily those of the Course Team or of The Open University.

If you are interested in studying this course or working towards a related degree or diploma please write to the Information Officer, School of Health and Social Welfare, The Open University, Walton Hall, Milton Keynes, MK7 6AA, UK. Details can also be viewed on our web page http://www.open.ac.uk.

Understanding CARE, WELFARE and COMMUNITY
A READER

Edited by Bill Bytheway, Vivien Bacigalupo,
Joanna Bornat, Julia Johnson and Susan Spurr

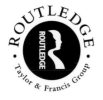

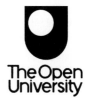

London and New York

First published 2002
by Routledge
11 New Fetter Lane, London EC4P 4EE

Simultaneously published in the USA and Canada
by Routledge
29 West 35th Street, New York, NY 10001

Routledge is an imprint of the Taylor & Francis Group

Typeset in 10/12 Sabon by Wearset Ltd, Boldon, Tyne and Wear
Printed and bound in Great Britain by Biddles Ltd, Guildford and
King's Lynn

British Library Cataloguing in Publication Data
A catalogue record for this book is available from the British Library

Library of Congress Cataloging in Publication Data
Understanding care, welfare and community : a reader / edited by
Bill Bytheway ... [et al.].
      p. cm.
   "This reader forms part of The Open University course Care,
welfare and community (K202)"–P. .
   Includes bibliographical references and index.
   1. Human services–Great Britain–Case studies. 2. Social
service–Great Britain–Case studies. 3. Socially handicapped–
Great Britain–Attitudes–Case studies. 4. Welfare recipients–Great
Britain–Attitudes–Case studies. 5. Human services–Cross-cultural
studies. I. Bytheway, Bill.

   HV245 .U53 2001
   361.941–dc21
                                                           2001052001
   ISBN 0-415-25859-6 (hbk.)
   ISBN 0-415-25860-X (pbk.)

CONTENTS

Preface   xi
Acknowledgements   xv

PART I
Power and Inequality   1

Introduction   1

1   Unsettled lives   3

    1.1   In exile   3
        AIT

    1.2   Places in between   5
        CAS ALLAND

    1.3   From community to institution – and back again   8
        DAVID BARRON

    1.4   Living in the borderlands of disability   11
        CAROL THOMAS

2   William and Teresa   13
    ALAN PERRY

3   The effects of poverty   20
    PETER BERESFORD, DAVID GREEN, RUTH LISTER
    AND KIRSTY WOODARD

4   Poverty and the social services   29
    MARK DRAKEFORD

5 **Witnesses to welfare**   38

    5.1   Ways of labeling the poor   38
        HERBERT J. GANS

    5.2   An end to welfare rights   41
        DAVID G. GREEN

    5.3   An unemployment assistance investigator in the 1930s   43
        GLADYS GIBSON

    5.4   Disabled people and disincentives to work   45
        CLIFF PRIOR

    5.5   Who are social services for?   47
        PETER BERESFORD AND SUZY CROFT

    5.6   The needs of strangers   50
        MICHAEL IGNATIEFF

6 **The history of community care for people with learning difficulties**   53
    JAN WALMSLEY AND SHEENA ROLPH

7 **Multiple oppression and the disabled people's movement**   64
    AYESHA VERNON

8 **Campaigning and the pensioners' movement**   69
    DAVE GOODMAN

9 **Settling in and moving on**   76
    JAN REED, VALERIE ROSKELL PAYTON AND SENGA BOND

10 **Paying for nursing home care**   83
    MARGARET FORSTER

PART II
Difference and Identity   87

Introduction   87

11 **Different communities**   89

    11.1 The communities of football and sickle cell   89
        GARTH CROOKS AND ROXY HARRIS

    11.2 Memories of a rural community   92
        MAURICE HAYES

11.3 Being part of a psychiatric community   93
KEITH SHIRES

11.4 They all help each other on the Island   95
JANET FOSTER

11.5 Communities on the move   96
KEVIN HETHERINGTON

11.6 The spirit of community   100
AMITAI ETZIONI

12 The regeneration of communities   103
STEVE CLARKE

13 Social change, networks and family life   112
CHRIS PHILLIPSON, MIRIAM BERNARD, JUDITH PHILLIPS
AND JIM OGG

14 Problematizing social care needs in minority
communities   121
KEN BLAKEMORE

15 A child's view of care in the community   130
MEERA SYAL

16 Community and stigma   138

16.1 The principle of normalization   138
WOLF WOLFENSBERGER AND STEPHEN TULLMAN

16.2 Stigma and social identity   143
ERVING GOFFMAN

16.3 Liberation and schizophrenia   145
DAVID COOPER

16.4 Critical psychiatry   146
PHIL THOMAS AND JOANNA MONCRIEFF

16.5 The sanatorium at Virginia Water   148
BILL BRYSON

17 Ageing, learning difficulties and maintaining
independence   151
ALAN WALKER AND CAROL WALKER

18 Whiteness and emotions in social care   158
YASMIN GUNARATNAM

19 On becoming a disabled person   168
    ANDREW HUBBARD

20 Remind me who I am, again   174
    LINDA GRANT

    PART III
    Rights and Risk   181

    Introduction   181

21 Risk and dangerousness   183
    ANDY ALASZEWSKI

22 Evaluating self-determination   192
    MICHAEL PRESTON-SHOOT

23 Out in the world   205
    JEAN

24 The prospect of residential care   209
    JABER GUBRIUM

25 Independence, privacy and risk   216
    ROSEMARY BLAND

26 Malignant social psychology   225
    TOM KITWOOD

27 Exposing abuse in care homes   232
    JOHN BURTON

28 Regulating informality: small homes and the inspectors   240
    CAROLINE HOLLAND AND SHEILA PEACE

29 Community care law and the Human Rights Act 1998   247
    LUKE CLEMENTS

30 Self-advocacy for people with learning difficulties   255
    SIMONE ASPIS

    PART IV
    Territories and Boundaries   263

    Introduction   263

31 Community care in the information age   265
    JOHN HUDSON

32 Providing support   274

    32.1 House calls   274
          CAROLE MCHUGH

    32.2 Organising voluntary support   276
          JOHN SWAIN AND SALLY FRENCH

    32.3 Being reorganised   280
          JULIA JOHNSON

33 Carework and bodywork   285
    JULIA TWIGG

34 European policies on home care services compared   299
    CAROLINE GLENDINNING

35 The boundary between health and social care for
    older people   313
    JANE LEWIS

36 Health and social care assessment in action   321
    ALLISON WORTH

37 The importance of housing and home   330
    CHRISTINE OLDMAN

38 Partnerships between disabled people and service
    providers   341
    FRANCES HASLER

39 Care as a commodity   351
    CLARE UNGERSON

40 Good companions   362

    40.1 Working as a 'Country Cousin'   362
          ALICE KADEL

    40.2 'Being a thing called a companion'   364
          DAPHNE DU MAURIER

    40.3 It's my party: personal assistants and your
          social life   366
          RUTH BAILEY

Index   369

PREFACE

Care. Welfare. Community. Three familiar and simple words that para-doxically take a great deal of understanding. In compiling this Reader, our primary objective has been to include a wide variety of writings that cast light on the associations which these concepts provoke and those areas of people's lives which they seek to describe and explain. Two basic questions thread through the Reader and have informed the selection of material included. These are: how do people experience and make sense of care and support, and how have we got to where we are today in organising and providing this.

The policy landscape has changed considerably since 1990. The NHS and Community Care Act 1990 had a major impact on the nature and delivery of community-based services. Further legislation, regulation and official guidance has followed with: recognition for carers, disability dis-crimination law, direct payments to care users, single assessments, and partnerships at all levels of provision between health and social care, as well as national standards of service posing new challenges and opportunities for practitioners and users of services alike. Policy flowing from central government is generating a new terminology, changing responsibilities and introducing innovatory practices. It is transforming understandings of where care is located on the wider map of social real-ities.

Not far below the surface of all these changes, some continuities persist. There are debates and dilemmas which will not go away, no matter how much the language changes or the focus shifts. So, we include key texts which address issues such as poverty, homelessness, racism and abuse that have a significance for society which reaches far beyond the detail of even the most tightly drawn regulations and guidance.

The story presented in this collection draws on a wide range of sources. We have included accounts written by the recipients of services, and by people involved in systems for providing care and welfare. In our view the very existence of such witness statements offers a dimension of hopefulness in a history which has been characterised, often appropriately, as cruel and indifferent.

The writings that make up this book come from many different disciplines, literatures and political orientations. Most have been written in the relatively recent past, but there are several which refer back to the first half of the twentieth century. Similarly, most relate directly to the existing situation in various parts of the United Kingdom, but there are also a few contributions which draw attention to policy and practice in Europe and in the USA. Cross-national comparisons add to our understanding and critical reflection on our own domestic preoccupations and assumptions.

The Reader is organised in four Parts, around the themes of: power and inequality, difference and identity, rights and risks, and territories and boundaries. Each part has a short introduction in which we discuss these themes and introduce the various chapters. We decided on the sequence of chapters in part by common links, but also by contrasting perspectives. So, for example, the analyses of risk and self-determination offered by Alaszewski and Preston-Shoot are followed by Jean's autobiographical account of living with risk and achieving a life of her own choosing. Similarly, Ungerson's review of how care can be paid for is set between Hasler's defence of direct payments and Chapter 40 which includes three very different accounts of paid companionship.

Throughout, our aim has been to create a broad basis for understanding how care and support is organised in relation to *care*, *welfare* and *community*. The themes with which we have organised the book draw out, for example, how institutions, social groups and individuals respond to *inequalities* and *power* differentials, and how *difference* is recognised and experienced and *identity* expressed and communicated. They illustrate the struggles of individuals seeking to assert their *rights*, whilst others may try to contain them in order to minimise *risk*. *Territories* and *boundaries* draw attention to how areas of public and private life are patrolled and owned, creating barriers as well as opportunities for shared experience in the organisation of care.

As editors, we hope that this Reader will provide you with the opportunity to explore these various key concepts 'at the ground level'. You may already have a good, indeed expert, understanding of some particular care setting or particular need for support. If so, we are confident that you will see some of this reflected in what you read, and that, taken together, the chapters will provide you with opportunities for comparison and reflection.

We wish to acknowledge the enthusiastic collaboration of the many contributors, the support of colleagues at The Open University, and not least the professional expertise of the staff at Routledge. Just one name need be mentioned: Dave Goodman died whilst the book was being edited. In our view, his chapter epitomises much that is excellent and forward-looking in the field of care, welfare and community. We dedicate the Reader to his memory.

Bill Bytheway, Vivien Bacigalupo, Joanna Bornat, Julia Johnson, Susan Spurr

ACKNOWLEDGEMENTS

The editors and publishers are grateful to the following for permission to include their material in this reader.

1.1   Ait, *iNexile*, pp. 14–15, Refugee Council, 8 January 2000.
1.3   David Barron, 'From Community to Institution and Back Again', from Brigham *et al.* (eds) *Crossing Boundaries: Change and Continuity in the History of Learning Disability*, BILD, 2000, pp. 10–13.
1.4   Carol Thomas, 'Living in the Borderlands of Disability', from *Female Forms: Experiencing and Understanding Disability*, Open University Press, 1999, pp. 54–5.
2   Alan Perry, 'William and Teresa', from *Music You Don't Normally Hear*, Alun Books, Port Talbot, 1998, © Alan Perry, pp. 35–42.
3   Peter Beresford, David Green, Ruth Lister, Kirsty Woodard, 'The Effects of Poverty', from *Poverty First Hand: Poor People Speak for Themselves*, CPAG, 1999, pp. 34–9, 89–108, 143–4, 205.
5.1   Herbert J. Gans, 'Ways of Labeling the Poor', from *The War Against the Poor*, pp. 14–18, Basic Books, 1995. Copyright © 1995 by Herbert J. Gans Reprinted by permission of Basic Books, a member of Perseus Books, L.L.C.
5.2   David G. Green, *An End to Welfare Rights: the Discovery of Independence*, Institute of Economic Affairs, 1999, reprinted by permission of Civitas, pp. 67–9.
5.3   Gladys Gibson (in the voice of), 'An Unemployment Investigator in the 1930s', from © Nigel Gray, *The Worst of Times*, Wildwood House, 1985, pp. 60–1, reprinted by permission of Ashgate Publishing Limited.
5.4   Cliff Prior, 'Disabled People and Disincentives to Work', published from 'Swallowed up by the system', *Community Care*, pp. 26–7, 29 July–4 August 1999. Published by permission of the editor of Community Care.
5.5   Peter Beresford and Suzy Croft, 'Who Are Social Services For?' from

Whose Welfare? Private Care or Public Services, Lewis Cohen Urban Studies Centre, pp. 42–4.

5.6 Michael Ignatieff, 'The Needs of Strangers', from *The Needs of Strangers*, Viking, 1984, pp. 9–12, first published by Chatto & Windus. Reprinted by permission of The Random House Group Ltd, (Territories, British Commonwealth) Sheil Land Associates Ltd for remaining territories.

6 Jan Walmsley and Sheena Rolph, 'The History of Community Care for People with Learning Difficulties', from *Development of Community Care for People with Learning Difficulties, 1913–1946* in *Critical Social Policy*, Vol. 21 (1), pp. 59–80. Reprinted by permission of Sage Publications Ltd.

7 Ayesha Vernon, 'Multiple Oppression and the Disabled People's Movement', from 'The Disability Reader: Social Science Perspective', Tom Sheakespeare (ed), Chapter 13, pp. 205–10, Continuum, 1998.

9 Jan Reed, Valerie Roskell Payton and Senga Bond, 'Settling In and Moving On', in *Social Policy and Administration*, 32 (2), pp. 151–65, 1998 © Blackwell Publishers Ltd

10 Margaret Forster, 'Paying for Nursing Home Care', adapted from an article in *The Independent Magazine*, pp. 26–7, 2 September 1995.

11.1 Garth Crooks interviewed by Roxy Harris, 'The Communitites of Football and Sickle Cell', from *Changing Britannia: Life Experience with Britain*, edited by Roxy Harris and Sarah White, New Beacon Books and the George Padmore Institute, 1999, pp. 29–30, 41–2.

11.2 Maurice Hayes, 'Memories of a Rural Community', from *Sweet Killough: Let Your Anchor Go*, Blackstaff Press, 1994, pp. 191–3.

11.4 Janet Foster, 'They All Help Each Other in East End Communities', from *Docklands*, UCL Press, 1999, pp. 190–1.

11.5 Kevin Hetherington, 'Communities on the Move', from *New Age Travellers*, pp. 80–6, Cassell, 2000.

11.6 From *The Spirit of Community* by Amitai Etzioni, pp. 30–6, copyright © 1993 Amitai Etzioni. Used by permission of Crown Publishers, a division of Random House, Inc, (territories: US, Canada, P.I., Open Market). Used by permission of HarperCollins Publishers Ltd, (territories UK, Canada).

13 Chris Phillipson, Miriam Bernard, Judith Philips and Jim Ogg, 'Social Change, Networks and Family Life', adapted from a chapter in Susan McRae (ed.), *Changing Britain: Families and Households in the 1990s*, Oxford University Press, 1999.

14 Ken Blakemore, 'Problematizing Social Care Needs in Minority Communities', from *Health and Social Care in the Community*, 8.1, pp. 22–30, 2000, © Blackwell Science

15 Meera Syal, an extract from *Anita and Me*, pp. 57–68, Flamingo, 1997, reprinted by permission of HarperCollins Publishers Ltd for rights in World territories excluding the USA. For rights in USA

© Meera Syal 1996. Reproduced by permission of the Author c/o Rogers, Coleridge & White Ltd., 20 Powis Mews, London W11 1JN.

16.1 Wolf Wolfensberger and Stephen Tullman, 'The Principle of Normalization', from *Rehabilitation Psychology*, 27 (3), pp. 131, 147, 1982, used by permission of © Springer Publishing Company, Inc., New York 10012

16.2 Erving Goffman, 'Stigma and Social Identity', from *Stigma: Notes on the Management of Spoilt Identity*, pp. 11–15, 17–18. Reprinted with the permission of Simon and Schuster, Inc. Copyright © 1963 by Prentice Hall: copyright renewed 1991 by Simon & Schuster, Inc.

16.3 David Cooper, 'Liberation and Schizophrenia', from *The Dialectics of Liberation*, Penguin, pp. 7–8, 1968.

16.4 Phil Thomas and Joanna Moncrieff, 'Critical Psychiatry', from http://www.critpsynet.freeuk.com

16.5 © Bill Bryson. Extracted from *Notes from a Small Island*, published by Transworld Publishers, a division of the Random House Group Ltd. All rights reserved for territories – United Kingdom and Commonwealth. HarperCollins Publishers Inc for territories – USA.

17 Alan Walker and Carol Walker, 'Ageing, Learning Difficulties and Maintaining Independence', from *Disability and Society*, 13.1, pp. 129–42, Taylor and Francis, 1998. http://www.tandf.co.uk/

20 Linda Grant, *Remind Me Who I Am, Again*, pp. 185–93, 233–8, 1998, with permission of Granta books.

22 Michael Preston-Shoot, 'Evaluating Self-Determination: An Adult Protection Case Study', from *Journal of Adult Protection*, 3.1, pp. 4–15, February 2001. Reproduced by permission of Pavilion Publishing (Brighton) Ltd.

24 Jaber Gubrium, an extract from *The Mosaic of Care: Frail Elderly and their Families in the Real World*, pp. 72–4, 88–92, used by permission of © Springer Publishing Company, Inc., New York 10012.

25 Rosemary Bland, 'Independence Privacy and Risk: Two Contrasting Approaches to Residential Care for Older People', from *Ageing and Society*, 19 (5) pp. 539–60. © Cambridge University Press.

26 Tom Kitwood, 'Malignant Social Psychology', from *Dementia Reconsidered: the Person Comes First*, pp. 38–42, 45–9, Open University Press, 1997.

27 John Burton, 'Exposing Abuse in Care Homes', from *Managing Residential Care*, pp. 222–31, Routledge, London, 1998.

30 Simone Aspis, 'Self-advocacy for People with Learning Disabilities', from *Disability and Society*, 12.4, pp. 647–54, Taylor and Francis, 1997. http://www.tandf.co.uk/

32.1 Carole McHugh, 'House Calls', *The Guardian: Society* 13 October 1999, p. 3.

32.2 This material first appeared in '*Confronting Disabling Barriers: Towards Making Organisations Accessible*' by John Swain, Maureen

Gilman and Sally French published by Venture Press and reproduced by permission of the British Association of Social Workers.

33   Julia Twigg, 'Carework and Bodywork', from *Bathing – the Body and Community Care*, pp. 42, 79–83, 88–9, 137–49, Routledge, 2001.

40.2 Daphne du Maurier, from *Rebecca*, pp. 19–22. Reproduced with permission of Curtis Brown Ltd, London, on behalf of The Chichester Partnership. © Daphne du Maurier 1938.

40.3 Ruth Bailey, 'It's My Party: Personal Assistants and Your Social Life', from *The Rough Guide to Managing Personal Assistants*, Sian Vasey, pp. 69–76, National Centre for Independent Living, London, 1998.

While the authors and the publishers have made every effort to contact copyright holders of the material used in this volume, they would be happy to hear from anyone they were unable to contact.

Throughout the Reader, ellipses have been used to indicate the omission of sections of previously published material and have been displayed in two ways. The exclusion of larger sections has been presented like this [. . .], while for smaller deletions . . . has been used.

POWER AND INEQUALITY

INTRODUCTION

In this section, Power and Inequality, we draw attention to the dynamics of relationships: between people, between organisations and between social groups. Even the most intimate of support relationships may involve oppressive or alienating feelings of powerlessness. Many policies relating to care, welfare and community are intended to challenge or alleviate some of the negative consequences of inequalities; for example, by ending discrimination, by empowering users, or by ensuring that priority is given to those 'most in need'.

In this first Part of the Reader, we begin with four personal accounts of 'unsettled' lives. These describe experiences of exile, mental illness, institutional life and physical disability. Although very different, they all reveal ways in which inequalities and power differentials in the care system affect interpersonal relations and life chances. In Chapter 2, a single autobiographical account describes how one couple, following family difficulties and migration, entered a state of abject poverty and fear. In Chapter 3, a Child Poverty Action Group team reports on a project that provided poor people with the opportunity to describe the effects of poverty in their own words and then, in Chapter 4, Mark Drakeford critically examines the post-Beveridge history of social security and social services. This reveals something of the power of central government, given its abiding concern with public expenditure, to limit the autonomy of local government and to determine the role of social workers.

Poverty and wealth have been the focus of much research and policy analysis throughout the twentieth century. There is a strong case for arguing that this particular dimension of social inequality is that most strongly associated with the need for care and welfare. So, in Chapter 5, we include a series of contrasting commentaries on the history of poverty and welfare. Some are based in the UK, some abroad. Issues of power and inequality and care and welfare in the community, underlie the observations of all these witnesses.

In Chapter 6, Jan Walmsley and Sheena Rolph report on their research into the history of a particular aspect of community care. They argue that the current idea that community care is new is mistaken and that there is much to be learned from studying how statutory agencies worked with – and against – families in the decades before the launching of the Welfare State. The inequality which disabled people continue to experience is detailed by Ayesha Vernon in Chapter 7. Here she articulates the anger that is widely felt by people with multiple oppressions.

Power and inequality are the driving force of political action. In Chapter 8, Dave Goodman describes his experience of campaigning and challenging current fiscal policies that directly affect the circumstances and welfare of older people. One important focus of political action is choice. In Chapter 9, we include extracts from a report on research into the moves that older people make, into and between care homes. Who has the power to determine who moves where and when? Chapter 10 is based on personal experience and provides some insight into this difficult process. Margaret Forster, the well-known novelist and biographer, vividly describes what was involved in negotiating the care of her father in the last years of his life.

CHAPTER 1

UNSETTLED LIVES

1.1 IN EXILE

Ait

Source: *iNexile*, Refugee Council, 8, January 2000, pp. 14–15.

I left my homeland Algeria in an attempt to flee persecution and horrendous acts of torture. In October of 1998 I arrived in the UK and was held in detention for the first four days after my arrival. On my release I was advised to contact the Refugee Council who would be able to advise me of my rights and provide me with accommodation.

I arrived in London on a Sunday with no money and nowhere to sleep and spent the night in Victoria station. I finally arrived at the Refugee Council on Monday morning and was sent to their One Stop Service. By this point I felt exhausted, distressed and disorientated, and after the experiences of the previous 24 hours I wished that I had remained in detention where I would at least have had a roof over my head and some form of security.

I was advised that there was no accommodation available in London and was made an offer of accommodation on a farm in Lincolnshire. I didn't want to leave London but in my emotional state coupled with my limited knowledge of English geography I agreed, reluctantly.

When I arrived in Lincolnshire I realised just how secluded the accommodation was. The farm itself was far away from the town centre. The landlord spent long periods away from the property and even when he was there it was hard for me to communicate with him due to my limited English. I started to experience the familiar feelings of loneliness and isolation, which deteriorated quite rapidly into a severe depression. My doctor advised me to return to London and with his written recommendation I left Lincolnshire and revisited the Refugee Council's One Stop Service.

By the time I arrived at the One Stop Service I was very distressed and crying. I was placed in a hotel for the first two days – then sent to a hostel for refugees where I spent the following two weeks. I was asked to leave the hostel due to the fact that I was taking medication and was advised that they do not have the facilities to cater for residents taking medication. I returned for a third time to the Refugee Council who placed me in church accommodation in North West London. All of the other residents in this accommodation were Kosovar refugees and I felt extremely isolated and uncomfortable as we could not communicate with each other. It became quite awkward for me to stay and I returned for the fourth time to the Refugee Council.

I was placed in my current accommodation, which is a room located in another church. Since my arrival I have found it very difficult to relax or rest here as there are church meetings throughout the week. This means that I cannot use my room because of the noise level and disruption caused by the music being played so loudly. This has forced me to stay out in the street during these times, which has often meant all day! I have been forced to stay in the cold without being able to use my room, which is in the middle of the main hall. Because of the noise, I have not been to sleep properly. The music keeps playing in my head, long after they have gone and I find my head spinning throughout the night. Sleeping pills have not helped me and my doctor said that he could not prescribe any stronger medicine. I cannot even rest during the day, especially when I have had such sleepless and stressful nights.

This noise level added to the fact that the room is unhygienic and has no adequate washing or bathing facilities exposes my life to unaccounted for risks. I have raised the problem with all those concerned, but I have not noticed an improvement or consideration for my health situation. My health is continuing to suffer due to having to take so much medicine without being able to recover at all. I am in a crisis situation. I do not think that it is right to leave me to undergo all this traumatising stress after all that I have suffered throughout all these many long years.

It has been nearly seven years since I departed from my homeland in Algeria and since that time I have not had anywhere that has felt like a base, a place where I have felt at ease and secure. I feel like a nomad and look forward to the time when I can once again have a space, which feels like a home, somewhere which is quiet and private. Somewhere which will contribute to my ability to recover from my traumatic experiences of the past and which will enable me to build upon for the future.

1.2 PLACES IN BETWEEN

Cas Alland

It is my view that periods of transition in our lives test to the utmost our own resourcefulness as well as that of the social networks in which we move. This is perhaps all the more so when, because of debility, we need to depend on agents outside our usual social spheres. My example is a personal one of my own transition from hospital to the community after a long illness. However I know, from the people who journeyed alongside me in similar states, that my experience is not unique. There are common themes and issues which, if left unresolved, make the problems of such transitions more traumatic.

I spent five and half months in a mental hospital. Being admitted to such a place is a shock, to me more so because I had spent ten years working in psychiatry. It is a humbling experience in which you appear to give up so much – not least the control to make decisions about your life. Your illness is the presenting picture and in the depths of despair the only hallmark that is seen by those helping you. They seldom have another reference point that indicates who you are separate from your illness. The roles you had are just labels that have their own stereotypes attached. There is little indication of your character strengths under such circumstances. If your illness is not incapacitating in itself then the sense that you are nothing more than your diagnosis can debilitate you further. The challenge is to retain a sense of who you are and convey it to others so that they have a key to give you the support that will most facilitate your recovery.

Over two months of my time in hospital was spent on a high observation unit whose objectives were to provide a high level of support and therapy whilst keeping me safe from my suicidal intentions. The unit was excellent. The boundaries were clear and the staff were confident about their role and worked well as a team. The help I received was unimaginable. I was lucky to find myself in such a place. It not only kept me safe but also allowed me to begin to deal with the issues which had brought me there. I was able to rediscover a commitment to life that I thought I had lost. It gave me the courage to face the depths of despair and challenged me to take back some control in my life. I was given permission to express myself and positively encouraged to make my own decisions and rediscover those lost reservoirs within. It is perhaps a paradox that a place that appeared to take away so much freedom helped me to be free.

A few weeks after I moved back onto the main ward I was asking to be discharged. With an impending date in sight the number of people involved in my situation increased and with it the confusion. Under the pressure to prove my need for help it was easy for me to lose touch with the progress I had made

During my period in hospital it became evident that my marriage had irretrievably broken down and for my health's sake it was inappropriate to go back to the marital home. I had been working part-time and was fortunate enough to be still receiving pay although by the time I left hospital I was being paid a quarter of a full-time salary. I was wrongly told by a social worker that I didn't qualify for any benefits because I had an income. I was informed that I was not entitled to housing because, as a single person with no dependants, I was low priority. From my own research my income was not enough to cover a private rent. After being advised to see a solicitor I discovered that I earned £10 too much to receive legal aid and could not afford the legal costs. The progress I had made was already being severely tested.

At my care programme discharge meeting there were three major areas of concern: the need to receive ongoing support and monitoring of my mental state following transition from the protected environment of hospital; the need for social support with the practical issues; and the need for long-term psychological therapy to continue working through the issues of my past. There were ten people at the meeting. If this wasn't intimidating in itself then the lack of motivation, from the community agents, to become involved in my care was devastating.

The Community Mental Health Team (CMHT) said I didn't fulfil their referral criteria and did not want to be involved. Although I work for a CMHT I don't know to this day why this was the case. They gave no explanation. The social worker said that technically I had a home and, although my consultant was adamant that returning home was not an option, said there was nothing she could do. I was told there was a waiting list of a few months for psychology or psychotherapy but that a consultant psychiatrist would see me on a regular basis. The first appointment to see a psychiatrist, which I received a few days later, was for two months after my discharge. A keyworker was not identified. The psychology service had already assessed me. It was agreed that whoever saw me from there would fulfil that role, at some unknown future point. The only other option was to attend a day hospital. Two days later I went for an assessment and was again told that I did not come under their referral criteria but, because there were no other avenues to explore, they would give me a place two days a week for a month until psychological support was in place.

I am fortunate to have a sister who cares a great deal. She offered me her home as a place to convalesce immediately after hospital. Unfortunately she lives in Spain and although her support was invaluable I was not able to sort out practical issues from such a distance until I returned home three weeks later. Again I was fortunate to have good support from friends and went to stay with a couple on a temporary basis. The friends in question were also going through a period of extreme crisis. The husband had been made redundant and his wife was seeing her mother through the last stages of cancer. The arrangement was not ideal, but their generosity was moving.

After discharge I received a letter from the psychology service offering me yet another assessment. At the assessment I was told it would more likely be a year before I could be seen. I couldn't help asking whether their waiting lists might be reduced had they not duplicated assessments. I was asked, hypothetically, what difference it would make if I were seen in the next month given that most of my concerns related to practical issues? It seemed impossible to convince them that to me it would make all the difference. I had been used to a high level of psychological help and was now receiving none. I had responded well to that approach. My ability to resolve my practical difficulties had been greatly facilitated by psychological intervention. Two weeks later they wrote explaining that they could not see me and had referred me to the CMHT – the same people who had already refused to be involved in my care. At the day hospital I was offered very low-level distraction groups that left me feeling paralysed. I felt unsafe about grappling the issues in my life without adequate and ongoing support. I was dependent on help being on offer. I did not want to turn anything down through fear of being labelled difficult and the help being cut off. However I was also aware that the support I was receiving was not matching my needs.

My mood deteriorated significantly. My recovery was in jeopardy. I was keen that everything possible should be done to prevent relapse. In desperation I saw my GP who was concerned enough to arrange an emergency appointment with a psychiatrist. Unfortunately I saw a locum who, very sympathetic to my situation, did what he could to pursue an urgent referral to the CMHT but was not around long enough to follow my progress. Two months on and I am still waiting for a response from them. Out of the blue I received an incapacity benefit form from my employer. Confused, following the advice that I was not entitled to any benefits, I made enquiries and was put in touch with the Welfare Rights Office. The help they provided was excellent and the guidance they gave invaluable. I realised that there were many sources of practical and financial help available to me. How sad that this was not made apparent at an earlier time and that agents did not work collaboratively to ease my distress sooner. However the very same situation forced me to find the strength to take some initiative. The lack of appropriate help provided the space where I had to rely on myself and realise my own resourcefulness.

I was, at the time of discharge, an emerging shoot, still delicate with fragile roots. I had found new strength and new ways of relating to people but in the vacuum of an institution. The challenge was to take these skills, together with my original character strengths, back into the reality of life. Old patterns die hard. Under pressure we all fall back on familiar if unhealthy habits that in a previous time had, perhaps, helped us to survive. My old roots were particularly stubborn. Depression and suicide had been constant companions for so long and sat alongside a learned helplessness that I had used to get support – albeit of the wrong kind. It masked my ability to tap into my own resources and was fed by the need of professionals and agencies to identify individual weakness as an appropriate reason for referral and help.

I fought hard against those patterns and spoke out. Becoming my own advocate was intensely empowering. Yet at the same time I felt my very ability to articulate clearly what I needed had become a hindrance. How much easier it is for us, as professionals, to provide for someone who has no idea what will help than for someone who can clearly identify what they need. How much less threatening it is to be able to tell someone that what we can provide is what they need rather than hear someone state clearly what they want and have to face our inadequacy in supplying it. How much more challenging it is to coordinate packages of care that involve multi-agency working than to stay within our insular professional frames of reference.

There appears to be a fine line between convincing community agencies that you have needs and showing your own resourcefulness to illustrate how your needs might best be met. Show too much of the latter and you are seen to be too articulate, too controlling, too much of a challenge to warrant help. It appears too much emphasis is placed on moulding an individual around resources already available, rather than identifying the resourcefulness of an individual (including their support networks) and providing appropriate and complementary help. The latter requires an ability to think laterally and cast the net wider than your immediate professional context. I believe that it has to be much more fulfilling (as well as cost-effective) to see people flourish under the right help and guidance than to watch the dependency that results when individual strengths are not recognised or worse, ignored. A flexible and collaborative approach which focuses on accessing the individual's resources and commitment to their own recovery has to be the creative way forward. Such an approach would undoubtedly have helped ease the trauma of my transition.

1.3 FROM COMMUNITY TO INSTITUTION – AND BACK AGAIN

David Barron

Source: Brigham L. *et al.* (eds) *Crossing Boundaries: Change and Continuity in the History of Learning Disability*, BILD, Kidderminster, 2000, pp. 10–13.

. . . And so this is how it went on. The biggest part of the time was when it was half term. I run away from my sadistic foster mother because of cruelty, the severe beatings, a scald. One day I came home three minutes late from school. My foster mother firmly believed in beating first, questions after, one foot in the hearth, one out, and I got a pan of boiling scalding stock down my left leg with a scald which I'll carry with me to the grave. So all these things were there, but the love was still there for my foster mother. I still accepted these things.

I ran away from my foster mother's home, and I slept in a park, and it was only then I really knew the true value and love of young people. Today I will let no one come to me and say they are tearaways, they are layabouts; as far as I'm concerned I owe my life to the young people of yesteryear. [. . .]

Eventually I was taken away from my foster mother because a prison warder came in and saw that I was being beaten up in the back yard, and he intervened, and I was taken away from my foster mother's home at the age of eleven-and-a-half years for being severely beaten over and over and over again. He used to sneak food into the attic. He used to go, 'Mum's the word' – that was the only food I got. The people came with a search warrant – I didn't know what it was – but they came, and eventually after the to-and-froing with my foster mother and another – someone she'd taken off the street – I was taken away from her. The same night I was taken in to stay with children my age, but what they should have done is left me there, but no, the next day my foster mother appeared in Court. Great! She appeared in Court. I got a kick out of being in Court because seeing people walking round with wigs on, I thought they were Indians – but that was me as a child. Then things were to change. I was never ever to see my dear foster mother again alive. I was taken away by two burly men – I was told by these people . . . that just simply because I was being severely beaten up where a foster mother was being paid to look after me, practically starving me to death, that's why I was put in this mental hospital.

In the mental hospital it had its good points. It was spotless and clean, but I can always remember the day on one ward in particular, I will remember that day until I go to the grave, after they got the formalities out of the way and the forms were signed I was taken – this attendant took me with a big long dog chain to Ward 1. Ward 1 to me when I first went in of course, I just looked round. There was dear souls sat around the ward. The windows had bars on every one. The doors were locked. I was taken for a bath; they must have thought I couldn't bath myself, even that was locked, but from my experiences I know now why bath houses are locked. I settled in and I tried to communicate with the people – and I'll use that word again which I used earlier – 'poor souls'. I tried to communicate but couldn't because there was a big age gap, some twenty-odd years. Some of those poor souls must have been born practically in Whixley [the hospital].

In Whixley you were not allowed to mix with the opposite sex. It was against the law throughout England, Scotland, Ireland and Wales that if a patient went out as a trustee it was all right for him to go and talk and mess about with his own sex but he must not go and be seen to talk – because I know from my documents – he must not go and be seen talking to a female because that's against the law, and that was the ruling and the law of the institutions at that time.

I'm now still back as a child, settled in, and we had a Superintendent there, and his voice became very familiar to me and it still is to this day; he came down to me and what did I cop? I got an occupation. I would go down, they would put me in the toilets, with a long corridor to scrub, to scrub the corridor, and when I'd finished start it over again, and the Superintendent came down and he said 'Hello David, you settling in all right, s'all right, ayh?' I got used to that word 'ayh' because that was his familiar saying, a posh word 'ayh', it came in all the time. Exercise – you had regular exercise, went out – but they also used the exercise yard as another thing.

Patients at that time, as we were called, if you did or said anything wrong, or you didn't please an attendant the way he wanted pleasing, he just put something in the Report Book and you were sent to Ward 1. Now Ward 1 was a notorious punishment ward. I as a child grew up and saw patients being brought into there for different things. One thing they had was the periodicals – privileges stopped. One of the main things I saw, was patients who smoked – I loved sweets, but I don't smoke, but they did, and they were desperate for getting cigarettes, so what they used to do they used to scoop dust off the floor just as a means of getting a sly smoke. A lot of those poor souls died with Yellow Jaundice, but it's a different wording medically in this book. Now, this was how it went on. I dreaded Ward 1 but nevertheless I was always in and out of there as I got older. I stayed in there, but I must admit it had its good points. If of course you did anything wrong, a patient would be sent out to scrub the concrete with a common house brick, half a bucket of cold water, regardless of the weather if it was freezing, and your ration of bread was cut from two slices of bread to half a slice of bread. If you pleased the attendants on the ward by going to bed with them, and all this kind of thing as it was done to me by force, well then brilliant! They'd give you maybe a little piece of extra bread, or something like that.

But let's look on the other side of the institution. It had its own tailor's shop, everywhere suits was made, mat shop, cobbler's shop, it had everything you could humanly think of in the institution, even to the laundry, everything was all under one roof.

The attendants had to have four qualifications: they had to know how to participate in sport; they had to have a form of religion whatever it was; they had to know how to use a bunch of keys; and they had to know how to use their fists. If they could do that they passed qualifications – there they were, they got the uniform, the lot. There was no male nurses in those days, only attendants. It wasn't all bad. We had one of the finest Scout bands throughout Yorkshire, and I used to love being in that. As I got older we used to go down to the village church once a month, and I used to brag being the youngest that our band was better than the ATC's band, and I am pleased to say that I'm still connected with some of the young people, who of course have now grown up, who lived in the village.

1.4 LIVING IN THE BORDERLANDS OF DISABILITY

Carol Thomas

Source: *Female Forms: Experiencing and Understanding Disability*, Oxford University Press, 1999, pp. 54–5.

I was born without a left hand, an impairment which I began to conceal at some point in my childhood (probably around 9 or 10 years of age). This childhood concealment strategy has left a long legacy: I still struggle with the 'reveal or not to reveal' dilemma, and more often than not will hide my 'hand' and 'pass' as normal. But concealment carried, and continues to carry, considerable psychological and emotional costs and has real social consequences. This hiding strategy was partly bound up with school life, but looking back I think a key influence was my association with the 'Roehampton Limb Fitting Hospital'. Once a year from a very young age I was taken by my parents to this hospital. My parents felt it was their duty to do this for my sake: to seek the advice of 'experts'. On these annual visits, my 'hand' was examined by a doctor who I remember as being very kind, and questions were asked about how I was 'managing'. As a result of these visits I was kitted out with a number of 'aides' like a strap which went around my left 'wrist' in which a fork could be inserted so that I could eat with 'two hands' like everyone else! The main 'prize' of these visits, however, was a series of artificial, or 'cosmetic' hands. These were ghastly, heavy and uncomfortable objects which I invariably relegated to the drawer soon after receipt. By the middle of my teenage years I had a gruesome collection of hands in the drawer. It was only some years later that I finally threw them away. I remember standing in front of a full-length mirror gazing at myself with the latest cosmetic hand on – how strange and unnatural it looked. Fortunately my parents never pressed me to wear these hands – leaving it up to me to make the decision. You could count the number of times I wore these on the fingers of one hand! However they did their work indirectly because the underlying message was clear. The experts were saying that my 'hand' was something to be hidden, disguised. I had to appear as 'normal' as possible. I found the easiest solution was to hide my 'hand' in a pocket, and I became very skilled at this concealment. Thereafter I always had to have clothes with a strategically placed pocket. So it was, and so it is.

As well as reflecting the gender narratives of my time, this account also tells us something about the public narrative that 'out of sight [is] out of mind'. I would suggest that this social narrative operates powerfully in relation to people who have impairments that can be, or by their very nature are, hidden, but it is a narrative of much broader significance in Western culture: conceal that which is 'bad' or shameful, make things appear to be 'normal'. In my case, doctors and others in 'caring' positions were conduits of this narrative because it was embedded in their own professional and personal identity narratives. My own ontological narrative, like those of the others discussed, has been retold through and in the new public narratives associated with the disabled people's movement. However, one of the difficulties in sustaining it, or rather in 'acting it out', is that the long history of 'hiding' my impairment has meant that it is 'second nature' to me now. There is thus a disjuncture between my sense of 'who I am' (a disabled woman) and the sense of 'who she is' held by most other people who know me. This means that much of the time I feel that I am in the 'borderlands' between the disabled and non-disabled worlds, and I suspect that this is a very common experience for people like me who have impairments which, for one reason or another, are not obvious.

CHAPTER 2

WILLIAM AND TERESA

Alan Perry

TERESA: I was born in County Mayo and I'm the youngest of a family of three. My parents had a small grocery shop and after my father died, we moved to Galway. I worked in the pub business there for ten to twelve years and that's how I met William.

WILLIAM: I too come from the West of Ireland. I had my own business there and I got divorced and lost the lot: the business, my home, my family. And then I met Teresa. She had nothing to do with my divorce. We met afterwards...

I was at the Hostel the day they arrived, four months ago. They looked worn out. All their clothes and luggage got soaked when they were forced to hitch-hike to Cork in an open truck a few days earlier and they needed somewhere to dry them. Since then, they've become frequent and popular lunchtime visitors. Softly-spoken and with a quiet dignity, William is in his early fifties. Teresa is small, dark and pretty and in her early thirties.

WILLIAM: We both come from two very well-educated, decent family backgrounds and when we met first I tried to revive my business but it didn't work. The market I was in got overcrowded and it didn't get off the ground. At the time, we were much better off than we are now. Without wishing to sound boastful, up to six months ago, we lived as good if not better, than the people in those luxury flats out there. We had our own caravan trailer and we came over here on holiday and toured around. We'd been up the coast to Holyhead but we'd never actually been through the Valleys. So I drove to Bangor, up through Merthyr and Portmadoc and it was beautiful and that's what eventually gave us the idea of coming back.

Source: *Music You Don't Normally Hear*, Alun Books, Port Talbot, 1998, pp. 35–42.

But we went back to Ireland first and settled about fifty miles away from where we actually lived. In this particular little town, we both had part time jobs and we were signing on and we were very happy. I was working for a local man as a coach driver doing local tours and Teresa was working in a rather famous pub owned by a well-known County Mayo hurler. But it was kinda seasonal work and we knew that eventually it would peter out. And then we found out we were expecting a baby and initially it was a bit of a shock, even though we'd often talked about it. There's a stigma attached to single, pregnant women in Ireland, so when our families were informed, a bit of hostility set in. And it was uncomfortable for us, particularly because a lot of the work I was doing took me into Galway City, where both her parents and my family live.

TERESA: I'd been out of work for three months before we left because the cellar work got too heavy for me. On the way to Cork our car broke down and we had to leave it behind. Then we had to spend three nights in a bed and breakfast because there was no sailing, so two days after we arrived in Swansea we found ourselves almost penniless. On the third day, we were walking through town and saw two girls and three fellas sitting in a doorway with two dogs and they directed us to Paxton Street. In the Hostel, we were introduced to Sheralee, one of the workers here, and she gave us soup and coffee and got in touch with the Emergency Housing Officer who immediately came down and interviewed us and arranged for us to be moved into one of the Homeless flats. I was nearly six months pregnant at the time. We got our luggage, which was six big black bags and she drove us out there. It was teeming with rain that particular day. We didn't know what to expect but when we saw the place, it was run-down and filthy. We carried the bags up four floors, only to be told when we got up to the fourth floor, that there was no electricity, that the roof had caved in and we'd have to move all the luggage back down another floor. There was no electricity in that flat either so she decided, after losing her temper on several occasions, to put us back into a bed and breakfast for the night. We'd had bad times prior to coming over here but it was always in a place where we had friends or family whereas now we were completely alone. This woman wasn't a bit understanding or helpful and seemed to think that we were out to use and abuse the system and we were in a situation where we had no *choice* but to do as she said. So we went back to the bed and breakfast and were advised to ring the caretaker on the Monday. He told us to come back out before four o'clock and he moved us into a flat and helped us with our bags. When we went into Housing on the Wednesday, the woman didn't even realise we'd been out in the flat for two days. She assumed we were still in the bed and breakfast. She told us we'd have to stay there for eight weeks, instead of which, we've been there nearly sixteen.

WILLIAM: It's three and a half miles there and three and a half miles back and it takes an hour to an hour and a half to walk it. Most of the windows are boarded up and you wake in the morning and you don't know whether it's day or night because the room's blacked-out.

TERESA: We never see daylight and we're too afraid to pull the curtains. One of our biggest expenses out there is electric light bulbs, cause we leave the lights on twenty four hours a day, for security.

WILLIAM: They have a mania for breaking glass up there and you can't go out the front door because of it. If the houses are vacated *today*, the windows are all smashed *tomorrow*. Milk bottles, mineral bottles: the place is like a Diamond Field with glass. When the sun is shining you can *see* it: not just one bottle, a continuous, sheer carpet of broken glass. So we use the back door, but then you have to climb a grass bank cause there's a steel building frame bent across the path. Teresa's slipped quite a few times.

TERESA: A lot of the bells upstairs don't work, so there's always kids banging our front window to open the door to let them in.

WILLIAM: There's fourteen or fifteen of them upstairs. They kick the door, throw rubbish, smash bottles – and everything lands on the bottom landing. Their parents don't seem to care. Some of them never seem to be there. There's constant noise from about eight in the morning to two or three the following morning. And these are all children ranging between the age of three and twelve. It's an absolute nightmare! The police have been up and down the stairs three or four times in the last week and people come knocking at the doors at all hours asking for cigarettes or tobacco or cigarette papers. One fella came at *twenty past one* in the morning, during the New Year, looking for a *bucket*.

The other day, some kids lit a fire outside our bedroom window and the fire brigade were called. I saw the flashing lights and heard the noise and went out and saw this bloody big bonfire outside the window.

There's a man across the road, runs the corner shop – Mr Singh. And when we went there first we thought he was a right bastard, cause he was so stand-offish but after a while we realised he was a lovely, lovely man who just had so much *crap* to put up with. And from young kids – teeny-boppers – not adults or teenagers. He has a son, twenty-six, and there were kids outside there one day intimidating his dog and he chased them off and one of them shouts back to him: 'Sure, you're only an old black bastard, anyway!'

TERESA: There's nothing to do all day but look at a darkened, boarded-up window. The only pastime we have is that we take Jesse, our little Jack Russell, for walks. We've been keeping him illegally in the flat because our case worker made us sign a form saying no pets, no animals – no nothing.

WILLIAM: But the funny thing was, bad-minded and ill-mannered as our case worker was, she actually drove him around for three and a half hours that wet Sunday afternoon and didn't even know he was in the car because we keep him in that little rucksack there. We call it the Squawk. I even took it into Singleton Hospital to see Teresa when she had to go in for a week because she'd gone off eating and lost weight and needed building up.

Teresa was letting the dog out on Christmas night and the crowd upstairs were throwing empty bottles out the window. She was lucky they didn't hit her. She came into me, white as a sheet. On the other side of the building, above our sitting room window, they were throwing out dirty nappies. Some crowd made chips in another flat and poured all the oil down the sink, clogging up all the outside drains and when the kids were coming in and out, the hallway was like a bloody skating rink! And the smell! I came out there one morning and there was eggs – hard-boiled eggs – shelled and halved, left neatly on the mat outside our door and it only dawned on me after that it was to see if we'd come out and slip on them.

WILLIAM: In the beginning, it took so long for our Income Support to come through – what with forms being sent back because there was a stroke of a pen or a dot over an 'i' missing – that we had to walk everywhere: in rain, hail or sleet. We were classed as a married couple and our giro was for thirty five pounds each. So we couldn't afford to take twelve pound out of that for two weekly bus tickets, even though Teresa was over seven months pregnant.

TERESA: On top of which, being concerned, we used to ring home every week and that was as much as five pounds a call. I was expecting a very small cheque from an insurance company after cancelling what was left to run on the car and I suppose we spent a quarter of that on trying to get through to this company in Ireland.

WILLIAM: So from then on – living in this emergency flat for the homeless with people urinating through the letterbox, kicking the doors at nights, trying to get in cause we're on the ground floor – we've suffered a terrible time. At one point I went to Bangor to a friend of mine to see if I could get some work and when I got there he was on the point of going to France with a coachload of people on a tour. There wasn't any work and I didn't have any money to get back, so I rang Teresa and she was after getting the Maternity Grant, so she got a train and came up to Bangor to bring me back. And while I'd been gone our case worker had collared Teresa and put the flat in her name and I became what's known as N.F.A.: No Fixed Abode. Basically, what it meant was, I could visit Teresa in the flat but I couldn't live there. Mind you, I *was* living there, and still am.

Teresa, being pregnant, could have been excused for being depressed but I can assure you I was getting very depressed, too – and I wasn't pregnant – and very annoyed and frustrated about it. But we were told by the staff here to come in every day and have soup and sandwiches and whatever, and it gave us great comfort and a kind of boost.

TERESA: And, whereas we were filling in forms and getting a letter back from somebody we'd never *seen* upstairs in the Social Welfare Offices, Sheralee *knew* the person to contact and she really put herself out for us.

WILLIAM: So it went on and on and the case worker was mucking us about so much that I got very annoyed one day and told her in no uncertain terms what I thought of her and her outlook towards people. I told her she could stick her flat where Jack stuck the nine halfpennies. And the sun doesn't shine *there*, either!

WILLIAM: We have a lovely doctor but he was missing the day Teresa was getting pains. She wasn't getting the usual kicks that you get from a baby and we got a bit concerned. We went to our practitioners and there was a locum there and he wasn't very helpful or courteous. He wouldn't get an ambulance for us, so we had to find our own way to Singleton Hospital and that upset us because we had no money. We had a single fare over but not enough for a return. But we went over anyway and she was put on the ultrascan and we were told that the baby was dead. If she'd like to stay she could but she said no, she'd like to go home. They're beautiful people out there. He said 'That's fine, that's okay. You can go home and come in tomorrow in your own time.' And there was this lovely nurse there and she said 'Have you a car? and I said 'No,' and she says 'Where are you going to?' and I said we had to get to Blaenymaes and she said 'Oh, I'll check the buses,' and I said 'There's no need. We don't have the bus fare. We came down here in a hurry and we didn't bring any money with us,' 'cause I didn't want to say the position we were in financially. So she says 'I'll be back in a minute,' so she goes out and comes back and says 'That's all I've got in change,' and out of her *own* pocket, she gave us four pound, which was enough to get us home and back to Singleton the following day. Now that, to me, was what I call a little bit of Christian charity, without expecting any gains in return. So we came back the next day and they had a double room with a double bed for the two of us and they treated us the same as if we were in a Five Star Hotel. I was present for the birth and they took the baby away and dressed it up – I'm going on about this but it was a great traumatic time for us – and then they took it back. When the baby was born, Teresa rejected it. She didn't want to see it. But when they took the baby back all dressed up, she took the baby in her arms and it was so natural that you'd think it was going to move any second.

But, anyway, after we buried the baby, we offended some people that we thought were genuine. They came and took us to the funeral and were very nice and took us for coffee afterwards but what we didn't realise at the time was that they were a religious sect and that I was expected to *join* them. There was a *price* for their friendliness. So that was *another* thorn in our side because we have our own religion and we don't interfere with anyone else. And then Teresa had a bit of a bad run. She was depressed and had to go into hospital twice. And, if the truth were known, I should have been taken in with her, cause I was *worse*, but I hide it. But through all these bad times, we still came into the Cyrenians and got our soup and sandwiches and little parcels of food to keep us going. We always come in clean: I'd be shaved, clean shirt, sometimes a collar and tie. We speak well and act well and none of the Staff ever turned their back on us or looked on us as two down-and-outs. I remember coming in the day the baby was born and telling some of the people here – and their genuine shock and concern was unbelievable. So human. These people never knew us from Adam and they had befriended us so much and been so kind to us in so many ways and I've seen cases of people here who are *worse* than we are. And we haven't forgotten that and we *won't* forget it, either.

WILLIAM: On Christmas Eve, we were told that there was a house available but that we couldn't move into it because there was no furniture or gas. So we were advised to leave it until the New Year, to put in for a grant and to go back down to Housing Options to see if they could provide a little bit of furniture. We got the keys of the flat on the 30th of December and came back down to the Cyrenians, who helped us fill in the forms. When we went up to Housing Options to see if they had any furniture, we were told that there was no furniture and that we'd have to go on another waiting list. So we're still waiting.

We've got the house but we can't move into it because of problems with Benefits over a grant. I think they're going to have to give it to us, though, because Alan Morgan did a wonderful job of filling in the forms. If ever I need to get into heaven, I'm going to get *him* to write the letter for me.

Without the Cyrenians, we wouldn't have a friend in Swansea. Where we live, we go in in the evenings and we lock the door. And the only time we come out is to run across the road to the shop. I wouldn't tar *everywhere* up there with the same brush. We meet some people on the bus and we meet the odd person going in and out of the shop and there are some lovely, lovely people up there but we have never really spoken to anybody in Blaenymaes. There's nobody to talk to. We're in a boarded-up cage.

TERESA: When you stay in the Homeless flats, you won't get a job because the minute you mention them you're automatically classed as being trash or somebody who can't be trusted or somebody who's going to be drunk on the first day of work. I've worked for ten years and I'm quite capable of doing a job *well* and I'm not *stupid* but because you're homeless and you don't have money, people assume that you don't *want* to work and you're somebody that wouldn't understand plain English.

WILLIAM: We never say that we're living in Blaenymaes now. We say we're living in Robin Close, where the new house is. Because one evening just before Christmas, we were going home and we went into a particular takeaway food shop on the Kingsway and there was a notice in the window said 'Kitchen Staff Wanted'. Well, we're not proud. If we get paid for a job, we'll do it. So we both went in and asked about the work and this young lady said 'Fine, I'll give you the forms.' So we filled them in and handed them over on the spot. She picked them up, looked at the name and address and said '*Penmaes Place*. Oh!' Unfortunately there's a *stigma* attached to it. Teresa had another interview for a job in another restaurant also in the Kingsway and the Manageress asked her if she'd done that sort of work before and she said she'd done bar and catering work all her life. But when she told her she lived in Penmaes, the Manageress said 'I'm sorry, the job has gone.' Now, *twice* in the one street is too much of a coincidence. And when we went to a surgery in the Kingsway, to sign on with a doctor, the receptionist took our particulars but when she got to Blaenymaes she said 'I'm sorry. We don't treat patients from Blaenymaes. It's not our area.' I don't know what became of the Hippocratic Oath. As far as I'm concerned, it's Hypocritic!

We're at the stage now where we're picking ourselves up. We're on the move. We're back to eating normally. We were drinking a bit heavily there for a couple of weeks after the baby died but that's finished now and we're getting some counselling for people recouping from a still-birth. There's a lady comes to see us and we talk to her and she's given us great support. And once we get ourselves a bit better organised, we're going to offer to do a bit of voluntary work. We *did* try to give a hand in the kitchen on New Year's Eve and New Year's Day and, thankfully, we didn't poison anyone!

I've applied in person to the South Wales Transport Company and been given an application form, which I'm not going to fill in until we're at our permanent address. Then I'm going to put Robin Close. An awful lot of people working for that Company, live up there, so there shouldn't be any problems.

We have talked seriously about another baby. Teresa wants another one and the circumstances will be a lot better next time because if you're living in a house, however bad a house is, soap and water will clean a lot of it. And another thing is, you can go in your front door and you can go upstairs, downstairs, out the back and into a nice garden.

TERESA: I'm thirty three years old now and I can honestly say I have learned more in the last three months about life and people than I think I've learnt for the past thirteen years...

CHAPTER 3

THE EFFECTS OF POVERTY

Peter Beresford, David Green, Ruth Lister and Kirsty Woodard

A growing dissatisfaction with traditional approaches to the analysis of poverty is now ... emerging from some poverty academics and there is a search for new theories of poverty (Jordan 1996). These have, however, largely maintained the traditional social relations of inquiry, with commentators and analysts offering their own ideas and proposals. But there is also beginning to be recognition that such an exclusive approach to analysis may actually be part of the broader problem of poverty, which itself may be better understood in terms of the social relations of power and the unequal distribution of power, rather than of material goods (Becker 1997). Members of the disabled people's movement, in the related context of disability research, have also highlighted the destructive effects of traditional research relations.

The key objectives of the Poverty First Hand project were to enable the fuller participation of people with experience of poverty and to make it possible for them to speak for themselves, rather than just inform the analysis and arguments of others. Thus the project was crucially different in purpose and process to traditional poverty research, while located in the growing tradition of participatory and emancipatory research. [...]

We adopted the method of group discussions. We had considerable experience of this method and we knew that it helped put research participants in a stronger relationship to the research process through giving them the confidence and assertiveness that comes from being with each other and because it helped them to develop their own discussion, bouncing views and ideas off each other. [...]

We carried out a series of twenty group discussions with people who

Source: Adapted from *Poverty First Hand: Poor People Speak for Themselves*, CPAG, London, 1999, pp. 34–9, 89–108, 143–4, 205.

had current or previous experience of poverty. [...] We tried to identify and include groups in the project in as systematic and representative a way as possible, to reflect the diversity of people included as poor. Most were existing groups, rather than groups brought together for the purpose of this project, so they had their own identity and history. Groups were identified by a range of criteria which were relevant both in reflecting the diversity of people who experience poverty and the different reasons for which people who are poor may come together. [...]

A total of 137 people took part in the project, of whom ninety-six were women and forty-one men; 122 white and fifteen black and members of minority ethnic groups, and fifteen disabled.

The psychological and physical effects

These took a number of forms which could affect different people and the same people at different times. Twelve of the twenty groups discussed the psychological pressures involved in living on low incomes. [...]

> *Poverty strips your dignity. You can't have any dignity with poverty. Where I come from you've people, like they go to the supermarket, they haven't got enough money to pay for what they need. And how does that person go home and say to the children that they haven't got enough food in to feed them?*
>
> *(Women's discussion group)*

> *It has a major impact because money is power basically. If you've got money, you've got the power to do what you want when you want. If you've not got that money, you've not got the spendability, you feel powerless because you can't do a lot of things, you can't live up to the expectations that people have. I'm kind of criticising myself, but I'd like these jumpers and all the fancy names and that. Folk have expectations and trying to live up to it and all that though you're powerless and you've got no money.*
>
> *(Anti-poverty youth group)*

> *Constantly worrying, twenty-four hours a day about money and having to manage for the rest of the week, month, year, whatever.*
>
> *(Lone parents' group)*

> *I think also it's the stress that's overlooked – the actual stress that this causes. I think especially at the times when people are trying to do*

something for their children like birthdays and Christmas, you find you're just about managing on your budget, try to do something extra. Whatever you're on, you still want to provide for your children – well in our family you want to.

(Rural tenants' group)

About half the groups thought that living in poverty resulted in depression.

Sometimes I wake up and think, 'Oh, this is so boring'. It's the boredom of poverty and the boredom is what wears you down and makes you despondent in the end. I try to find jobs and I look around and then I think there's no point, they're not out there, the salaries are not out there, the child facilities are not out there.... It's deadly boring having to penny pinch all the time.

(Member of Local Exchange and Trading System group)

Some might get depressed about thinking all day, sitting in the chair thinking all day, how am I going to pay the gas bill, the electricity bill, the water bill, the TV licence? How am I going to shop? Where's the next meal coming from? And it goes on.

(Women's discussion group)

More depressed ... because you know you can't afford to buy anything. I mean Christmas and birthdays is when you dread most because you know you haven't the money.

(Group for low income families)

It's a multitude of things that are just going on in your head, churning over. I remember when my kids were little I couldn't sleep at night. I literally had a nervous breakdown when my children were little and I ended up in a psychiatric unit a few times ... I couldn't cope with it.

(Women's discussion group)

A lot of people go without food, definitely. I would say that the majority of young people that come in here don't eat properly. And when they do they just go for bags of chips and things like that, cheap things.

(Young people's project)

You're more tired. I mean just the thing that being poor is so much work, your whole life. You see people going into a shop, they buy what they want and they leave. But you're there, you're having to calculate how much money you've got as you go round, you're having to look at one brand then another, and meanwhile the store detective is looking over your shoulder which is also work having to cope with that kind of scrutiny, because you're poor they expect you to take something. . . . There's that pressure all the time.

(Groups of women involved in campaigns)

Effects on personal relationships

Half the groups who took part in the study thought that being poor had destructive effects on personal relationships between partners and within the family.

My daughter and her husband and family had a good living and a nice home and her husband lost his business – it went to the wall – and they split up. The kids went haywire and one left home and the other one got pregnant. . . . My daughter, she lost everything, and I mean it, after twenty years of marriage. She's now living on £42.00 a week and she's really, really finding it hard and she just had nothing.

(Group of disabled people)

The isolation . . . that in itself means that you have more chances of your relationships not working because you're isolated.

(Group of women involved in campaigns)

You don't pay one of the bills and you get into debt and the whole stress of this cycle that builds up then has repercussions in your relationships with other people.

(Group of homeless people)

We did not ask people specifically about stigma. We deliberately did not use the word. But it was an issue to which they repeatedly turned. Almost every group discussed stigma as a key consequence of being poor. Stigma shaped, overshadowed and was the context for their relationships with other people, particularly their relationships with non-poor and official agencies.

Even in the church which I belong to, when they were collecting, somebody said, 'we're collecting for "you people"'. I thought all of a sudden I have become 'you people', you know, whereas before, my husband, my ex-husband, and I were in all these groups and we were quite up on the upper thing and now I've become 'you people', that's how it affects you.

(Group of unemployed people)

A lot of single parents have actually worked and are paying their share. A lot of people seem to think we're scroungers who've never done anything in our lives . . . we've all contributed to the Chancellor's pocket, we're only surviving on what we deserve to survive on . . .

(Lone parents' group)

When you go to the DSS to sign on you're treated like a criminal, as if you're going to cheat the country out of a fiver and stuff like that. . . .

(Lone parents' group)

I've been to the social security and they make you feel exactly as if you're dirt. People who make you feel as if you're nothing. I've always worked, now I can't work. I can stand up for myself but there's thousands of people out there who can't stand up for themselves and are made to feel as if they're nothing. They're not even allowed to have the luxury to have a bit of pride in themselves because it's knocked out of them.

(Lone parents' group)

The media campaigns during the middle or late eighties, things about Costa del Dole and benefit fraud and so on and so forth. They gave their readership the impression that everyone who's claiming is unworthy. Maybe they did it for political reasons or for circulation reasons but it's a pretty miserable intention.

(Group of homeless people)

Some of the other participants singled out lone parents as victims of stigma. Lone parents themselves believed that they were a group who have been readily lumped together and labelled as deviant.

We've got a stigma that all our kids are going to grow up as child-murdering, glue sniffing, car joy riders and we're trying harder to make sure that they're disciplined, to get rid of that stigma.

(Lone parents' group)

I think single parents have a lot to prove because we're constantly being told that we're not a correct family; that we can't look after our children the same as a man or a woman in a relationship can look after children, a two-parent family. It's almost like we're desperate to prove that you can look after your kids the same, more, or better than if you were a two-parent family. I've never been into single parents' homes that were scruffy and I've met many single parents in poverty but they keep their houses nice, their kids really smart.

(Lone parents' group)

Practical effects

When we asked what they thought were the worst things about being poor, seventeen of the twenty groups talked about the restrictions and the lack of choices it imposed. [. . .]

There's also going in shopping and not having enough money and having to put half the things back and these are essential things. You get to the cashier and have you got thirty pounds because it comes to thirty pounds?

(Lone parents' group)

They're sitting in the dark. I mean I live in a complex where there are elderly people and they sit in the dark because they can't afford the electric.

(Group of disabled people)

It can mean restrictions on your social life. Several participants said that budgeting for a social life while living on a low income was very difficult. Most followed a fortnightly boom and bust cycle from receiving a giro to having to manage for two weeks before receiving the next one.

It curtails your social life definitely. . . . You can't go out when you want to, basically, and if you go out you're financially crippled for the next fortnight.

(Group of homeless people)

You're restricted to where you can go. Even to travel on the buses in and out of town, it's almost two pounds just to go in and out, and that's just one person. It's terrible for families.

(Community centre users' group)

You're all right if there's no birthdays, it's not Christmas and you don't want to go on holiday and you haven't got a car and you don't smoke. If you're a good budgeter you find you can live on it, but when things come up.... But there's always something crops up that you don't expect and it's, Oh, xxxxx hell, where am I going to get the money for this? Because you can't borrow, you can't get a loan – well, if you can you're going to pay treble what it's worth. Nine out of ten you've lost your credit rating because of things that happened in the beginning when you were first out of work.

(Lone parents' group)

Well you actually miss something else, say, like for example, if you buy like electric stamps, gas stamps or whatever, you'll say I'll miss that this week, we'll buy shoes, then say that the next week, the next week and then before you know where you are the bill's there and you just haven't got enough for the bill so you start missing something else to pay for the bills – it's a vicious circle.

(Rural tenants' group)

It means we don't have choices. We don't have the option to do what we want to do. We're very limited both in what you actually do and when you do it. If you don't have money you can't get anywhere, so I mean that can be down to things like it's difficult to choose where your children can go to school. You don't have options like people who have more money, or like getting out of the area.

It's a wider thing I think that whole thing about options, it's about having choices in life ... not being able to choose where you live, how you dress, what you eat even. Most of us would choose to eat better but can't afford it. Like you said, where your children go, education, and if you haven't got choices it limits your power around what you can actually do about it.

(Lone parents' group)

You can actually sit with your money and if you go through it with your older children, that's what you're paying out on bills and food every week, and for a few seconds they can understand it, why you don't have the money, but they really don't understand because they're still going out on the street and their friends have got Reebok boots, or what have you, and they don't understand. They know where your money's going and they know you've got very little but they don't understand why other people's children can have these things. Like one of mine was using a felt-tip pen on his shoes because he was writing Reebok on them, a pair of cheap trainers. . . .

(A lone parent)

The 'underclass' and labelling

Some people thought that labelling people as part of an 'underclass' could become a self-fulfilling prophesy.

But don't you think this could be part of a self-fulfilling prophesy as well that these kids are growing up being told by society, 'You are the dregs. We don't what anything to do with you'? And they think, 'Well, if that's how you are going to treat me, why should I be any different?' And that's creating a section of society that has nothing to lose, which is a very dangerous thing to do.

(Group of disabled people)

Many believed that, once you were labelled as 'deviant', or as part of the 'underclass', it was incredibly difficult to shake off the stigma surrounding these labels.

Say you get somebody coming in to this centre that's been to prison and done his sentence, his sentence doesn't begin until he comes out of prison and he gets dogged every other way because he's been in prison. He's not allowed to be a normal person again. He's always labelled as a parasite or he won't work, he's workshy and this, that and the other. It's really weird how people pin labels on when they only know a quarter of the summary.

(Lone parents' group)

Participants thought that many poor people, who had little other choice than to live in increasingly impoverished environments, where there was overcrowding and crime, were stigmatised by media amplification of the idea of the 'underclass'.

The media blow it out of proportion. I mean there's always been an element of crime and violence in housing schemes throughout Britain. I mean we have so many people, I mean, at one time. . . . You've got multi-stories and you've got maybe 80-odd families in a high block of flats, and at one time there was only a few families lived in that. And you've got your crowd, and you have it – there always has been and there always will be. But I think the media do now blow it completely out of proportion.

(Group of low income families)

It's propaganda put out by people that have got jobs. Lords and these MPs that talk out saying that, 'Well, he's just a dole scrounger.' They don't know what it is. Let's face it, you'll not hear anybody round here calling anybody the underclass because they're all in the same bloody boat.

(Group of unemployed people)

REFERENCES

Becker, S. (1997). *Responding to Poverty: the Politics of Cash and Care*, London, Longman.

Jordan, B. (1996). *A Theory of Poverty and Exclusion*, Cambridge, Polity Press.

CHAPTER 4

POVERTY AND THE SOCIAL SERVICES

Mark Drakeford

This chapter considers the relationship between poverty and social work. Any such discussion should begin with recognition of one over-riding fact: the large majority of social welfare provided in the community is supplied, not by organisations, but by families and, to a lesser extent, by friends and neighbours. The direct financial costs involved may be considerable, to individuals and families where paid work has to be foregone in order to undertake care, or where career prospects suffer through reduced opportunities for mobility and responsiveness in an increasingly flexible labour market. Nevertheless, and despite these very real costs, the bulk of community care is provided both free and freely within the immediate circles of those in receipt of it.

Caring relationships involve exchanges which go far beyond money. Costs and rewards are involved both in caring for another person and in receiving care. These advantages and disadvantages are emotional and practical as well as financial. Yet, there are very often cash-consequences which have to be negotiated within such relationships. These costs can sometimes amount to, or lead someone into, a life lived in poverty.

Formal services are, for most people, a recourse of the last resort. For some, the stigma of 'the parish' still clings to welfare, especially where a reliance upon state-sponsored services implies a culpable failure in personal networks. For others, the feared loss of independence is a barrier to seeking help outside the narrow circle of mutuality. More generally, a lack of knowledge and an apprehensiveness in dealing with official organisations, can stand in the way of looking for assistance.

As a result, for many individuals in need of help, the use of formal social work services is a struggle. That struggle also has an impact upon those who provide these services.

The boundary between social services and social security

The factor which has traditionally separated social services and social security has been money. The social security system exists primarily to provide cash – and sometimes vouchers or in-kind help – to those who need it. The social services, by contrast, have a long history of hostility to the idea that they, too, should be part of the business of income maintenance.

Traditionally, social workers have seen themselves working intensively with 'the individual person', covering a wide range of issues in that person's life and often involving other family members. Social services provide help through advice and guidance. When social workers make decisions these have involved a high level of professional judgement and discretion. Benefit Agency staff, by contrast, have been thought of as dealing only relatively briefly with individual claimants, and in a way which focuses narrowly on certain specific issues. When Benefit Agency staff make decisions these involve the application of a set of routines and rules which allow for very little autonomy or flexibility.

From the 1980s onwards, however, this distinction has become less clear-cut. In some cases, such as the Social Fund and Exceptional Hardship payments for teenagers, social security staff have taken on some characteristics of a social work role, investigating individual circumstances, contacting family members and making discretionary decisions. Conversely, social workers have become more like social security staff, directly rationing cash and cash-equivalent services to a range of dependent groups according to a set of formulaic procedures. The common ground over which this confusion hangs is poverty and the responsibility for addressing it.

Changes in social security policies since the war

The postwar welfare state settlement was shaped by the social and economic conditions in which the Beveridge Plan had been produced. Many of the assumptions and circumstances upon which it was based have changed radically in the years which have followed. The social security system, however, has not proved responsive to a number of these changes. In particular, the Beveridge ideal of a universal, insurance-based social security system has been overtaken by a return to means-testing as the basis upon which the mass benefits of the system are distributed.

Over the same period, encouraged by government, a new reliance has emerged upon private insurance provision for at least some welfare needs. This has been particularly pronounced in relation to private and occupational pension provision. For older people this has produced a growing inequality between those reliant upon the state pension only, and those who have access to additional income.

Well before the half-century anniversary of the Beveridge Plan, the social security system had come under attack from both left and right of the political spectrum. It was accused of failure to achieve social justice and equality on the one hand, and of creating dependency and economic damage on the other. In the years which followed the Conservative election victory of 1979, the critique developed by the new right in relation to social and economic policy came to exercise increasing influence upon social security policy making.

In the middle years of the 1980s a major review of the whole benefit system was undertaken, abolishing the supplementary benefits system and replacing it with Income Support. It also established the Social Fund. The reforms were said to have made the system 'fit for a new millennium'. Behind the fine words lay a series of purposes which Bradshaw (1992, p. 83) summarises as 'privatisation, selectivity, managerialism, incentives and last, but certainly not least, the needs of the economy'. In particular, the White Paper *The Reform of Social Security: Programme for Action*, set out the 'basic principle' that, 'social security is not a function of the state alone. It is a partnership between the individual and the state – a system built on twin pillars' (DHSS 1985, para. 1.5). The aim which lay behind this contention was to shift the responsibility between these pillars, with the state assuming less and, as a result, individuals having to assume more.

Change remained on the agenda again in the late 1990s and, in the words of Ruth Lister (1996), it amounted to a strategy of 'permanent revolution'. Underlying this was a combination of the long-standing Conservative belief that contemporary levels of state expenditure were economically unsustainable, and a more recent neo-liberal assertion that the social consequences of benefit dependency were so problematic in themselves that the system had become a cause of difficulty in its own right. Those who relied upon benefit were portrayed as a constant drain on the general economy and in need of a suspicion-driven surveillance to prevent fraud and abuse. The practical effect of this was to emphasise the difference between those who use state services and other members of the community. As Becker (1997, p. 5) suggests, social security claimants had come to be portrayed as a group apart, and one which the nation 'can no longer afford, nor should wish to maintain'. The emphasis, he pointed out, was on exclusion rather than inclusion. While those in receipt of community care as well as benefits were generally spared the worst of such rhetoric, the general climate took its toll upon those who, in sickness or old age, were obliged to rely upon the same system for their maintenance.

Moreover, those parts of the benefit system which are of particular importance to community care users were not left untouched by the reforms.
Social security arrangements for community care and residential care were
reformed in 1993, followed by radical changes in invalidity benefits and
housing benefit in 1995. To the very end of the Conservative government
in 1997 therefore, the social security system was undergoing constant
reform, the combined effect of which was, in essence, to reduce individual
entitlement and to narrow down the scope of state responsibility.

Changes in social services since the war

In the immediate postwar period, the connection between poverty and
social welfare appeared to be weakening. Undoubtedly the shaping of the
welfare state did much to ameliorate the conditions of physical and
material squalor which had been the lot of poorer families before the war,
while the universal state pensions improved the position of the poorest
retired people. It was assumed that the connection between poverty and
the personal social services had been severed, because the welfare state
would provide an income sufficient for all to be lifted out of poverty. Yet,
if the connection between poverty and welfare appeared to be weakening,
the sense of stigma (which continued to cling to usage of social services)
proved more difficult to eradicate. The solution proposed by the Seebohm
reforms of 1970 was the creation of a universal social service in which
contact with a social worker would be as normal and natural as visiting
the doctor or going to school. In the new era, social ills were regarded by
many as less the product of poverty and more the result of troubled family
life.

The initial optimism which underpinned such beliefs was overtaken by
economic pressures during the mid 1970s, both in terms of the enduring
nature of poverty itself and in terms of cuts within the public services. The
retreat from universalism was accelerated in the years after 1979, with a
new emphasis upon family and voluntary effort in the social services and
the introduction of marketisation into the provision of publicly funded services.

Running through the period were three trends which emerge as of
particular importance in studying the relationship between poverty and
community care.

Firstly, the re-discovery of poverty in the 1960s, the first postwar return
to mass unemployment in the 1970s, and the final abandonment of the
basic Beveridge principle that the social security system should rest on
insurance benefits, all combined to make it increasingly pivotal rather than
peripheral to the tasks which social workers were called upon to perform.

Secondly, within the provision of community care services, the emphasis
upon competition and contracting soon had an impact upon the working

conditions of those employed within them. Keeping prices down meant, in many instances, the creation of a low-wage, low-skill work force. Poverty, in social work, is often a condition of those who provide, as well as require, services.

Thirdly, and most importantly, the emphasis upon the power of service users which accompanied the community care reforms of the early 1990s, soon met the constraints of a cash-limited service. The Association of Directors of Social Services complained that the cash allocation from central government for the new community care services was less than half of the sum required to discharge the new responsibilities. Far from being led by the needs of consumers, the system fell back rapidly, in Becker's words, upon 'the use of assessment, prioritising and eligibility criteria ... to regulate and ration access to expensive forms of care, both residential, nursing and domiciliary, for users and carers' (1997, p. 136).

The limited resources available through state-provided community care led inevitably to a system of rationing. While local authorities are not obliged to charge for services such as home care, day care, meals-on-wheels or aids and adaptations, the Conservative government, in setting the level of annual central government grant which councils receive, assumed that charges for domiciliary services would be levied. The Local Government Anti-Poverty Unit (1995, p. 1) pin-pointed the essential dilemma which this produced for social services authorities: 'to raise revenue from charges to ensure that service levels are maintained whilst not impoverishing individual users. These two objectives are incompatible. All that local authorities can do is trade one off against the other.'

Social services and the growth in poverty

If the increasing association between poverty and becoming a user of social services had become apparent in the 1970s, the effect of policies pursued after 1979 was to make the connection entirely explicit. The evidence marshalled by Becker (1997, pp. 94–96; 121ff.) illustrates the extent to which, as the Thatcher years unfolded, the business of social welfare became the business of working with people in poverty. At the time of the first major post-1979 changes in social security, the reform of the supplementary benefit system, investigation in 1982 by the Policy Studies Institute showed that 20 per cent of all supplementary benefits claimants were in contact with a social worker, 30 per cent of whom had contacted a social worker only because of needing benefit advice. In 1985, research in the metropolitan areas found that more than 90 per cent of all social worker referrals were from 'economically inactive' people. In the same year 46 per cent of all referrals to social workers in the Strathclyde region of Scotland were found to be from the poorest sections of the population, those dependent upon means-tested benefits. Fully two-thirds of all new Strathclyde referrals to social workers were to do with financial and housing problems, and nearly two-thirds of this number were brought by women.

Nor did the figures show simply that individuals were turning to the social services for advice and information. A major 'snap-shot' survey conducted during the latter part of the 1980s suggested that between 6 and 10 per cent of all new financial referrals made to social workers in the participating social work teams, were simply requests for money. The survey also identified a new problem in the battleground between poverty and the social services. The introduction of the Social Fund in 1988 lowered the baseline conditions for people living in the greatest poverty. It provided its much diminished assistance on a cash-limited basis, eked out through loans rather than grants. In doing so, the Fund created a category of claimant hitherto unknown in postwar social security policy, the person *too poor* to be helped. Where an applicant was assessed by Fund officers as deserving of help, but so impoverished as to be unable to repay the loan which might be offered, an offer of help was to be denied. Craig (1998, p. 53) estimates that, less than ten years into the Fund's operation, considerably more than half a million applicants were refused help because of this 'inability to pay' condition.

Social services departments prepared for the introduction of the Fund in 1988 by sharper policing of the boundary between social work and Social Fund staff. Yet, within a very short period, more than a quarter of the new poor clients were people who had made one or more applications to the Social Fund. Poverty on this scale and in this concentration is not without the most serious consequences in the lives of social work clients.

Nor was the Social Fund the only mechanism through which direct connections between poverty and community care services came together during this period. The White Paper, which preceded the NHS and Community Care Act 1990, described the financial hub around which community care services were to be provided. Case managers – as social workers were described in the Paper – '*should* take account of the wishes of the individual and his or her carer' but '*will have to* take into account what is available and affordable' (Department of Health 1989, emphasis added). Resources are finite, people are malleable, and the poorer they are, the more malleable they would need to be.

Additionally, as noted earlier, the pressures generated by the income generation requirements which Government attached to the Health and Social Services and Social Security Adjudications Act 1983, were exacerbated once community care responsibilities were transferred to the local authorities. The impact upon users of services was twofold. On the one hand, as Becker (1997, p. 144) suggests, increasing charges led to 'user resistance to paying'. On the other, Becker also found that the result was to distort demand 'deterring poor people who need home care from applying for it and deflecting services to more wealthy elderly people who need them less'. The charity *Scope* has reported that almost one in five disabled people had to turn down the offer of care from social services because they could not afford to meet the charges.

The detailed decisions which local authorities have subsequently made about charging policies have had a major impact upon individuals. Policies which exempt claimants of base-line benefits from charges, for example, are clearly more sensitive to poverty issues than those which impose flat-rate charges regardless of income. While means-testing for community care services may result in highest charges for those who can best afford them, it is also worth remembering the argument that such complex systems are off-putting and can lead to 'residualisation'. This occurs when charges prompt those with money of their own to opt out of public services and look elsewhere. The services which remain become confined to poorest users and, in the argument of Richard Titmuss, services which have 'Reserved for the Poor' hung on their door stand in imminent danger of becoming poor services. Where the cost balance between private and public may be closely matched, the dangers of residualisation may well be more acute.

By the first half of the 1990s therefore, a combination of circumstances had drawn the staff of social services departments far closer into a cash-based role than had ever previously been the case. On the one hand, social workers gave out money to families in need on an unprecedented scale. On the other, the same departments were responsible for the collection of cash for services provided.

A number of general issues of principle arose from this new alignment of social work and poverty questions.

Firstly, both in relation to providing cash and services, the system depended upon rationing by social workers, who were expected to select out those applicants who appeared most vulnerable or needy. Such judgements are inevitably discretionary and subjective. Applicants have few ground-rules upon which they can base an application and almost no rights-based access to having unfavourable decisions reviewed or over-turned.

Secondly, the system varied considerably between local authorities. If individual social workers were bound to vary in their assessments, so too, on a wider scale, were councils, allocated different amounts of money to these purposes and set different rules under which access to them might be obtained. Thus, the chances of receiving help were cast into the lottery of geography, as well as the mercy of individual discretion.

Thirdly, given the level of demand, even the most generous local authorities were forced to adopt systems focused more on deterring than meeting applications. In such a context, success depends both on individual determination and a willingness to parade the poverty which makes an application necessary. Success may be unlikely but the price of any achievement is quite certainly high in terms of personal dignity and distress.

Social work after 1997

In the great debate between public and private provision, which had been so acute during the Tory years, New Labour declared itself agnostic. It preferred a policy of 'modernisation', based on 'what works', which, it claimed, put practicality above ideology (see Drakeford 1999 for a more extended account of these arguments). As time went on, however, the government often appeared to be impatient with the pace of change in public services and to use the threat of transfer to the (implicitly better) private sector as a lever to alter performance. Ambivalence, rather than agnosticism, came to be the hallmark of New Labour's attitude to public services.

In relation to poverty, the new government adopted a radically different approach to that traditionally adopted by previous left-leaning administrations. Rather than redistribute what the soon-to-be Chancellor, Gordon Brown, referred to as 'mere money', New Labour set about the redistribution of what he called 'the golden currency of opportunity'. A twin-track approach developed, in which those individuals willing and able to take advantage of the practical measures favoured by the government – the New Deal, the Working Families Tax Credit, and so on – were treated with conspicuously greater generosity than had ever been available under the previous regime. For those who failed to take advantage of the government-sponsored opportunities, however, a more harshly authoritarian response emerged than could ever have been contemplated by previous Labour governments. Across the field of social policy the same dichotomy emerged: considerable help for those who, in the Prime Minister's words, 'played the game', and a repressive intolerance of those who did not.

Conclusion

Where did all this leave social work? As argued in more detail elsewhere (Butler and Drakeford 2001; Jordan 2001; Jones 2001), the New Labour years were not wholly happy for the profession. When the government acted in generous mode – in the Sure Start scheme for disadvantaged children, to take just one example – the term 'social work' almost never appeared in official discourse, even where the tasks to be undertaken – advice, guidance, practical help and so on – appeared very close indeed to social work itself. Only when the government turned to authoritarian mode – in its treatment of 'anti-social' children, the regulation of the family, or the compulsory treatment of the mentally ill – did the place of social work seem secure.

I earlier referred to the residualisation which occurs when services become reserved only for the least well-off and least powerful sections of the community. Under New Labour this took a new turn for social work. As the government embarked upon its ambitious programmes for the eradication of child and pensioner poverty, and the tackling of poverty amongst people of working age, there emerged a real prospect of improvement for large numbers of individuals and families. For those who remained outside this circle of inclusion, however, increased regulation, surveillance and penalisation were positively advanced by government ministers as necessary goads to improvement. This chapter began by noting the stigma and sense of deterrence which has remained wrapped around social work services, even at times of policy-determination to resist such attributions. Under New Labour that determination had lapsed. Rather than 'Reserved for the Poor', now the message hung on the social work door seemed more and more to be 'Only for the Undeserving'.

REFERENCES

Becker, S. (1997) *Responding to Poverty: the Politics of Cash and Care*, London, Longman.

Bradshaw, J. (1992) 'Social Security', in D. Marsh and R.A.W. Rhodes (eds) *Implementing Thatcherite Policies: Audit of an Era*, Buckingham, Open University Press, 81–99.

Butler, I. and Drakeford, M. (2001) 'End of the Line for Social Work?', *Journal of Social Work*, 1:1.

Craig, G. (1998) 'The Privatisation of Human Misery', *Critical Social Policy*, 18:1, 51–76.

Department of Health and Social Security (1985) *Reform of Social Security*, Green Paper, Cmnd 9517, London, DHSS.

Department of Health. (1989) *Caring for People*, London, HMSO.

Drakeford, M. (1999) *Privatisation and Social Policy*, London, Longman.

Jones, C. (2001) 'Carrying out State Social Work Under New Labour', *British Journal of Social Work*, special issue 31: 4.

Jordan, B. (2001) 'Social Work and New Labour', *British Journal of Social Work*, special issue 31: 1.

Lister, R. (1996) 'Permanent Revolution: The Politics of Two Decades of Social Security Reform', Paper presented to the DSS Summer School, King's College Cambridge.

Local Government Anti-Poverty Unit (1995) *Survey of Charges for Social Care 1993–95*, London, Association of Metropolitan Authorities.

CHAPTER 5

WITNESSES TO WELFARE

5.1 WAYS OF LABELING THE POOR

Herbert J. Gans

Source: *The War Against the Poor: the Underclass and Antipoverty Policy*, Basic Books, New York, 1995, pp. 14–18.

Labels with which to stigmatize the poor have probably existed since the emergence of hierarchical societies, but it suffices to look back to the end of the medieval era to understand the historical context of today's labels. Since then, the poor have regularly been dichotomized, at least by critics of the poor and formulators of laws about poverty, into two groups. The first encompassed the sick and old, as well as the working poor, and was considered good or worthy of help, while the second, able-bodied nonworking poor people, have been deemed unworthy.

America has inherited much of its labeling tradition from England, which seems to have invented the modern version. The first users of the distinction between worthy and unworthy poor people have never been identified, but it began to be applied regularly when responsibility for the English poor was given over from the centralized church to locally governed parishes starting in about the fourteenth century. The words 'deserving' and 'undeserving' were actually invented much later, again in England, in connection with discussions concerning the 1834 Poor Law.

Not surprisingly, labels for the various kinds of deserving poor are virtually nonexistent, although at this writing 'working poor' is becoming an increasingly positive label in mainstream American culture. Conversely, the supply of labels for the undeserving poor, as of that for stigmatized racial and ethnic groups, is plentiful.

My historical survey of the labels for the undeserving poor is cursory and meant to be merely illustrative. The label with the greatest longevity may be 'pauper', although over the years it underwent several changes in meaning. In the fourteenth century it was used to describe the mobile poor. Then it became a synonym for deserving poor women; later the women became undeserving, but in the nineteenth century the word was also used to label the impoverished men and women who would, in today's medical vocabulary, be considered depressed, and in the punitive vocabulary lazy or shiftless.

I will list here only some of the other prominently used labels of the past, with the help of a nineteenth-century classificatory scheme for the undeserving poor: 'defective, dependent, and delinquent'. The trichotomy is not mutually exclusive, for some of the labels that classified the poor as culturally, morally, and biologically defective also treated them as criminal (or delinquent) and vice versa.

Despite the hostility the better-off classes have long felt toward poor people who were not supporting themselves, there are not many words for those solely or primarily dependent; in rough historical order, these include 'paupers', 'hard-core poor' (although people with this label are also viewed as stubbornly, almost delinquently poor), and (today) 'welfare dependent' and 'illegal immigrant'. The latter is a good example of a term that has become a label.

The largest number of labels seems to have been invented for the various kinds of poor people deemed defective. These include, again in approximate historical order: paupers (as shiftless); debauched, hopeless classes; 'ne'er-do-wells'; dregs; residue; residuum; feebleminded; morons; white trash; school dropouts; cultural deprived or disadvantaged; and poor in the culture of poverty. To this list must be added the class of labels that view the defective poor as dangers to public health, referring to their ragged and dirty state, their living in slums, and the like. This set of labels was particularly important before and during the nineteenth century, although some overtones of past labels survive in today's AIDS victims and needle-using substance-users.

The delinquents include the politically threatening: the dangerous classes, *Lumpenproletariat*, and sometimes, rabble and mob. Charles Loring Brace used the term 'dangerous class' in America for homeless children, also called street urchins or street arabs, because he feared what they would do politically when they were adults. The remainder of the labels for delinquents mainly describe street people, criminal and otherwise, although this informal survey found few older words for this label. Today's are all familiar, and include 'bums', 'substance abusers' (including the earlier 'dissolute' and 'debauched'), 'gang members', 'muggers', 'beggars', and 'panhandlers' – although some of these also double as descriptive terms. In the 1980s, 'babies having babies' became popular, and in the 1990s, 'illegitimacy' was revived to call particular attention to the poor single-parent family.

Two further types of labels deserve separate attention. The *mobile* or *transient* poor have been considered delinquent since at least medieval times, on the assumption that, being mobile, they were free from local social control, and thus expected to turn to crime, mostly economic but also sexual and political, during their wanderings. The list includes 'vagabonds', 'vagrants', 'bums' once more, 'street urchins' or 'street arabs', 'tramps', 'shiftless', 'lodgers', 'hobos', 'drifters', 'loiterers' and, more recently, 'the homeless'. The mobile poor were particularly threatening in the centuries before the invention of the police, and most European languages include labels for them.

The other label type might be called *class failures*, for some labels, including a few already listed above, treat the undeserving poor as being below, or having fallen out of, the class structure. Among these are 'residue', 'residuum', 'dregs' and 'lower-lower class'; but the label that banishes the poor from the class hierarchy most literally is 'the underclass'.

All of the labeled are inevitably charged with the failure to adhere to one or more mainstream values by their behavior, but this is why they are considered undeserving in the first place. The labels lend themselves to many other kinds of analyses and distinctions, for example whether they pertain to individuals, such as school dropouts, or to collectivities, like a mob.

A more significant distinction that deserves systematic study is the extent to which labels are either race-blind or racially pejorative. Although most labels for the poor are literally neutral with respect to ethnicity and race, they have actually been meant mainly for immigrants and dark-skinned people in the United States and elsewhere, even if most of those fitting the labels probably came, and still come, from the majority population. In the nineteenth century, a high proportion of those labeled in England were Irish, while the Americans who were labeled were immigrants, many initially also Irish. Later in the century the labels were transferred to Southern European Catholics and Eastern European Jews, who were typically described as 'swarthy races', while Italian immigrants were also called 'guineas' because of their dark skin. Even before these immigrants had been administered the intelligence tests that were newly invented to stigmatize and exclude them, many were deemed of low intelligence or even feeble-minded by the eugenicists, who were almost all white Anglo-Saxon Protestants (WASPs). But WASPs were not the only ones to conduct racial labeling; a nineteenth-century American magazine intended for German-Jewish readers described the newly arriving Eastern European Jewish immigrants as 'miserable *darkened* Hebrews'.

Although some labels have cut across gender, criminal and mobile ones have been mostly, if not completely, reserved for men, while women have been labeled with economic, familial, and sexual failings. Mothers have to be supported with tax funds as paupers or welfare recipients, but despite the existence of home relief for men, poor men are rarely thought to be welfare dependents. There is not even a regularly used label for their inability to be stable breadwinners, probably because the better-off fear them mainly as potentially violent street criminals. Conversely, although the young men are periodically blamed for failing to pay child support, they are rarely labeled for being unmarried parents, perhaps because of the traditional sexual double standard. Those men who impregnate several adolescent women are sometimes labeled 'studs', but the women involved have always borne the brunt of exclusively pejorative labeling.

5.2 AN END TO WELFARE RIGHTS

David G. Green

Source: *An End to Welfare Rights: the Discovery of Independence*, Institute of Economic Affairs, London, 1999, pp. 67–9.

Annual income £20, annual expenditure £19 19s 6d, result happiness.
Annual income £20, annual expenditure £20 0s 6d, result misery.

When Dickens put these words into the mouth of Mr Micawber in *David Copperfield* he reminded us of the obvious but easily forgotten truth that, whether people are poor or not, depends on their expenditure as much as their income and that some expenditure is discretionary. It has become common to treat individuals as if they were the victims of circumstance and the policies of the Blair Government continue to reflect this view. But just how much responsibility can individuals be expected to assume and at what point and in what manner should the community step in? The first step in devising a new welfare system is to define what we can reasonably expect of each other.

Perhaps who wish to be free and responsible members of a community require a lifetime plan of action to allow them to be self-sufficient and thus able to make a positive contribution to the wealth and well-being of the society. People who have decided to take command of their own affairs would reasonably expect to make provision for the normal expenses of living, and for periods when expenditure will be high – most notably when children come along – or when income is lower, especially during retirement. Provision also needs to be made against misfortunes such as the early death of a partner, or illness, which may both reduce income and increase expenditure.

If a person plans to have children, then the lifetime plan will need to include a partner to allow for the children to be both cared for and supported financially. Theories which assume that people are largely, or to a significant extent, victims of circumstance, or at the mercy of 'barriers', tend to take 'income' as a given fact not under the control of the individual and to accept that a household is poor if income does not match expenses. However, it may be useful to state the obvious: that at any one stage of life, whether people have enough to live on will depend on four main considerations: their income; their expenditure; their earlier decisions about how best to organise their household; and their earlier provision against contingencies and lifecycle events.

Policy makers often speak of 'low pay' as if it were something entirely outside the influence of individuals. It is true that income is partly dependent on competition in the labour market, but we are not powerless. The rate of pay depends in part on skills acquired and willingness to move jobs or to change locality in order to command a higher wage. And the number of hours worked can be increased either through overtime or a second job, or another household member taking a job. The vast majority of people who escape poverty do so because they work hard and use their freedom to make the most of the conditions they find themselves in. One of the chief defects of many welfare benefits is that paying them can reduce work effort, a tendency to which family credit and working families tax credit are especially prone.

A certain amount of household expenditure is inevitable for simple survival, but some is discretionary, as earlier researchers like Rowntree recognised. The squalid conditions in which some people live are often the result of unwise expenditure. According to deterministic theories, however, to say as much is to 'blame the victim'. Household structure may also be the cause of low income and it, too, may be outside individual control, for example, when a partner is widowed or deserted. But often lone parenthood is a choice made by one or both parents, without proper consideration of the consequences for the children. Finally, we have become accustomed to relying on the state to provide against contingencies such as the death of the breadwinner or disability, and for lifecycle events such as the reduction of income during old age. However, income during retirement above the basic state pension has long been a personal responsibility with significant consequences for the standard of living.

With due allowance for factors beyond individual control, is it reasonable to expect individuals to take personal responsibility for improving their income, controlling their expenses, selecting an economically and socially viable family structure, and providing against both misfortunes and lifecycle events?

The welfare state was built on the assumption that it was not reasonable to expect anything like that degree of personal responsibility. Indeed it was built on very low, paternalistic, expectations and, step by step, it took responsibility for decisions that would have been better left to individuals. Provision against sick pay, the cost of primary medical care, and unemployment (for some) ceased to be voluntary in 1911. From 1920 most people had unemployment 'insurance', which was not insurance in the strict sense. Pensions followed under the 1925 Act.

During the 1920s and 30s it became possible to be better off out of work than in, though the impact was mitigated by the wage stop, which was introduced by the Unemployment Assistance Board in 1934 and not abolished until 1975.

From 1948 large families were subsidised, when people who could only afford a couple of children would have been better served by limiting their family. Personal responsibility for housing expenditure was diminished, at first by subsidising council rents and later by paying cash benefits. In 1967 a national scheme of rate rebates was introduced followed by a national scheme of rent rebates and allowances in 1972. In 1983 rent rebates and allowances became housing benefit.

In the 1940s and 1950s it was taken for granted that most men would work, and that couples who planned to raise children would get married in order to be self-sufficient as a family unit. However, it became possible during the 1970s to have a child outside marriage and to have enough to live on. Planning ahead in the sense of marrying a partner suitable to be a good father or mother and saving (the bottom drawer) became less important.

5.3 AN UNEMPLOYMENT ASSISTANCE INVESTIGATOR IN THE 1930s

Gladys Gibson

Source: Gray, N., *The Worst of Times: an Oral History of the Great Depression in Britain*, Wildwood House, London, 1985, pp. 60–1.

When I went to the Unemployment Assistance Board my position was difficult. My colleagues, one woman and a number of men, all came in from the suburbs. They thought I was mad to live in Stepney. I was not happy in the atmosphere at the office, where there was not much sympathy for the unemployed. The constant cry was 'Don't forget it's public money these people are getting.' Some people we visited were resentful of our right of entry into their homes, but most took it as a matter of course. One man told me to fill up my bloody form in the street but it did him no good. He had to go to the office to be ticked off.

I suppose the investigators were the lowest in the hierarchy in our office. The area officer once said to me, 'You surely don't want to be a common investigator all your life?' The porter, an Irishman, had been an N.C.O. in the British Army and when he had nothing to do he whistled a martial air and went through his drill, an imaginary musket on his shoulder. It was his job to see to the men in the waiting room, some called up for interview, some to report a change in their circumstances. He was anti-semitic, believing, against all the evidence, that no Jew ever fought in a war. One day he came with blazing eyes to tell me that one of my men, Jewish of course, was trying to get out of having me call by pitching a yarn about a visit to hospital. 'A nasty type. Cheeky. Know the feller? He drags a leg.' As he limped across the room to show me, I looked at the yellow card without which an unemployed man would be lost. 'It's an honourable limp,' I said. 'He draws a disability pension for it.' 'What! That cock sparrer? Who's the girl he's after seeing?' 'His daughter, in a sanatorium. His wife died of T.B. Please return his card, say I'll make another appointment and give him my best wishes.' I doubt whether the man got my good wishes but he caught his bus.

The office was usually crowded with people reporting changed circumstances or simply asking for more money. Occasionally a man twirled a razor blade on a string or clung to the legs of a table or chair. Most of the cases of threatening behaviour took place in the registry, a large room where there were several desks and a table for interview. I don't think I actually saw any violence though I heard scuffling and shouting when an offender was being hustled out by the porter. I came back one afternoon to write up my reports and found a broken window and some ruffled tempers. I was told that the porter was not to be found at the time. 'Where were you when the affray took place?' the area officer asked him. 'Sure I was like the Bobby when there's a bit of trouble. I was just around the corner.'

The morning the men barricaded themselves into the waiting room was exciting. They came in a body when the office opened, handed their yellow cards to the porter, hustled out the few men not involved and barred the door. We in our room heard singing, mostly music hall songs such as *Lily of Laguna*. There was consternation among the officers because our book of rules gave no instructions that met the case. The porter could hardly be restrained from battering in the door. The area office rang up a higher authority for instructions. The men inside wanted to send out a delegation of three to discuss their demands and the porter was delighted to bawl a refusal through the door. We had to go on our way but we heard later how the door had been lifted off its hinges and the contingent bundled out, laughing.

One of my colleagues was a plump, lugubrious little man whose parrot cry was 'Roll on Friday'. He said he was paid for only half the week. He had sailed the China seas selling whisky, but all good things come to an end. Most of the people were terrified of him. He said to me, speaking of a man I knew well, 'Why doesn't that young chap get himself a job?' 'He has a duodenal ulcer. Last time he was doing his stint on the Borough he collapsed.' 'They all say that,' he grumbled.

An older, well educated man who had been a geologist was very popular. The people liked him for his courtesy and his even temper. They referred to him as a nice old gent, a proper gentleman. He regarded himself as a cut above his colleagues and, when asked to go on an office outing, he replied, 'I wouldn't be seen dead among such people.' These words, often quoted, caused no resentment.

5.4 DISABLED PEOPLE AND DISINCENTIVES TO WORK

Cliff Prior

Source: 'Swallowed up by the system', *Community Care*, 29 July–4 August 1999, pp. 26–7.

Karen hears voices and suffers from panic attacks in public places. The voices feed the panic, terrifying Karen who is forced to retreat to the safety of her one-bedroom council flat in Bournemouth. She insists that she would never go out unless she had the safety net of enough money in her pocket to get a taxi home when the panic attacks strike.

'I would have to stay indoors,' she says. 'Knowing that I have enough money to get home means that I can combat the voices and stave off the panic attacks. The money is a must for me – it is part and parcel of maintaining and improving my mental health.'

Karen heard on the radio that the government was cutting benefits to disabled people and feared that she would be forced to retreat from the world and back into her small flat. She receives Incapacity Benefit and lower rate Disability Living Allowance to help with her care and mobility. In fact, Karen's benefits are safe. But only as long as she remains unemployed.

It is a deep irony that the government has built into its welfare-to-work plans a disincentive for people like Karen to seek work. Backbench rebellions and loud protestations from disability pressure groups forced the government to retreat from plans to cut Incapacity Benefit for all new claimants. People like Karen will be able to reclaim benefits at their old levels if a new job fails in the first twelve months. But, after that, if their job folds or their mental health worsens, they can be put on a lower rate of benefits. It is a real problem for people with a severe mental illness who may have successfully controlled their illness with the help of health and social support for many years.

Gerard was diagnosed with schizophrenia at the age of 18 and managed to carve out a successful career in spinal injury nursing for nearly twenty years before a 'young psychiatric registrar decided that I was too well to be a true schizophrenic'. His medication was stopped. 'I became mentally very ill because of the deleterious effects of this and was hospitalised for a period of two years.' Gerard is just the kind of person who, after two years hospitalisation, moves back to the community only to discover that he will be confined to the new lower rate Incapacity Benefit, despite two decades of national insurance contributions. The government says that Incapacity Benefit was abused by the last Tory government who turned it into an early retirement scheme to massage the unemployment figures. That is not the way Gerard sees it. 'I felt that I had to stop work after several attempts at resuming my job.' He is incapacitated and wants the government to recognise the fact.

Maureen had stayed out of hospital for seventeen years before a change in medication led to a breakdown. 'People I thought were my friends ignore me in the street and now my life is lonely,' she says. 'I am not well enough to hold down a job but I am doing some voluntary work and trying to learn something about computers.' She does not want the pressure of compulsory interviews and the threat of benefit cuts when she knows that she is not well enough to hold down a full time job.

Pressure and schizophrenia do not mix. People may feel well enough to work only to discover that the stress of holding down a job throws progress into reverse. Gerard says that while he was working as a nurse 'I was accepted, supported and treated as a normal person.' Unfortunately, Gerard's experience is far from the norm.

Annabelle has been in and out of work over the years and insists 'there is a block against people like us with a disability. I want to work, be accepted in society and pay my way. But, because of my illness, I have suffered verbal abuse at work and this caused me considerable distress and financial loss.' A recent ruling that schizophrenia is a disability for the purposes of disability discrimination legislation opens the way to greater employment protection, but there is nothing in the government's Welfare Reform Bill to match it for benefits protection.

People with a severe mental illness should not be confined to a life on benefits. However generous, they are no substitute for the financial and social rewards that can flow from paid employment. But, with unemployment rates approaching 90 per cent for people diagnosed with schizophrenia, identifying suitable work, getting over the catch-all mental health questions on the application form and convincing a prospective employer that you can cope is a huge task.

Experience from the National Schizophrenia Fellowship's 52 employment and training projects around the country tells us that the government's New Deal initiative for disabled people will create opportunities for people with a severe mental illness who have previously been prevented from working. The NFS has been awarded £170,000 of New Deal money to help people with a severe mental illness into sustained employment in the London and Essex areas.

NSF is serious about helping people get back to paid employment and other meaningful occupations. Employment lifts the social isolation experienced by many people with a severe mental illness and it puts money in their pockets. However, ministers have misunderstood the nature of severe mental illness in drawing up separate rules that will force disabled people to negotiate an obstacle course of employment and benefits interviews before being able to claim financial assistance if their work plans fail. [...]

5.5 WHO ARE SOCIAL SERVICES FOR?

Peter Beresford and Suzy Croft

Source: *Whose Welfare? Private Care or Public Services,*
Lewis Cohen Urban Studies Centre, Brighton, pp. 42–4.

[The authors are a partnership who have personal experience of being welfare recipients. They have become leading spokespersons, as academics and activists, for people who use services. The book from which this extract comes draws together evidence from people in one area of Brighton and, when it was published, was important on at least two counts. It investigated the reality of the localisation of public services following the turn to the more generic social work practice recommended in the Barclay Report of 1982. But perhaps more significantly it demonstrated it is essential to talk to those who are the recipients of care services.]

But other ideas and assumptions about social services held by members of the sample raise much more complicated issues. Some clearly saw social services as provided for particular groups, or people with particular problems.

You always think of social services helping the old and the poor, but not the average person, I suppose.

They are some sort of use, I suppose up the rougher areas of Brighton where you have families breaking up.

I think really it is mostly the older people who do need social services. I may need them as I get older as well.

I understand they are to provide a service of support and assistance for those who can't help themselves for a variety of reasons.

As well as the fourteen who made such explicit comments there were a few more ambiguous observations along the lines of 'Presumably they're good for the people who need them', where it was not clear whether people had in mind a particular kind or class of people for whom social services were intended, or circumstances or problems that might befall anyone.

A much larger number of people (34 out of a sample of 100) overlapping these, expressed the same attitude in a different way, saying or implying they did not see social services as being for people like them (19) or themselves as having any needs for social services (17). Again the two overlapped.

I have no needs relating to social services.

It doesn't affect me.

My idea of social services in my own life is nil.

I haven't any problems they'd want to cope with.
                                    (Unemployed young teacher)

I don't need help from social services.... I've never needed it or wanted it.
             (Young man who had been unemployed for 18 months and in trouble with the police)

I'd have thought they have enough without worrying about what problems I've got.
                                    (Young woman expecting a baby)

Only that it's stupid that people in our age group (66) – we've had a tough life – don't get help. I suppose they do their best for those who require it.

It couldn't offer me very much as I'm not really the sort of person who needs social services, not at the moment anyway.
                                    (Teacher in his 30s)

The woman part-time teacher was an exception who said 'I think of social services to be called on in moments of need'. What people seemed to be saying was 'I'm not the sort of person', or 'I haven't the kind of problem or need for social services to deal with' or perhaps, 'that I would take to them'. What was not always clear though was whether they meant they did not *at present* have needs to take to social services, but might one day, or that they could never envisage such a course of action for themselves. A couple suggested that it was something they might think about again or find out more about, when they were older. People's low expectations – their reluctance to burden social services – seemed to underlie some comments. In some cases the implication also seemed to be that people wanted or expected to keep clear of social services. Six people made explicit their desire to keep away from them, although their comments might also have meant that they were anxious to avoid the *reasons* for coming to social services' attention and not just social services themselves.

> *I'm glad they're there, but I don't want to have to use them.*

> *Any experience of them? No, not if I can help it.*

> *I don't need them, thank God.*

One woman, however, at the end of her interview expressed a feeling about welfare that many people have shared from the poor law to the present:

> *I'm sorry I don't know much about social services. I like to get on with my life. ... I don't like people telling me what to do. I suppose some people do need them though.*

The number (42) who seemed to see social services as for others and not for themselves was matched closely by the 41 who when asked, said they would not like to have closer contact with social services. They were also more likely to be included in this category than the rest of the sample. People categorised as working class were under-represented and those categorised as middle class were also over-represented among them.

While some of the people surveyed seemed to want to keep social services at arm's length, others as we have seen, appeared to think that social services were not intended, or didn't offer services for the kinds of needs they had. Some of those who said that they didn't think social services had

any understanding or interest in the kind of issues and problems that concerned them, didn't seem to expect them to, saying, for example, 'there's
no need for them to', 'I don't expect that' and 'It doesn't really apply'.
What is also not clear is whether people's disassociation of social services
from their own needs sprang from their own choice or self-perceptions, or
as many of the responses when people were asked whether they thought
social services had any understanding or interest in their needs, suggested,
because of their perceptions of social services' orientation and nature. Elsewhere in her interview, one woman said:

> In my circumstances, I don't think I'd ever get any help from social
> services as I've no children and I tend to associate them with families.
> My marriage has broken up and I've been through a very traumatic
> period, but I don't think they would have helped.

The question for us is whether this woman *should* have expected social
services to be concerned with the kind of problems she had faced, or those
facing the unemployed young teacher, or the young man who had got into
trouble with the police when he was out of work. Were people like these
mistaken in thinking that social services were not for them? Were others
right to see them as for certain stigmatised or disadvantaged groups rather
than 'for people like me'?

5.6 THE NEEDS OF STRANGERS

Michael Ignatieff

Source: *The Needs of Strangers*, Viking, London, 1984, pp. 9–12.

I live in a market street in north London. Every Tuesday morning there is a
barrow outside my door and a cluster of old age pensioners rummage
through the torn curtains, buttonless shirts, stained vests, torn jackets,
frayed trousers and faded dresses that the barrow man has on offer. They
make a cheerful chatter outside my door, beating down the barrow man's
prices, scrabbling for bargains like crows pecking among the stubble.

    They are not destitute, just respectably poor. The old men seem more
neglected than the women: their faces are grey and unshaven and their
necks hang loose inside yellowed shirt collars. Their old bodies must be
thin and white beneath their clothes. The women seem more self-
possessed, as if old age were something their mothers had prepared them

for. They also have the skills for poverty: the hems of their coats are neatly darned, their buttons are still in place.

These people give the impression of having buried their wives and husbands long ago and having watched their children decamp to the suburbs. I imagine them living alone in small dark rooms lit by the glow of electric heaters. I came upon one old man once doing his shopping alone, weighed down in a queue at a potato stall and nearly fainting from tiredness. I made him sit down in a pub while I did the rest of his shopping. But if he needed my help, he certainly didn't want it. He was clinging on to his life, gasping for breath, but he stared straight ahead when we talked and his fingers would not be pried from his burdens. All these old people seem like that, cut adrift from family, slipping away into the dwindling realm of their inner voices, clinging to the old barrow as if it were a raft carrying them out to sea.

My encounters with them are a parable of moral relations between strangers in the welfare state. They have needs, and because they live within a welfare state, these needs confer entitlements – rights – to the resources of people like me. Their needs and their entitlements establish a silent relation between us. As we stand together in line at the post office, while they cash their pension cheques, some tiny portion of my income is transferred into their pockets through the numberless capillaries of the state. The mediated quality of our relationship seems necessary to both of us. They are dependent on the state, not upon me, and we are both glad of it. Yet I am also aware of how this mediation walls us off from each other. We are responsible for each other, but we are not responsible to each other.

My responsibilities towards them are mediated through a vast division of labour. In my name a social worker climbs the stairs to their rooms and makes sure they are as warm and as clean as they can be persuaded to be. When they get too old to go out, a volunteer will bring them a hot meal, make up their beds, and if the volunteer is a compassionate person, listen to their whispering streams of memory. When they can't go on, an ambulance will take them to the hospital, and when they die, a nurse will be there to listen to the ebbing of their breath. It is this solidarity among strangers, this transformation through the division of labour of needs into rights and rights into care that gives us whatever fragile basis we have for saying that we live in a moral community.

Modern welfare may not be generous by any standard other than a comparison with the nineteenth-century workhouse, but it does attempt to satisfy a wide range of basic needs for food, shelter, clothing, warmth and medical care. The question is whether that is all a human being needs. When we talk about needs we mean something more than just the basic necessities of human survival. We also use the word to describe what a person needs in order to live to their full potential. What we need in order to survive, and what we need in order to flourish are two different things. The aged poor on my street get just enough to survive. The question is whether they get what they need in order to live a human life.

The political arguments between right and left over the future of the welfare state which rage over these old people's heads almost always take their needs entirely for granted. Both sides assume that what they need is income, food, clothing, shelter and medical care, then debate whether they are entitled to these goods as a matter of right, and whether there are adequate resources to provide them if they are. What almost never gets asked is whether they might need something more than the means of mere survival.

There are good reasons for this silence. It is difficult enough to define human need in terms of basic necessities. These are, after all, relative and historical, and there has always been fierce controversy over the level at which basic human entitlements should be set in any society. How much more controversial must be the definition of need as the conditions for human flourishing. There is not just one good human life, but many. Who is to say what humans need to accomplish all the finest purposes they can set for themselves?

It is also notorious how self-deceiving we are about our needs. By definition, a person must know that he desires something. It is quite possible, on the other hand, to be in need of something and not know that one is. Just as we often desire what we do not need, so we often need what we do not consciously desire.

If we often deceive ourselves about what we need, we are likely to be deceived about what strangers need. There are few presumptions in human relations more dangerous than the idea that one knows what another human being needs better than they do themselves. In politics, this presumption is a warrant to ignore democratic preferences and to trample on freedom. In other realms too, the arrogation of the right by doctors to define the needs of their patients, of social workers to administer the needs of their clients, and finally of parents to decide the needs of their children is in each case a warrant for abuse.

Yet if we are often deceived about our own needs, there must be cases in which it is in our interest that someone speaks for our needs when we ourselves cannot. There are people who have had to survive on so little for so long in our society that their needs have withered away to barest necessity. Is it wrong to raise their expectations, to give them a sense of the things they have gone without? Is it wrong to argue that the strangers at my door should not be content with the scraps at the barrow? Any politics which wants to improve the conditions of their lives has to speak for needs which they themselves may not be able to articulate. That is why politics is such a dangerous business: to mobilise a majority for change you must raise expectations and create needs which leap beyond the confines of existing reality. To create needs is to create discontent, and to invite disillusionment. It is to play with lives and hopes. The only safeguard in this dangerous game is the democratic requirement of informed consent. One has no right to speak for needs which those one represents cannot intelligibly recognise as their own. [...]

CHAPTER 6

THE HISTORY OF COMMUNITY CARE FOR PEOPLE WITH LEARNING DIFFICULTIES

Jan Walmsley and Sheena Rolph

In this chapter, we present some of the findings of our research into the history of community care for people with learning difficulties because we argue that it is important to examine how previous generations have wrestled with the sort of questions presented by the needs of people who need long term care or support. What role should families be expected to play? Can some of the costs of welfare be defrayed by encouraging participation in the labour market? How can a balance be struck between care and control, protecting the community and protecting the individual? In this chapter we seek to illuminate these questions by reference to past policies for people with learning disabilities.
[. . .]

The early twentieth century saw a sustained successful campaign to promote institutional care for 'mental defectives', culminating in the 1913 Mental Deficiency Act. Eugenic fears of criminality, violence, a rising tide of illegitimacy and racial degeneracy, all attributed to the 'feeble minded', coupled with more humanitarian concerns about neglect and abuse of vulnerable individuals produced enough impetus for a Royal Commission (The Radnor Commission) which sat from 1904 to 1908. The Act which followed set up machinery to identify this problematic group and to inhibit its numerical growth by segregation. Although best known for promoting institutional care, it also set up a framework for development of formal provision in the 'community'. Thomson sees this as the state appropriating

Source: 'The development of community care for people with learning difficulties 1913–1946', *Critical Social Policy*, 2001, 21, 1, pp. 59–80.

community care with the explicit intention of more effectively controlling 'mental defectives', thus dating the inception of formal community care far earlier than the 1950s (Thomson 1996).

The 1913 Act made it a duty of local authorities to ascertain, certify and, where necessary, institutionalize mental defectives. It introduced three types of formal 'care, supervision and control': institutional care, guardianship and supervision. These are described in turn.

Institutional care was seen, not as an end in itself, but as a means to an end, namely the provision of instruction and training, and to stabilize and socialize inmates and if possible fit them for life outside:

> *The modern aim is to restore such a person to the community pro-*
> *vided adequate steps can be taken to avoid his falling into misconduct*
> *or becoming a parent.*
>
> *(Shrubsall and Williams 1932: 177)*

A system of licensing patients to work or to be cared for outside was insti-tuted. Such licences were always conditional on good behaviour, and the patient could be returned to the institution without further formalities if there was concern about behaviour. Thus official policy explicitly visual-ized institutional care and community care as part of a continuum, with individuals expected to move from one to the other.

Guardianship provided for the placing of an individual in the control of a suitable person, a guardian whose powers were such 'as could be exer-cised by the parent of a child of under fourteen years' (Tredgold 1947: 445). If a guardian was appointed the local authority could provide finan-cial assistance, whereas without it no payments could be made outside the Poor Law framework. It was possible to make parents into formal guardians, thus enabling local authorities to pay allowances.

Statutory supervision consisted of the visiting and overseeing of defec-tives in their homes by salaried officials, health visitors, school nurses or local voluntary organizations. Visitors reported quarterly to their local Mental Deficiency Committee, and were to draw its attention to cases where proper control was not being exercised so that the defective could be placed under guardianship or institutional care.

The 1927 Mental Deficiency Act made it the duty of local authorities in addition to ensure that any necessary training was provided for all defec-tives. For those outside institutions, this meant Occupation and Industrial Centres, forerunners of the modern Adult Training Centre.

There were many gaps in implementation, but in principle the 1913 and 1927 Mental Deficiency Acts created a framework of formal community care. However, rather than being seen as an alternative to the institution, community care in the interwar years was an adjunct to it, providing for individuals before entering institutional care, after leaving it and, indeed, for those who never experienced it.

Some contemporaries had a clear vision of community care and its role. This is the vision of Evelyn Fox, Secretary of the Central Association for Mental Welfare:

> *Community care should vary from the giving of purely friendly advice and help to the various forms of state guardianship with compulsory power ... It should include the power of affording every kind of assistance to the defective – boarding out, maintenance grants, the provision of tools, travelling expenses to and from work, of temporary care, change of air – in a word, all those things which will enable a defective to remain safely in his family ... If the state has undertaken the duty and responsibility of active interference in the life of an individual by supervision, compulsory attention and so forth, it must undertake the corresponding duty of making his life as happy as possible.*
>
> *The effective control of a defective at home does inevitably mean a restriction in his complete freedom to go in and out as he pleases, to make what friends he chooses, to select what type of employment he likes out of those that are open to him. To impose these limitations without at the same time giving compensating interests is to court disaster.*
>
> *(Fox, 1930: 71)*

Fox's vision illustrates the complementarity of care and control. One notes the taken-for-granted role of the family as a place where he can remain 'safely', with the proviso that 'effective control' is exercised, alongside the impetus to positive provision to offset the 'loss of freedom'.

The role of the family

Fox placed the family at the centre of community care. In effect, families were to be co-opted to supply 'effective control'. If they did not, then institutional care was imposed. In practice a large proportion of people certified as 'defective' remained with their families. In 1939 Board of Control statistics show 46,054 in institutions, with 43,850 under statutory supervision (quoted in Tredgold 1947). As hostels were rare (Jones 1972), it seems safe to assume that large numbers lived with family members.

Families where a 'mental defective' had been certified were subject to regular critical scrutiny for their ability to care for and, above all, control their relative. Families were means tested for contributions to the cost of keeping their relatives in institutions. They also had to pay towards the cost of attending an occupation centre, where one was available. Visitors were required to respond to questions about the family's ability and willingness to prevent defectives from associating with the opposite sex:

> *Frequent visits should be paid by an experienced visitor and any tendency to form friendships likely to lead to marriage or immorality should be reported at once, in order that recall to the Institution or a change of Guardianship can be effected in time.*
> *(Somerset Mental Deficiency Committee, 1925)*

When decisions were made about allowing discharge, home leave from institutions, or suitability for licensing, the family was scrutinized. For example in 1937 Florence O.'s brother wrote to the Bedfordshire Mental Deficiency Committee requesting that she be allowed home for a holiday: 'I am the only one who gose [sic] to see her. I thought a change would do her good to being in there.' The letter prompted a visit by the voluntary visitor who reported:

> *The rooms were not only untidy but in a very dirty condition. . . . In my judgment it is highly undesirable that a defective who has at the present time the benefits of living in clean and healthy surroundings should be granted leave of absence to these premises.*
> *(Bedfordshire Mental Deficiency Committee, 1914–1940: Vol. 23)*

The request for home leave was refused.

[. . .]

Family resistance to institutional care was cited by the Bedfordshire Mental Deficiency Committee when asked by the Luton Education Committee in 1932 why less than half the children and young people certified by them as mental defectives had been provided for: their reply indicated that fifteen of the thirty-two parents were unwilling for them to be institutionalized (Bedfordshire Mental Deficiency Committee, 1914–1940: Vol. 23). The absence, in this local authority, of any midway point between quarterly supervision or full scale institutional care meant that provision for those who were not deemed to be a danger to 'the community' was minimal.

Although the word 'abuse' is not used, at times concern for the safety of the individual prompted action in their own interest. Walmsley *et al.* (1999) cite an instance of a woman's return to an institution after a period on licence because of 'an incestuous relationship with her father'. Again, this is far from an isolated instance, though careful reading of the evidence is necessary to infer abuse because of a tendency to blame the victim in official reports.

Family 'respectability' was influential. Visitors' Reports from Bedford-shire in the 1930s shows that, on the whole, the Visitor was prepared to support families, occasionally interceding with the Committee for small grants. But some families drew the Visitor's attention as being in need of more than supervision. Poverty and poor management were factors. The 'S.' family of Marston Morteyne was one such. The Visitor reported in March 1937 that 'the home is a poor one, though there does not seem to be a lack of money'. The Reports became more critical over the following year: 'an unfortunate family', 'mother is a delicate person of very simple intellect', one daughter 'certainly deficient', another 'definitely not normal'. It was decided to institutionalize one of the daughters to help the family cope with 'the remaining borderline defective children' (Bedfordshire Mental Deficiency Committee, 1914–1940: Vol. 23 passim).

Another factor appears to have been the absence of a mother. George C., aged 17, lived with his father and worked on his farm. In March 1937 the Visitor reported that she had visited and believed 'the lad would benefit from training' as there was no mother, and he was left alone a lot of the time. George's father was duly persuaded it would be in his best interests to go to the local colony, Bromham, where he remained for twenty-three years (Bedfordshire Mental Deficiency Committee, 1914–1940: Vol. 23; Atkinson 1997).

Care, control (and neglect)

As noted, the formal position was that all certified mental defectives were to be provided for, whether inside or outside the institution. In practice, there were huge gaps. Some local authorities developed quite sophisticated provision. Middlesex had twelve occupation centres before the Second World War, and arranged for home tuition to groups, but Bedfordshire did not open its first occupation centre until 1947 (French 1971).

Somerset had five occupation centres in 1929 (Walmsley et al. 1999). These were seen as: 'one of the most satisfactory means of keeping in touch with defectives living in their own homes or under guardianship' (Darwin 1926). Residential accommodation outside of institutions was a rarity, though where it existed it had an important bridging role (see later discussion).

One way of assessing the adequacy of provision is to look at the perspective of those on the receiving end. Oral history evidence (Rolph 2000) gives insight into one family's experience. Mrs R.'s uncle, born in 1900, had learning difficulties and epilepsy. Until he was 30 he was cared for by the family, initially his father, and later his brother, her own father. She recalled:

Strange thing was we had a very small cottage and mother had us three children in three years, but we managed somehow. . . . Of course it was the recognised thing in those days that you did look after your family . . . you all helped each other.

When he was a man of 30 he had to go into the Poor Law institution. [The market garden business failed and] my parents emigrated to Canada with us in 1930 and the sisters couldn't look after him. He went into the Poor Law, and of course that was like an institution.

There is no mention of help from community care facilities. It also illustrates some factors which caused the breakdown of a family's capacity to care – poverty caused by economic recession.

The voluntary sector had a part to play in enabling local authorities to exercise care and control, and to some extent prevent neglect. The National Association for Promoting the Welfare of the Feeble Minded (founded 1896) had campaigned for the 1913 Act, and subsequently played an important role under its new name, the Central Association for Mental Welfare. It lobbied for change: as early as 1921 it was urging local authorities to begin 'friendly supervision' for 'borderline cases'. In Bedfordshire, Buckinghamshire and Somerset its members were the Visitors who undertook supervisory visits, and wrote the Reports. Our examination of the records of six local authorities indicates that the stronger the Voluntary Association, the greater the level of community care activity. Buckinghamshire formed its branch in 1914, and there was a Visitor in every parish. Visitors were active in reporting suspected defectives: the number they reported regularly exceeded the number of subsequent certifications. Members, mostly women, visited Poor Law institutions, organized home tuition, advertised for guardians and maintained links with people out on licence. For those under statutory supervision the voluntary Visitor was the primary link with the family, and the Visitor had the duty of balancing care and control, providing some support, but also reporting people who appeared either neglected or inadequately controlled.

Little evidence has yet come to light about how families perceived these visits. Peggy, sister of a woman with Downs Syndrome born in the 1930s, recalled visits from:

a rather large florid lady – I believe she was a retired district nurse – who always rode a bicycle. . . . This person came one day to our home when Kathleen was still very young, and after her visit our mother was very worried and upset. The woman came a second time when our father was there and he ordered her out, shouting and swearing, telling her to go away and mind her own business. From the following undercurrent, I gathered she was 'trying to take Kathleen away from us'. She never came again, but whenever I saw her afterwards I felt afraid, and came to regard her as a big black witch who wanted to steal my sister.

(Personal communication, 9 May 1999)

Such testimonies remind us both that families could resist officialdom, and that the machinery of community care could be quite threatening.

Some voluntary sector initiatives made inroads into the absence of residential provision. The Guardianship Society, Brighton (BGS) was founded in 1914 to 'board out the Mentally and Physically Defective and other cases under the Deficiency, Lunacy Act or otherwise', and to supervise such cases. Its 1914 publicity stated: 'Emphasis is given to individual care in family life against institutional care and treatment' (Aloisio, 1995: 1). The BGS founded the first class for training 'the mentally handicapped' outside of large institutions in 1914. Although it initially served the Brighton area, from 1916 other local authorities began to contract for their 'mental defectives' to be cared for by Guardians recruited and supervised by the BGS. The Society advertised itself thus in 1916:

The procedure is to place the patient under the care of a respectable family, generally of the working class. Suitable employment is sought: if found, most of the wages are used to defray maintenance charges.

(Letter from BGS filed in Bedfordshire Mental Deficiency Committee, 1914–1940: Vol. 3)

By 1933 it had contracts with forty local authorities and 1076 clients and had developed training farms and occupation centres (Aloisio 1995). The BGS emphasis on family-style care as early as 1914 is a harbinger of attitudes which came into prominence much later, for example in the 1971 White Paper, *Better Services*.

Work and its significance

Whereas there was no discernible rhetoric in the philosophy of early-twentieth-century community care to echo the modern aim of enabling people to live as independently as possible (Department of Health 1989), enabling people to earn their keep was seen as desirable. Being in work did not prevent people from being taken into institutions if sexual control was at stake. Sixteen-year-old Grace H. of Luton was institutionalized in 1936 despite having a job in a box factory, and despite the objections of her family, because she was staying out all night. But in the same year, in the same local authority, it was decided not to certify Samuel E., aged 17, described as 'a quiet well behaved boy' with a mental age of 10 who 'may settle to a job of a simple nature, and his aunt is endeavouring to find him a suitable post' (Bedfordshire Mental Deficiency Committee, 1914–1940: Vol. 23).

Obtaining a job for 'mental defectives' was an explicit aim of some community care services. Eaton Grange, a hostel for women in Norwich set up in 1930, sought employment for women as domestic servants in local homes. This had a dual purpose – it defrayed some of the expenses of care because a proportion of the wages was appropriated by the local authority, and it furnished daytime occupation in a controlled environment (Rolph 2000). Similarly, patients going out on licence from institutions were placed in settings where they could be fully regulated. In 1940 there were ten women out on licence from Bromham Hospital, Bedfordshire, all of whom were in domestic service, or doing domestic work in hospitals or sanitoria (Bedfordshire Mental Deficiency Committee, 1914–1940: Vol. 40).

Work had a role in enabling local authorities to exercise control. They were exhorted by the central authority, the Board of Control, to develop community care. A 1937 circular encouraged local authorities 'to promote harmony in the workings of the Mental Deficiency Acts' by the use of 'community care' – licensing, occupation centres, finding guardians – but at the same time warned against letting people out who were 'unsuitable' (Board of Control 1937). Situations where people lived in, and where employers could be expected to report misdemeanours, were attractive. From the point of view of the individual, the opportunity to work was often valued, and it could be a positive experience. Rolph (1999), for example, cites the case of Alice who, after a life in institutions, found a surrogate family life in her role as a domestic servant to a Norwich family. But it also opened the person to exploitation. Oral history evidence shows that some of the women in domestic service in Norwich were worked extremely hard 'doing the rough', and that hostel authorities failed to protect them from this (Rolph 2000).

Conclusion

We have shown that in the early twentieth century there existed a statutory system of community care which occupied a significant place in managing the space between the family and the institution, in supervising those outside the institution, in providing the evidence for commitment to an institution and in managing those out on licence.

Of what significance is this for an understanding of modern social policy developments? In part, it is simply a matter of correcting some prevailing assumptions, putting the record straight and placing the institutional era in context. Institutions were never the only answer to care for or to control people with learning difficulties. They were too expensive, impractical and in many cases unnecessary.

The thrust of much feminist research of the 1980s was to point out that community care shifted the burden onto families (see Pascall 1986, for example). This point was well made, but understates the extent to which families have always been expected to manage long term care. In the early twentieth century families were officially seen as objects of suspicion, likely to allow their defective children to multiply if not carefully supervised. But in practice rule of thumb judgments were made and 'good' or even adequate families left to manage with some minimal support from supervisory visits, or occupation centre where available. Families were charged for services. The post-war development of providing care free of charge begins to look like the aberration. This is not to justify initiatives to charge people for services like residential care or day services. It is to say that such practices are a reversion rather than an innovation.

Another point of significance is that the 1913 Mental Deficiency Act made it a duty of local authorities to exercise both care and control for all 'mental defectives' in their area. Although in practice this duty was not always carried out, it is a contrast to the situation which prevailed after the 1959 Act. As Marais observed in the 1970s, 'there is no mandatory duty laid upon the social services departments requiring them to have knowledge of, let alone remain in contact with, all the mentally handicapped people within their catchment areas' (Marais 1976: 227). Seen in this light, 'neglect' is more a hall-mark of the present than it was of the pre-1959 system.

Current welfare policy encourages people to work: 'the new welfare state should help and encourage people of working age to work when they are capable of doing so' and increasing the number of disabled people able to work is a specific policy objective (Welfare Reform Group 1998: 2, 6). Enabling people with learning difficulties to work through schemes like supported employment is seen as progressive, offering both an income and a valued social role (National Development Team 1992; Beyer 1995). The late-twentieth-century belief that paid work for people with learning difficulties is a good thing for enhancement of individual self-esteem has no real echoes in early-twentieth-century rhetoric, but encouraging people into manual or domestic labour, for minimal wages, was seen as a constructive objective because it both defrayed the costs of care and furnished an additional element of control.

In contrast to notions of community care in the 1990s – to 'enable people to achieve maximum independence and control over their lives' (Department of Health 1989) – the early-twentieth-century ideology was to use community care alongside institutional care to exert control over 'defectives' and their families. This is an important difference. However, debates around sterilization continue (Stanworth 1989), particularly in relation to genetic screening (Shakespeare 1998). Not only this, recent developments in mental health care have reintroduced routine surveillance as a dimension of community care (Royal College of Psychiatrists 1996; Brindle 1998). Whereas in the early twentieth century 'mental defectives' represented dangerousness, now it is people with mental illness.

Our historical survey shows that formal community care has long had elements of care and control. A combination of protecting the community and protecting the individual motivated the legislators of 1913. Community care developed alongside institutional care, an adjunct and an alternative. Local authorities sought to manage the system with a view to minimizing public resistance, but with an eye to the threat of allowing people perceived to be 'dangerous' to roam large. In view of current preoccupations with managing care in the community for people with mental health problems, it is salutary to recall that such a policy has longer antecedents than has generally been thought.

REFERENCES

Aloisio, F. (1995) *Grace Eyre Foundation: The Founder and the Foundation.* Brighton: Grace Eyre Foundation.

Atkinson, D. (1997) *An Auto/Biographical Approach to Learning Disability Research.* Ashgate: Avebury.

Bedfordshire Mental Deficiency Committee (1914–1940) *Mental Deficiency Papers Volumes 1 to 40.* (The records are kept in the Bedfordshire County Record Office.)

Beyer, S. (1995) 'Real Jobs and Supported Employment', in T. Philpot and L. Ward (eds) *Values and Visions: Changing Ideas in Services for People with Learning Difficulties.* London: Butterworth Heinemann.

Board of Control (1937) *Circular 835.* London: Board of Control.

Brindle, D. (1998) '£1bn to End Care in the Community', *Guardian,* 25 July, p. 1.

Darwin, R. (1926) 'The Proper Care of Defectives Outside Institutions', Paper presented at the 1926 Conference on Mental Welfare, Taunton, Somerset quoted in D. Atkinson 'Learning from Local history: Evidence from Somerset', in D. Atkinson, M. Jackson and J. Walmsley (eds) *Forgotten Lives: Exploring the History of Learning Disability.* Kidderminster: British Institute of Learning Difficulties.

Department of Health (1989) *Caring for People.* London: HMSO.

Fox, E. (1930) 'Community Schemes for the Social Control of Mental Defectives', *Mental Welfare* xi(3): 71.

French, C. (1971) *A History of the Development of the Mental Health Services in Bedfordshire.* Bedford: Bedfordshire County Council.

Jones, K. (1972) *A History of the Mental Health Services.* London: Routledge and Kegan Paul.

Marais, M. (1976) *Lives Worth Living: the Right of all the Handicapped.* London: Souvenir Press.

National Development Team (1992) *Survey of Supported Employment Services in England, Scotland and Wales.* Manchester: NDT.

Pascall, G. (1986) *Social Policy: A Feminist Analysis*, London: Routledge.

Rolph, S. (1999) 'Enforced Migrations by People With Learning Disabilities: a Case Study', *Oral History* 27(1): 47–56.

Rolph, S. (2000) *The History of Community Care for People With Learning Difficulties in Norfolk*, PhD research in progress. Milton Keynes: Open University.

Royal College of Psychiatrists (1996) *Report of the Confidentiality Inquiry into Homicides and Suicides by Mentally Ill People* (Boyd Report) Royal College of Psychiatrists for the Confidentiality Inquiry into Homicides and Suicides by Mentally Ill People.

Shakespeare, T. (1998) 'Choices and Rights: eugenics, Genetics and Disability Equality', *Disability and Society* 13(5): 665–83.

Shrubsall, F.C. and Williams, A.C. (1932) *Mental Deficiency Practice.* London: University of London Press.

Somerset Mental Deficiency Act Committee (1925) *Annual Report.* Taunton, Somerset: Somerset Mental Deficiency Act Committee.

Stanworth, M. (1989) 'The New Eugenics', in A. Brechin and J. Walmsley (eds) *Making Connections.* London: Hodder and Stoughton.

Thomson, M. (1996) 'Family, Community and State: the Micro Politics of Mental Deficiency', in A. Digby and D. Wright (eds) *From Idiocy to Mental Deficiency: Historical Perspectives on People with Learning Difficulties.* London: Routledge.

Tredgold, A.F. (1947) *A Text Book of Mental Deficiency (amentia)*, 7th edn. London: Baillière Tindall.

Walmsley, J., Rolph, S. and Atkinson, D. (1999) 'Community Care and Mental Deficiency 1913–1945', in P. Bartlett and D. Wright (eds) *Outside the Walls of the Asylum.* London: Athlone Press.

Welfare Reform Group Green Paper Consultation Team (1998) *New Ambitions for our Country: a New Contract for Welfare* (Consultation Document) London: Department of Social Security (DSS).

CHAPTER 7

MULTIPLE OPPRESSION AND THE DISABLED PEOPLE'S MOVEMENT

Ayesha Vernon

[...] In recent years there has been a number of polemical writings expressing a general dissatisfaction that the differing experiences of disabled women (Lloyd 1992; Morris 1991, 1996) and disabled Black people (Hill 1994a; Stuart 1993) are overlooked by social model theorists because of an overwhelming desire to proclaim commonality in the experience of disablement. For example, Morris (1996) has commented:

> the experience of disabled women has been largely absent from feminism's concerns and within the disabled people's movement has tended to be tagged on as a special interest ... Our encounters with both groups have often made us feel powerless for we have either been treated as invisible or our experiences have been defined for us. (p. 1)

Campbell and Oliver (1996) assert that the disabled people's movement has not so much ignored these issues out of a deliberate attempt to marginalize the experience of any one group. Rather it has been a 'pragmatic decision' to concentrate on an issue which has been so completely overlooked by other social movements – namely, how society disables people who have impairments. This may, indeed, be the case. However, it is also true, as Morris (1991, p. 178) points out, that 'Disabled people and their

Source: T. Shakespeare (ed.) *The Disability Reader: Social Science Perspective*, Continuum, London, 1998, Chapter 13, pp. 205–10.

organizations are no more exempt from racism, sexism and heterosexism than non-disabled people and their organizations ... both women and ethnic minorities are distinctly under-represented and issues around racism, sexism and sexuality have tended to be avoided.'

Similar critiques also exist with regard to other social movements, particularly the feminist movement (Adams 1994; Bhavnani and Coulson 1986; Carby 1982). Barnes (1996a) has responded to the criticisms made of the disabled people's movement by asserting that:

> *We live in a society centred around patriarchy, inequality and elitism, and it is inevitable that these traits should be present in our own organizations. But in my experience the British disabled people's movement has done far more than most to address these issues ... the movement has, in fact, been dominated by women ... women have held and continue to hold key posts in most of the organizations up and down the country. (p. 56)*

However, the real concern is not whether the disabled people's movement has enough numbers of disabled women or Black people in its organizations. Although, if they are grossly under-represented in proportion to their representation in the surrounding community, then that should also be a legitimate cause for concern. It is the fact that in all the numerous discussions and textbooks on disability, issues of 'race', gender, class, sexuality and age have been either omitted as irrelevant to disabled people's lives or added on as an optional extra.

Hill (1994b) argues that disabled Black people should 'keep faith with the Black voluntary sector' rather than with the disabled people's movement. However, this is far from satisfactory (Vernon 1996). The assertion that pragmatism dictates a need to concentrate on one oppression at a time is also prevalent in the Black community where the sole emphasis is on overcoming racism, as Macdonald's (1991) experience of his family's reaction demonstrates: 'to fight for the rights of black people is one thing; to fight for the rights of disabled people is something else, there is not enough time and energy to fight two different wars.' Such attitudes present a real dilemma for those who are rendered a multiple Other because, if you cannot be sure that the other Xs, Ys or Zs are going to accept or understand the extra dimension of your additional identity as a V or a W, which aspect of your identity do you prioritize and which do you leave out? The experience of those who are subjected to several forms of oppression cannot be compartmentalized as though they are quite distinct and separate from one another.

Barnes (1996b, cited by Campbell and Oliver 1996) has commented:

The politics of disablement is about far more than disabled people; it is about challenging oppression in all its forms. Indeed, impairment is not something which is peculiar to a small section of the population, it is fundamental to the human experience. Disability – defined by the disabled people's movement as the social oppression of people with impairments – on the other hand, is not. Like racism, sexism, heterosexism and all other forms of social oppression it is a human creation. It is impossible, therefore, to confront one type of oppression without confronting them all and, of course, the cultural values that created and sustain them.

This is indeed true. The politics of eradicating any oppression must take into account the whole oppressive nature of society and challenge all forms of social oppression, not least because of the mutual supporting interaction between different ideologies of oppression (Miles 1989; Williams 1995), but also because individuals are seldom affected by only one form of oppression.

However, the reality is rather different in that the politics of disability has only ever focused on disablement (the oppression of people with impairments). This is not unique to the disabled people's movement. The fundamental problem is that each oppressed group is really focusing only on a single system of oppression, the nearest to its heart, believing it to be the primary cause of all human suffering. An example is the feminist analysis of patriarchy seeing men's domination of women as the primary oppression and Black people seeing racism as the primary oppression etc. (King 1988); therefore, overlooking the significant feature of human oppression which is the interlocking of the different ideologies of oppression (Hill-Collins 1990), especially because individuals seldom fall into one neat category (for example, disabled women, Black middle-class men).

The experience of multiple oppression is treated as though it is an issue which concerns only a minority of disabled people. However, the majority of disabled people inevitably consists of disabled Black people, women, gay men and lesbians, older people and those from the working class, all of whom experience the negative effects of being rendered a multiple Other in consequence of deviating from the established norm in several ways. Consequently they are rejected for several reasons and from several quarters including those with whom they share some commonality (Vernon 1996). For example, Dragonsani Renteria, a deaf lesbian from the Hispanic community, has succinctly captured this reality in her poem 'Rejection' (1993, p. 38).

Thus, whilst disability may be the only aspect of disabled white heterosexual men's experience of oppression, the same cannot be said of disabled Black people, women, gay men and lesbians, older people and those from the working class. They can point to no single source for their oppression. For them the potential for discrimination is greater in all situations because of the increased likelihood of one or another aspect of their stigmatized identity being an 'undesired differentness' (Goffman 1968).

Their experience is commonly characterized by multiple rejections, discriminations and fragmentation of their identity even within the equality movements, including the disabled people's movement.

Despite some obvious differences between the experience of disabled Black people and white people, as well as between disabled women and men, etc., there is one critical similarity in the experience of all disabled people arising from the stigma of impairment which often overrides all other boundaries of 'race', gender, sexuality, class and age (Vernon 1996).

Because of this, the social model of disability has significance for all disabled people despite the fact that for many disabled people it does not account for the whole of their experience. However, the fault does not lie with the social model of disability, which is an excellent framework for ultimately eradicating the oppression of people who have impairments and, as such, must remain non-negotiable. Rather the problem lies in how the social model is being applied. That is, if the ensuing discussion does not take account of the fact that for the majority of disabled people their experience of oppression is shaped by additional dimensions of their lives, then the application of that methodology needs to be examined, for it represents only a partial picture. For example, if disabled people achieve full civil rights (enshrined in an anti-discrimination legislation which the disabled people's movement is tirelessly campaigning for), we will no longer be barred from entering public buildings, travelling on public transport, denied a job or educational opportunities on the basis of our impairment as we are now. But those of us who are Black, female, gay, etc. will continue to be denied jobs and experience (or live under a constant threat of experiencing) verbal and physical abuse.

There is an underlying assumption which is that the other experiences of disabled people such as racism, sexism and heterosexism are taken care of by other social movements. This would be true. Except that disabled people, because of the stigma of being impaired, are also excluded from the movements of 'race', gender and sexuality. Therefore it is all the more important that the disabled people's movement should not exclude or marginalize the experience of disabled people who are a multiple Other. Furthermore it is all the more important that the experience of disabled Black people, women, gay men and lesbians, older people and those from the working class is fully integrated to take account of the fact that the experience of disability is often exacerbated by the interaction of other forms of oppression. The politics of eradicating disability, therefore, must take into account the whole oppressive structure of our society and be careful to challenge all forms of oppression wherever it is found. It is not enough merely to acknowledge that, because inequality is rife in society at large, it is inevitable that disabled people will have absorbed these practices too. To do so is to condone and perpetuate all forms of inequality. As Read (1988) points out, in a society that is riddled with oppression there is no neutral ground.

REFERENCES

Adams, M.L. (1994) There's no place like home: on the place of identity in feminist politics, in M. Evans (ed.) *The Woman Question*. London: Sage.

Barnes, C. (1996a) Disability and the myth of the independent researcher, *Disability and Society*, 11, 1, 107–10.

Barnes, C. (1996b) The social model of disability: myths and misrepresentations,
Coalition, August, 25–30.

Bhavnani, K.-K. and Coulson, M. (1986) Transforming socialist-feminism: the
challenge of racism, in M. Evans (ed.) *The Woman Question*. London: Sage.

Campbell, J. and Oliver, M. (1996) *Disability Politics: Understanding Our Past,
Changing Our Future*. London: Routledge.

Carby, H. (1982) White woman listen! Black feminism and the boundaries of sis-
terhood, in Centre for Contemporary Cultural Studies (eds) *The Empire Strikes
Back: Race and Racism in 70s Britain*. London: Hutchinson.

Goffman, E. (1968) *Stigma*. Harmondsworth: Pelican.

Hill, M. (1994a) 'They are not our brothers': the disability movement and the
black disability movement, in N. Begum, N. Hill, and A. Stevens (eds) *Reflections: The Views of Black Disabled People on Their Lives and Community
Care*. London: CCETSW.

Hill (1994b) Burn and rage: Black voluntary organizations as a source of social
change, in N. Begum, N. Hill, and A. Stevens (eds) *Reflections: The Views of
Black Disabled People on Their Lives and Community Care*. London:
CCETSW.

Hill-Collins, P. (1990) *Black Feminist Thought: Knowledge, Consciousness and the
Politics of Empowerment*. London: Unwin Hyman.

King, D.K. (1988) Multiple jeopardy, multiple consciousness: the context of a
black feminist ideology, *Signs*, Autumn.

Lloyd, M. (1992) Does she boil eggs? Towards a feminist model of disability, *Disability, Handicap and Society*, 7, 3 (October), 207–21.

Macdonald, P. (1991) Double discrimination must be faced now. *Disability Now*,
March.

Miles, R. (1989) *Racism*. London: Routledge.

Morris, J. (1991) *Pride Against Prejudice: Transforming Attitudes to Disability*.
London: Women's Press.

Morris, J. (ed.) (1996) *Encounters with Strangers: Feminism and Disability*.
London: Women's Press.

Read, J. (1988) *The Equal Opportunities Book*. London: Interchange Books.

Renteria, D. (1993) Rejection, in R. Luczak (ed.) *Eyes of Desire: A Deaf Gay &
Lesbian Reader*. New York: Alyson Publications.

Stuart, O. (1993) Double oppression: an appropriate starting point? in J. Swain,
V. Finkelstein, S. French and M. Oliver (eds) *Disabling Barriers – Enabling
Environments*. London: Sage.

Vernon, A. (1996) Fighting two different battles: unity is preferable to enmity, *Disability and Society*, 11, 2, 285–90.

Williams, F. (1995) Race/ethnicity, gender, and class in welfare states: a framework
for comparative analysis, *Social Politics*, Summer, 127–59. Chicago: University
of Illinois.

CHAPTER 8

CAMPAIGNING AND THE PENSIONERS' MOVEMENT

Dave Goodman

North Staffs is a compact area centred on the city of Stoke-on-Trent. In a population of around half a million, it is estimated that the number of men and women of pension age is of the order of 100,000.

Before 1991 there was no campaigning pensioner organisation in North Staffs, only a large number of local groups whose activities were purely social. Tea and biscuits, bingo, an annual Christmas dinner and day outings during the summer: these were the order of the day, and many of the groups continue to offer these very useful services to their members. What has changed since 1991 is the development of a campaigning organisation with a very high profile, the North Staffs Pensioners' Convention. This is a component part of the National Pensioners' Convention, an umbrella body which is recognised by the Government and other interests, as the main organisation representing Britain's 11 million pensioners.

The restoration of the pensions–earnings link

In the local government elections of May 2000, each candidate of the ruling Labour Party in Stoke-on-Trent distributed an election address which strongly featured the Party's concern with pensioner issues. Its front cover, headed 'You're better off with a Labour Council', gave 'helping pensioners' as a reason. Inside, a prominent panel declared 'Your Labour Councillors support the North Staffs Pensioners' Convention in their campaign for a better deal for pensioners'. The key demand of that better deal was the subject of another panel which proclaimed 'Your Labour City Council supports the restoration of the pensions–earnings link'.

Over the years, the Convention has established a dialogue with all five local MPs. Meetings with them are held at intervals, either in the MPs' constituency offices or in the premises of the Convention. The object of the dialogue is to persuade the MPs to back the policy of the National Pensioners' Convention rather than that of the Government. Differences between the MPs and the Convention have been resolved in the course of these discussions, and this has been followed by the MPs, collectively as a North Staffs group, making representations to Pension Ministers in support of Convention policy. In the Commons debate on restoring the earnings link, forty-one back-bench Labour MPs defied the Government Whip and went into the rebel lobby. They included the three Stoke-on-Trent MPs.

A high point of the national campaign was a Day of Action on 7 November, 2000. This followed a victory for its policy at the Labour Party's Annual Conference. This was the first ever defeat of the platform for New Labour. On the Day of Action, a national petition of over half a million signatures, addressed to the Queen, was handed in to Buckingham Palace. The North Staffs Pensioners' Convention contributed 20,000 signatures to this petition. There followed a large rally in Westminster Central Hall sponsored by the *Sunday Mirror*, after which the action moved to the House of Commons. Here another rally was held at which Jack Jones, Barbara Castle and other leading campaign figures, reported on meetings they had had that day with the Prime Minister and Chancellor of the Exchequer. The Day ended with a Lobby of MPs.

Hundreds of pensioners from all parts of the country took part in the day's events. Amongst them were forty from the North Staffs Pensioners' Convention who travelled by coach. Because of the relationship that has developed with the MPs, they obtained access to the House without queueing and met the North Staffs MPs in the Grand Committee Room for a constructive and friendly exchange of views. Their level of commitment was demonstrated by the fact that each paid £9.00 towards the cost of the coach which left Stoke-on-Trent bus station at 7.45 a.m., returning fourteen hours later at 9.45 p.m. (added to which was the time spent travelling between home and bus).

Further evidence of the influence of the local Convention is that all three Local Authorities have unanimously adopted, and forwarded to the Government, motions which call for the restoration of the pensions–earnings link so that pensioners can share in the country's growing prosperity.

My retirement and the origins of the North Staffs Pensioners' Convention

It was in 1979 that I retired from a post in a residential adult education college. Some years later I got round to a project that I had saved for my retirement. This was a study of the forgotten history of how the old age pension was won in Britain in 1908. Contrary to the widely held view, the credit for this socially historic landmark should not be given to David Lloyd George, the Chancellor who piloted the measure through the House. Those to whom the principal credit is due are the pioneers who initiated a hard fought ten-year campaign and saw it through to a successful outcome. The Liberal Government was persuaded, reluctantly and grudgingly, to concede the Old Age Pension Act. The campaigners included Liverpool ship owner and pioneer of research into poverty, Charles Booth, the chocolate manufacturer, George Cadbury, the Warden of the Browning Settlement in South East London, Rev. Francis Herbert Stead, and the Organiser of the National Pensions Committee, Frederick Rogers. Also involved were leaders of Organised Labour (as the trade unions were then known) and Church leaders of all denominations.

It was their story that I told in a book, *No Thanks to Lloyd George*, published in 1988 for the 80th anniversary of the Act. The book, with a Foreword by pensioners' leader Jack Jones, resulted in my receiving invitations to speak at meetings of pensioner organisations in many parts of the country. Fulfilling these engagements introduced me to Britain's pensioner movement, its policies and activities. It also brought home to me that, while there were established organisations based in Birmingham and Manchester, there was a big gap in between.

The first step was to test whether the demand for such an organisation existed in North Staffs. Jack Jones agreed to speak at a public meeting. The experience of organising that meeting, without any financial resources, revealed that there was much latent goodwill in the area. Local people were concerned about pensioners' problems. An approach to the City Council for the free use of the Lecture Theatre of the City Museum and Art Gallery, an excellent venue with a capacity of 300, resulted in a solid yes vote. Age Concern North Staffs agreed to sponsor the meeting and volunteered some of their office facilities to help with publicity. A local MEP was able to draw on the funds of the Socialist Group of MEPs to fund the printing of posters and leaflets. The local press and radio provided some valuable advance coverage of the event. A strong supporting platform for Jack Jones included the Bishop of Stafford as Chair, the Lord Mayor of Stoke-on-Trent and some North Staffs MPs.

Every seat was filled when the meeting was due to start, and there was a further 300 people gathered on the Museum concourse. So two meetings were held, with the speakers using a loud hailer to address the overflow. There was great enthusiasm for the idea of launching a North Staffs Pensioners' Convention and several hundred names and addresses of potential supporters were collected.

The next step was to invite these supporters to another meeting called specifically to launch the Convention. The free use of a school assembly hall was volunteered for the meeting and over 200 came and unanimously voted in favour of setting up the Convention. At that meeting a list of volunteer activists signed up and from them, at a subsequent business meeting, a Secretary, Chair, Treasurer and Committee were elected. There was now a fledgling organisation in place, if not quite up and running.

Thanks to the local Council of Voluntary Service, the free use of a committee room was provided for six weeks. During that time the City Council were asked to come up with permanent accommodation for the use of the new organisation. Very suitable premises in the city centre were duly forthcoming for a peppercorn rent, together with basic furniture, phone and photocopier. The new pensioner lobby was now in business. None of this would have been possible had not the pensioners' cause resonated widely throughout the community.

Another crucial factor was the relationship which developed with *The Sentinel*, the regional daily paper, which circulates widely in Staffordshire and Cheshire. The spectacular response to the Jack Jones meeting made a splash story with pictures. An assistant editor invited me, as newly elected Chair of the Convention, to discuss with him the role of the newspaper in its future activities. My suggestion of a regular column was agreed and that was the beginning of a weekly full-page feature, *Grey Power*. Now into its tenth year, *Grey Power* is a platform for the policy of the National Pensioners' Convention, the activities of the North Staffs Pensioners' Convention, and any other issues of interest and concern to the older people of North Staffs. It is very widely read. There is regular feedback from readers, including relevant cuttings and stories which help the page to be topical and lively. At the editor's suggestion there has been added, once a month, a page of readers' letters titled *Grey Power Forum*. Initially a small fee was agreed for writing the page, that has been substantially increased over the years. It is paid directly to the Convention.

At the end of its first year of activity, officers of the Convention met the Leader and officers of the Stoke-on-Trent City Council to report on its work and to request continued support from the Council. This practice has continued annually with additions to the shopping list for assistance generally receiving a positive response. The Council agreed the free use of a venue for a monthly public meeting, as was the occasional use of a larger hall for an annual rally and a Christmas Fayre. An initial cash grant was followed by a successful request to fund a paid Coordinator for the Convention. At first this was for 18 hours a week but income from the *Grey Power* page has enabled this to be stepped up to 30 hours. The advert for the first Coordinator produced a large number of applicants, many of them with impressive qualifications and a 21-year-old graduate, fresh from university, was appointed who proved to be an excellent choice. The North Staffs Pensioners' Convention has always stressed that pension provision is an inter-generational issue and its striking banner includes the message 'Us Today, You Tomorrow'.

In 1999, responding to a UN lead and organised jointly with Age

Concern North Staffs, a new venture was launched: an annual celebration of 'the older person'. It combines a keynote speech with a programme of entertainment by community groups demonstrating the varied talents of the older generation. Very large and enthusiastic audiences have been attracted to this event.

Current activities

Although the main thrust of national campaigning has been on the issue of pension provision, the National Pensioners' Convention has articulated a range of concerns relevant to older people. These are set out in a 'Statement of Intent' which declares that 'every pensioner has the right to choice, dignity, independence and security as an integral and valued member of society'. The central aim of an 'adequate pension to enable retired people to be able to pay their own way' is followed by other issues on which concessions are sought. These relate to health, housing, transport, education and leisure.

When, in the mid-1990s, Chancellor Kenneth Clarke proposed to increase the rate of VAT on fuel bills from 8 per cent to 17.5 per cent the National Pensioners' Convention ran one of its most successful campaigns. It resulted in enough back-bench Tory MPs rebelling against their own Party Whip to ensure the defeat of the measure, compelling the Chancellor to scrap the proposed increase from the Budget. Subsequently, when Labour won the 1997 Election it carried out its Manifesto promise to reduce VAT on fuel bills to 5 per cent, the lowest level permitted by the European Union. When Gordon Brown first introduced a Winter Fuel Allowance for all pensioner households in 1998, he said it was a direct response to the pensioner lobby. The same could be said of the introduction of free TV licences for the over-75s, though the pensioner movement is seeking both enhanced pensions for the over-75s, and free or much-reduced fees for TV licences for all pensioners.

Similarly, the Government is introducing national guidelines for concessionary local half-price bus travel for pensioners. These will mainly benefit two million pensioners in areas where local authorities presently have no concessionary travel schemes. Here again, however, Government policy has fallen short of the objective of the pensioner movement which is a comprehensive nationwide scheme of free travel, on the lines of that in force in the Irish Republic.

The activities of the North Staffs Pensioners' Convention are wide ranging and include participation in national events. Coach-loads regularly go to London for special occasions and to Blackpool for the annual Pensioners' Parliament. At the local level, pensioner campaigning is part of coordinated national campaigning on priority issues.

One of the more dramatic actions of the local Convention was the 'hijacking' of a bus. Banner-bearing pensioners boarded the bus and occupied the window seats, from which posters were displayed protesting against the April 2000 increase of 75p in the basic state pension. Outstanding and friendly media publicity was given to this exercise in direct action.

On specific issues that arise in the locality, the most important local issue in recent years has been the plans of the North Staffs Health Authority to close over 250 long-stay beds, 60 per cent of existing provision. Other features of its plans have also been subject to objection but bed provision has been the central issue.

The plans of local Health Authorities are subject to public consultation and the Community Health Council, 'the people's watchdog', has a key role in the consultation process. It has the statutory power, in the event of it objecting to Health Authority proposals, to refer them for decision to the Secretary of State for Health. The proposals, if referred, cannot be implemented pending the decision of the Secretary of State which may, of course, uphold the objection. In North Staffs, the Community Health Council had never previously used this power. It held public consultation meetings and these were lobbied with the aim of securing a decision to refer objections to the closure of the beds to the Secretary of State for Health. The North Staffs Pensioners' Convention played an active role in the consultation process and launched a 'Save the Beds' campaign. Support was won from the local MPs. The campaign included a petition, large turnouts of protesters with banners at consultation meetings and much media publicity from both local press and regional TV.

The outcome was a breakthrough. It led to the formation of a broad 'NHS Care for All' lobby chaired by the prospective Labour candidate for a local constituency. The Community Health Council then decided that the Health Authority was not responding to the objections it had made to the plans and that it would, for the first time, make a referral to the Secretary of State. Health Minister Yvette Cooper, responsible for following up the referral, appointed a team of 'independent experts' to report on the situation in North Staffs. As part of its work, the team undertook a consultation which included the 'NHS Care for All' group and the North Staffs Pensioners' Convention. In the report to the Minister, there was reference to the 'fierce opposition' to the Health Authority's proposals and tribute was paid to the role of the protest movement.

Retrospect

The work of the North Staffs Pensioners' Convention is limited by the resources at its disposal. It has over 500 paid-up individual subscribers and around thirty organisations are affiliated to it. With the exception of the part-time coordinator, all activity is carried out on a voluntary basis. By comparison with charities like Age Concern which provides services to older people, the core funding of the North Staffs Pensioners' Convention is minimal. As a (non-party-political) campaigning organisation it has never sought charitable status.

The Committee of twenty members consists of committed activists and the level of attendance at its meetings is extremely high. This is the more impressive in view of its age range which goes up to the high 80s. A quarterly Newsletter goes out to all members and affiliated organisations and also to local Councillors.

In 2001, the North Staffs Pensioners' Convention is now established as part of the local scene. It has had a significant impact on public opinion and especially on the older generation. Many who are not involved on a regular basis follow reports of its campaigning in the local media. The views of the Convention are regularly sought when news items affecting pensioners arise. For example, when the annual Budget statement is made, and when the recommendations of bodies such as the Royal Commission on Long Term Care are published, the local press and radio interview the representatives of the Convention and publicise its views.

For those who are actively involved in planning and carrying out the campaigns of the North Staffs Pensioners' Convention, a positive and new dimension is added to the lives of those who are no longer part of the workforce. They acquire a sense of purpose, become part of a like-minded group, and find meaningful scope for their energies and abilities. This solidarity helps to sustain their commitment in the face of disappointments when progress towards realising objectives seems painfully slow. These disappointments are balanced against the significant partial gains that have been won. The long-term goals remain and, though there is an awareness that there is no shortcut to achieving them, there is a conviction that one day men and women in retirement will be able to live 'as valued and integral members of society'.

CHAPTER 9

SETTLING IN AND MOVING ON

Jan Reed, Valerie Roskell Payton and Senga Bond

[. . .] There is a certain amount of evidence to suggest that decisions made about moving into a care home are subject to re-evaluation over time. Allen, Hogg and Peace (1992), for example, found that 16 per cent of the private home residents that they interviewed had come from another home, which they interpreted as evidence of the greater choice and freedom enjoyed by those in private homes. Corden (1988) traced moves between homes and found that 14 per cent of residents in North Yorkshire and 10 per cent of residents in Somerset had moved between homes. The moves were over very short distances, and were not necessarily related to increasing dependence – over 50 per cent were between homes providing the same level of care or to homes which provided less care. As Corden points out, these figures raise many questions about the processes by which these moves take place. . . .

The questions about the reasons for these moves remain unexplored, and also the impact on the individuals who have moved. For those who expected their move into a care home to be a final decision, the process of making a subsequent move may have been an unwelcome one (Eley and Middleton 1983). [. . .]

The study reported in this chapter, then, develops this knowledge, and places the policy and practice debates about assessment and placement in the context of the experiences of older people moving into residential and nursing home care. While the findings discussed here raise some questions about the accuracy and validity of assessments and about the processes of placement, we are more concerned to present an alternative view to the

Source: Reed *et al.* 'Settling in and moving on: Transience and older people in care homes', *Social Policy and Administration* 32, 2, June 1998, pp. 151–65, Blackwell Publishers, Ltd.

one that regards the technological development of assessment as a primary objective, and to suggest that a much more crucial issue is about the way in which services are structured and regulated.

The fieldwork

The study involved following forty-two older people through the process of moving into a care home, with the aim of developing an understanding of how older people accommodate both the idea and the experience of this life change. A series of four in-depth interviews were carried out over a six-month period, beginning before the move, and ending approximately six months afterwards. These interviews were loosely structured around an interview agenda which covered areas such as the decision-making process, expectations of the care home, early experiences there and processes of building up a new life. We also spent periods of participant observation in the six homes in our study, sometimes as volunteer helpers and other times as simple visitors in the sitting rooms. Relationship maps, where we asked participants to describe and draw their social and family networks, and photographs, where we asked people to choose important images and scenes from their own home and the care home, provided supplementary information and aids to promote interview discussions.

The study involved six care homes chosen to reflect the range of types of provision available in one local authority area in the North of England, as detailed in Table 9.1.

The homes were all of a similar size, with 30–40 residents. The local authority-run homes were in buildings which were less than thirty years old, and the privately-run homes were in converted large houses.

The homes were selected from lists supplied by local inspectors who were asked to identify places where the care was, in their opinion, of a high standard. The decision to select such homes was based on the realization that it was only in places where practice was well developed that staff would be able to contribute to discussions about moving into care homes based on their awareness of this process. Given the small sample, notions of random sampling were inappropriate, and the concern of the sampling

Table 9.1 Type of homes in the study.

Provision	Management	No. of participants recruited to the study
Residential home	Private	6
Residential home	Local authority	6
Dual registered	Private	9
Nursing home	Private	6
Nursing home	Private	7
Residential home	Local authority	7

strategy was to maximize the collection of data relevant to the study focus, rather than to produce a survey of the range of practices available in the care home sector. Potential research participants were selected from the waiting lists for these homes, and were contacted prior to arrival via their local authority care managers or, in the case of self-funding residents, through the home managers. At this point they were asked if they would like to discuss the study further with the researchers. The target sample size was thirty residents (five from each home) but as attrition rates were likely to be high, given the age and frailty of the sample, we recruited forty-six participants to the study (including five people who gave us retrospective interviews approximately one year after moving). From this group, five withdrew and one participant died. Of all prospective residents those who were able to understand the purpose of the interview/study and who could converse without serious difficulty were invited to participate.

Because the study was undertaken over a period of time we have had one significant advantage, the opportunity to examine the processes involved in making moves. We have been able to consider the dynamics of decision-making not only from the residents' point of view but also against a backdrop of professional and organizational considerations.

The process of settling in

Adjusting to life in a care home is a complex process, requiring a range of social skills. Adjustment is required not only to the physical environment but also to the social environment, the people who also live and work there. Observing social conventions, while at the same time meeting needs for companionship and social contact, involves new residents in a complex negotiation of their new social world. One of the conventions which they have to manage is that of being intrusive, of being seen to 'push' themselves on strangers. One of the participants in the study demonstrated this convention by talking disapprovingly of another resident:

> *She talks to everyone, that one, doesn't matter who they are, she's always pestering.*

One way round this problem, of talking to strangers, was overcome by some of our residents by a strategy which we have called 'constructing familiarity', in other words, the active use of quite often sparse information to make a home and its occupants seem known.

Using this strategy, residents would interpret information about others as evidence that they 'knew' them, and this would therefore permit conversation. One woman for example, claimed to know another resident because he had lived close to a relative, even though she had never spoken to him, and had not identified him herself:

Oh yes, I know him, he lived in the same street as my cousin, I found that out when my niece came in to see me. She saw him as she was coming in, and told me he was there.

This initial building up of networks 'broke the ice' for new residents, and allowed them to engage in conversations with other residents. This could lead to supportive relationships developing between residents, which were very much valued. As one man described it:

Oh yes, when I first came here, John [another resident] and I took to each other straight away and he showed me around and he helped me to settle. Now since Gladys came, well she had nobody at all, so we moved in and talked to her and made friends. We took her down to the dining room and helped her to settle in ... We help one another, best way we can, you see.

While not all relationships were supportive, and some could be acrimonious, relationships with other residents were an important feature of life in the home, for many of our participants, and of the thirty-six people we were able to complete the full series of interviews with, thirty-one mentioned another resident as being important or close to them in their final interviews.

The importance of these friendships was not always made explicit by residents without some further probing by interviewers, and could escape the notice of staff and care managers. There seemed to be a convention under which these relationships were less formally acknowledged than those with family: for example one woman who had talked extensively about a friend that she saw every day, still placed relatives (some of whom she had not seen for years) before her friend in the relationship map. When asked about this she replied:

Well, family should come first, it's only right.

Nevertheless, when asked about whether they had 'settled in', residents who affirmed that they had, cited as evidence of this the relationships that they had formed with the people that they lived with. One woman expressed in this way:

Oh yes, I've settled in, the people here are so nice, we're just like sisters. I wouldn't want to be anywhere else.

For some of the participants in the study, however, the relationships that they had built up were disrupted by moves to other institutions when their health changed, and this forms the second part of our discussion.

Subsequent moves

When updating our records and visiting the care homes in the study, we became aware that some of the residents in the study had moved to another home. We pursued this systematically, and traced all of the residents in the study at a point twelve months after data collection had begun, which meant that participants had been recruited to the study between six and twelve months previously. We found that following arrival at the initial care home thirteen of the forty-four residents in our study had experienced a second move, the period of stay in the first home varying from ten months to two months (see Table 9.2).

Reviewing the information we had collected about participants' lifestyle before their move into the home, we found that many participants had moved from hospital or another care home (see Table 9.3).

Moving to residential or nursing care was preceded by a hospital admission for twenty of our participants and was especially common for those people who enter nursing home facilities. In effect this meant that these

Table 9.2 Movement of study participants to other accommodation during the period following arrival.

Residential to nursing	5
Nursing to residential	2
Residential to own home	3
Residential to other residential	2
Nursing to elderly mentally ill accommodation	1
Total	13

Table 9.3 Origin of participants.

Placement:	Nursing home	Residential home	Total
Original location:			
Own home	2	17	19
Hospital	13	7	20
Other care homes	1	2	3
Total	16	26	42

individuals are unable to make the normal preparations for departure from their own homes. It also indicates that, at the point of arrival in the care home many older people will already have had to accommodate at least one, often rapid, change in lifestyle. For some of our participants, these changes were even more complex, involving moves from family houses to specially adapted accommodation for older people, to sheltered accommodation before hospital admission and the move into the care home.

[...]

One of the points that we have tried to demonstrate is that the existence of a two-tier (residential/nursing) system for care homes can be divisive and lead to fragmented experiences for older people when and if their needs change. The results of our study indicate that such movement is not unusual, and that older people may be required to undergo the process of settling in and breaking friendships and forming new relationships several times as their care needs move from one category of provision to another. As we have shown above, constructing a sense of familiarity demands the considerable efforts of these older people at a time when they are already vulnerable because of poor health. To duplicate this process as needs change is to add further to the work that they must do in an effort to settle in.

These points suggest that it would be useful to explore ways of organizing care so that services move to older people rather than older people having to move to the services. This might involve more flexible registration of homes and the development of a system which is capable of responding to the changing needs of care home residents *in situ*. The provision for dual registration of all care homes appears to be one way of addressing the problem. In the home in our study, however, dual registration took the form of treating the building as housing two separate facilities, with separate staff teams, living rooms and bedrooms. Segregation of residential and nursing clients was justified to us by the home manager and care managers using the argument that it prevented the medicalization of life for residential clients in care homes. Managing dual registration in this way, however, with formal moving of residents from one wing to the other as needs change, does not seem to ameliorate some of the problems associated with moving on, although there is the potential for a less rigid form of management. [...]

Concerns about matching needs tend to confuse care with accommodation in a way which the Wagner Report (1988) warned against. Care should rather be informed by the principle that care homes are first and foremost places for living rather than, like hospitals, places for receiving care. Adopting this principle may make it possible for us to develop services which match people, rather than trying to match people to services.

REFERENCES

Allen, I., Hogg, D., and Peace, S. (1992), *Elderly People, Choice, Participation and Satisfaction*, London: Policy Studies Institute.

Corden, A. (1988), *Supplementary Benefit Claimants in Residential Care and Nursing Homes in North Yorkshire and Somerset*, Working Paper DHSS 494, University of York: Social Policy Research Unit.

Eley, R., and Middleton, L. (1983), Square pegs, round holes. The appropriateness of providing care for old people in residential settings, *Health Trends*, 15, 68–70.

Wagner, G. (1988), *Residential Care: A Positive Choice*, Report of the Independent Review of Residential Care, London: HMSO.

CHAPTER 10

PAYING FOR NURSING HOME CARE

Margaret Forster

My father was born in 1900. In 1995 he was admitted to a nursing home after a great deal of trauma – his, mine, my sister's, my brother's. It is a trauma not much written about.

All of his family feared the moment when my father would no longer be able to look after himself in his own home. He, on the other hand, did not worry. 'I'll leave here feet first and no other way,' he was fond of announcing. Actually, he did, but alive and on a stretcher, not dead and in a coffin. He fell and hurt himself. He'd been falling regularly but whatever the damage, however bad the cuts and bruises, he always angrily shook off help and said, 'I'll manage.' Manage he did, with a little help from the social services and support from his family and his kind next door neighbours. Then suddenly he could not manage any more. He was taken to hospital. At 94, he had never been in hospital and was terrified of it, seeing it as some kind of workhouse. But, blessedly, he loved it.

Maybe if he had taken so easily to being in hospital he would adapt, against all expectations, to being in a home. But no. He was adamant. He wanted to go to his own home. To his fury, the social workers and doctors said he would have to prove to them that he could look after himself before they would sanction his return. It was, in his opinion, a damned cheek.

My sister and her husband stayed to see him back in to his home and then returned to their own, after six weeks' heavy duty. It was my turn

Source: Adapted from an article published in *The Independent Magazine*, 2 September 1995, pp. 26–7.

again. He talked non-stop about being in hospital and boasted he'd go back any time. Unfortunately, when he had to, only a week later, after another, and this time disastrous, fall, he hated it. Now, indeed, it seemed to him more like the workhouse. No cubicle this time. He was in a geriatric ward and loathed it. 'Get me out of here!' he stormed, and 'It's a disgrace, I want to go home!' But that was exactly where he could no longer go. He was highly at risk. The social workers said so, the doctors said so, we (reluctantly) said so and in the end he grudgingly said so himself.

He couldn't keep his balance, he was incontinent and, though his mind was as sharp as ever, he had all sorts of physical ailments. 'Put me on a cliff and push me over,' he said wearily.

And now, as well as being heart-breaking, the situation started to get interesting, if in a worrying sort of way. We thought it was a case of us finding and getting him into the best home we could discover existed and then, if such a place turned out to be more expensive than the amount the Welfare State pays for the care of the elderly frail, topping it up. We duly found the best nursing home available and were relieved and comforted by how good it seemed. 'They're terrible places,' my father said, but we told him this was another myth about to be exploded.

We put his name down on the waiting list and when within two weeks a room became vacant, we accepted it eagerly, especially since the hospital made it plain they wanted rid of him. He was in any case becoming disorientated and it was terrifying to witness this new mental deterioration. And then the complications began. We suddenly learned that my father would have to be assessed before the local authority, whose responsibility it now was, would pay any fees at all. If they decided he needed residential care only, then they would contribute nothing whatsoever to his nursing home fees. His place would have to be privately funded. So, forty-eight hours before he was due to move into the nursing home (and if we had lost that place, it might have been months before another was offered), my father was assessed and rated as not in need of nursing.

The day before he left hospital we were told that £330 per week would have to be paid by us. We could appeal, and we were told how, but even if we won the appeal, it would take a long time and there would be no back payments made.

Now, this was tricky. I was in the position of being able and willing to pay but, apart from the fact that my sister and brother were not, and did not want me to do the Lady Bountiful act, there was the matter of justice. My father had never owned a house, never got anywhere near being able to buy one in spite of working hard as a fitter in a factory all his life. He had no savings. He had never been on the dole. Suddenly, he needed the support he was entitled to from our Welfare State, so what was I doing – a card-carrying member of the Labour Party, someone who had never resorted to private education or private health care – saying I would pay? So I decided to appeal, stating that I only wished for the local authority to contribute the £224 per week towards the higher nursing home costs, the sum they had agreed to pay if he was in a residential home.

There was a prettily designed leaflet explaining the appeals system. The lengthy procedure started with a formal letter of complaint to the authority's complaints officer. The next stage was the appointment of an independent investigator who interviewed everyone concerned. That took four weeks. His report was then made. In it, he upheld the decision of the social services to assess my father as in need of residential and not nursing care but recommended this case should be treated as an exception because, at the time we selected a nursing home, there were no written guidelines stating the council's policy.

Two weeks later, the social services rejected this recommendation – it seemed they could do this, even though they had paid for the investigation. I thought there was little point in doing this unless its outcome was going to be heeded.

The next, and final option was for me to appear before an independent review panel of three people (all chosen by the complaints officer). It was explained this was not a formal court and that I would not be able to bring a solicitor. I prepared my case with the greatest care, combing through my by now bulging file of letters from the social services[1] for inconsistencies and weaselly words. There were plenty. I based my case purely on timing: if, at the very beginning of my father's second stay in hospital, we had been informed of the criteria on which assessments were made, and of council policy, we would never have got into this situation. The three members of the review panel were attentive, most polite and seemed in possession of all the facts. Also present were the independent investigator, the complaints officer and the spokesman for the social services together with the care team manager. Quite a gathering. They were all anxious that I should not feel intimidated but the tension came from the social services guy. Defensive wasn't the word.

It all, it appeared, hinged on what the central government has said the local authorities must do. They must fund elderly frail patients *only* in accordance with their own assessments.

Choice? Ah, that was problematic. The elderly frail person and their family had a choice of home only if the cost of it came within the amount allocated by the authority, if the social workers agreed it was suitable, and if the home agreed to their terms and conditions. But choice was even further restricted by the matter of registration. If the home selected was registered only as a nursing home, it was only inspected as such and may not therefore be fit to reside in though fit to be nursed in.

But the local authorities were strapped for cash and could hardly be blamed for sticking to the letter of the law. It seemed to me no good at all to treat social workers, and those administering policies forced upon them and far from clear, as enemies. The 'grey area' my case fell into was the fault of the then new regulations and I had always been verbally warned that I might have to fund my father's placement.

It was a long, hot afternoon of argument and explanation but a model for how such things should be conducted. I left, that June day, thinking that even if I lost the appeal I had had a fair hearing. I won. The local authority subsequently paid £224 of my father's £330 per week costs.

NOTE

1   This file included: fourteen letters from two Finance Administrators of the Social Services, eighteen letters from the Senior Social Worker, seventeen letters from the Representations and Complaints Officer, and two from each of the following: the Independent Chair of the Review Panel, the Head of Corporate Services (of the council), the independent investigator, the Principal Officer (Community Care), and a Department of Health Inspector (from the Social Care group).

PART II

DIFFERENCE AND IDENTITY

INTRODUCTION

In exploring issues of difference and identity in this Part of the Reader, we draw primarily on literature concerning community and the different ways in which this idea is experienced and expressed. In the immediate postwar period, the British welfare state was developed on the back of an assumption that the population was composed of individuals who lived within 'the family', which in turn was located within 'the community'. It was also assumed that there was a set cradle-to-grave course to life, including marriage, work and child-raising.

Fifty years later, there is a recognition that Britain has become a multicultural society of many different communities and many different life courses. As a consequence, identity has become a burning issue. Community and campaign groups meet to consider their particular needs and rights and what actions they should take. Policies on a wide range of services, from housing to education, are increasingly tailored to the needs and expectations of specific groups or communities. Caring increasingly entails a negotiation over what kind of help and support is appropriate for whom.

Chapter 11 is a collection of extracts from a variety of sources, each describing life in particular communities. Running through them are issues of identity: who belongs and what do they share? In the last extract Amitai Etzioni discusses the moral basis of community, and this is then explored further in Chapter 12 where Steve Clarke assesses a Welsh initiative in the regeneration of communities. In Chapter 13, a research team reports on what they found when they returned to the settings of some classic sociological studies of postwar family life and community. They record some striking changes as well as unexpected continuities. One of the key issues was ethnicity, which is explored in more detail in Chapter 14 by Ken Blakemore. He uses some national surveys to illustrate some of the complex differences between minority ethnic groups and the implications these might have for family-based care. Concluding this examination of the significance of difference and community, Chapter 15 is a long extract from Meera Syal's popular autobiographical novel *Anita and Me* based on life in the Wolverhampton area in the 1960s.

For over thirty years, 'normalisation' has been an important objective in work with people with learning difficulties, and much of this has been aimed at tackling stigma. Chapter 16 begins with extracts from the classic work of Wolf Wolfensberger and Stephen Tullman and of Erving Goffman. It is interesting to return to their arguments and descriptions and set these first against the more radical action taken by David Cooper (and others) and, more recently, the campaigning of the Critical Psychiatry Network. Bringing issues of community, identity and difference down to earth, at this point we offer you Bill Bryson's colourful description of the changes he witnessed in the sanatorium at Virginia Water. In Chapter 17, Alan Walker and Carol Walker develop the possibilities of work based on normalisation by considering the support of older people with learning difficulties. Their concern is to develop integrationist practice which avoids the ageist assumption of increasing dependence in later life.

With Chapter 18 we return to matters of personal experience and how people working in care and support services handle matters of difference and identity. Here Yasmin Gunaratnam analyses in detail how white women employed as hospice social workers handle issues of race and cultural difference. Then, in Chapter 19, Andrew Hubbard writes about his experience of becoming visually impaired and of joining a course for trainers on Disability Equality. Both experiences were turning points in his life and, in describing them, he poses important questions regarding social identity and impairment. To conclude this Part, in Chapter 20 Linda Grant, a journalist and novelist, writes about the care of her mother, drawing important links between a whole-life biography and illness and care towards the end of life.

CHAPTER 11

DIFFERENT COMMUNITIES

11.1 THE COMMUNITIES OF FOOTBALL AND SICKLE CELL

Garth Crooks and Roxy Harris

Source: R. Harris and S. White (eds) *Changing Britannia: Life Experience with Britain*, New Beacon Books, London, 1999, pp. 29–30, 41–2.

GARTH CROOKS: [. . .] my mother and my father, regardless of what you might hear from me and regardless of what you might see in me, are very black and very Jamaican. That's the term, they're very Jamaican. My father's command of the English language is as bad today as it was 25 years ago, yet my mother had this enormous capacity to adapt to almost anything. And of course she was a nurse when she first came here, so it's hardly surprising that she was capable of adapting, bearing in mind the things that they asked her to do, and many people like her.

So I suppose that for me, growing up in Stoke represented a number of firsts in terms of experiences. You become part of their community. What does that mean? I open supermarkets. I have to go and do articles in the press, but am I really a part of their community? I'm from Stoke, but a few years ago I wasn't welcome. When I decided I wanted to move on from Stoke and go to a bigger club to try and find out just how good I was as a professional footballer, suddenly, there was a backlash. Many people in Stoke were asking 'who's this little upstart who was born in Butler Street? How dare he?' I found that very interesting. I couldn't believe that the very people who yesterday were celebrating me, were saying these things about my colour and what or who I now was or had become, because I wanted to better myself and not just my situation, but my family's situation. And these were working-class people, people that I grew up with, I understood these people. There was nothing middle-class about me at that time. Some people say there's not very much that's middle-class about me now. But certainly at that time and I became very upset with people who came from that background and had those attitudes, and to this day I still have a distrust of certain sections of the working-class community. [. . .]

GARTH CROOKS: Well, I sit now and I get paid to sit and pontificate and theorise about the game. I'm no longer at the sharp end but I can sit and I can theorise. It's safe where I sit. It's not safe where Ian Wright sits, it's not safe where John Barnes sits. I mean, they're on the cutting edge. They're on the cutting edge of not only the white community, but the black community. You know whatever they do is magnified by both sections of the community. But the great problem I had to cope with was racial abuse. In those days there was no possibility of someone coming on the football field and attacking a player, or indeed a player attacking the fans and that's not out of the question as you well know these days.

But I remember going to Anfield in 1978. Keegan was running things at the time. John Toshack, Emlyn Hughes, Tommy Smith, Steve Heighway, fantastic side. And what I wanted to do was to play. Peter Shilton was in goal for Stoke and I played with Alan Hudson – he'd arrived in Stoke and was doing very well, but we were never in the Liverpool class. We had one or two internationals who played for the Home Countries but very few played football that often for England, not even Hudson and he was, in my view, a great player. I remember going to Anfield, about 1978 I think it was, and *King Kong* the movie had just come out, and Scousers are renowned for their wit. There was nothing funny about this because the entire Kop for some reason, as I walked on to Anfield for the very first time in my life, thinking, 'This is Anfield, this is one of the temples of football', – the entire Kop started to cry 'King Kong! King Kong!'. And I was on that part of the field, the only black player on that field. They couldn't have been talking to anybody else. Well, it would have been strange if they had. It's funny the things that stay with you. I'm sure if I was to walk into a group of Scousers and I relayed that experience, they'd think 'Of all the things that you've done Garth, what a strange thing for you to remember and recall'. But when someone hits you across the back with a stick it marks you, and their sentiments that afternoon were across my back like a stick. [. . .]

ROXY HARRIS: I just want to finish my part by asking you questions about your work for Sickle Cell Anaemia Relief (SCAR). One of my relatives first told me that you were involved in this years ago. You seem to have stuck with it. There's got to be a reason, a good reason why.

GARTH CROOKS: I'll tell you why I've stuck with it: because they won't let me out. I can't get out and I've tried to get out. It's one of those things that, and maybe this is common experience. You start something and it becomes successful, you think. 'Well, thank you very much, I've done my bit'. They say 'You can't leave now, we've just started. You can't leave now, we've done this, we've done this, we've got all this to do. You can't leave now'. And it doesn't help if you go home and your wife says 'Well, what are we doing all this for anyway?' You know, she takes you down that route.

So, we've made some horrendous mistakes but it probably brought me in contact with my community more than anything else that I've ever done, because football in this country is still not embraced by the black community for very good reasons. I don't see why any black person should go in an enclosed environment to hear their heroes abused. So, football perhaps isn't the entity for black people, that it should be and that they would like it to be. But in SCAR we raise money in one of the best ways our Committee knows, and that's by having a party, and a bloody good party. I just thought it was quite strange that, when very good mainstream charities like cancer and cystic fibrosis were tapping into our community and raising huge sums of money for their organisations, I thought I'd quite like to help and I was quite justified in asking them if they could spend a bit of time in Sickle Cell and they were more than happy to do so. Plus the fact I got irritated with members of our community saying that people who've taken an awful lot out of our community don't put anything back. I don't think that's true. I don't agree. They put more than their fair share back. It's personal and Sickle Cell for me has been a great testing-ground for that. At a moment's notice they're prepared to drop stuff and help out or make donations and sponsor a child's education at a minute's notice.

So, I've been heartened by a lot that's gone on in Sickle Cell. At the moment, we've got sufficient money to sponsor 30-odd kids for further education and prepare for private teaching those who have to be in hospital for eight weeks or more, having blood washed as they say, to come back to school and go to Saturday schools and have their education supplemented. We pay for that. It's expensive but it's paid for and we think it's worth it. The children benefit, the parents benefit and the particular school and children in the classroom benefit. You haven't got a disruptive child who's losing interest, with low self-esteem. The parents are often at their wits end because they see all of those things that I've just explained but feel good because something is being done about their child, and their child is understood. The teacher understands now because someone's helping the child and it's not just an element that she doesn't quite understand. He or she's prone to say 'Well, is it as serious as you say it is?' But, because we've identified an area that is useful i.e. it's almost like short-term research as opposed to looking down a microscope. That's all excellent work, but we're told that the best breakthrough for sickle cell will come from bone marrow transplants and all that sort of genetic research. So we felt justified, when we spoke to top consultants and professionals in the field, that we should try and help the community now.

11.2 MEMORIES OF A RURAL COMMUNITY

Maurice Hayes

Source: *Sweet Killough: Let Your Anchor Go*, Blackstaff Press, Belfast, 1994, pp. 191–3.

Killough was transformed by the summer visitors, who increasingly justi-fied its existence. There were those who owned houses, available all the year round, but generally closed up and shuttered throughout the winter. Opened up for Easter, they would start to be used at weekends and then fully during July and August, when the population would swell to treble its usual numbers. Then there were those who took a house for a month, usually July or August, often returning to the same house year after year. Or those who came to lodge with local families for a week or two, and those who returned each year to holiday with relatives, from Belfast or Glasgow or Dublin or Liverpool, and campers and tenters and day-trippers. All moving and changing from category to category: starting as lodgers, progressing to renters, then finally buying a house, bringing new and different people to the village. Some of the village families gave up their own houses for letting in the summer and moved out into sheds in the back. You always knew that summer was coming when you saw beds being shifted from house to house, and likewise the sight of mattresses being manhandled back again signified that the holidays were over and winter was on its way. Killough didn't wake up again until the next Easter, when the village children were given a great new repertoire of friends and playmates. It was like having a large extended family for the whole community, with honorary membership for those who came year after year, like the starlings and the swallows, to the same nests, at the same time. Most of those with houses were professional people or shopkeepers or bankers or civil servants, mainly from Belfast. The family stayed put for the season and the fathers commuted by train, some every day, and some coming down only at weekends. Young Johnston McClure got into trouble with his mother for shouting bad names at a visitor, a girl called Gladys Bell. He denied any offence: 'I just said "Hello, Glad Ass".'

Killough drew most of its visitors on the railway line, and the location of the County Down station in Belfast meant that in July each year a large part of the population of the Markets decanted to Killough and spent the summer there and thus avoided the provocations and temptations of the Twelfth in the city. This exodus included many of the campers, and those who arrived *en masse* on bicycles with their tents, but increasingly, people who bought houses and began to set down the roots of a secondary home. Generally they brought fun, new games, and plenty of activity to the village. But sometimes there was a darker side, an echo of troubled and less tranquil times elsewhere. I remember, once, seeing a line of people with bundles of bedclothes over their shoulders, pushing prams, carrying babies or trailing youngsters behind them, crawling wearily up the foot-path from the station, some of them knowing where they were going, others knocking at doors asking to be let in, children crying and frightened and bemused by the whole confusion. These were refugees – the first I had experienced – people fleeing from the riots of Belfast. The riots themselves, or what caused them, were not really discussed but there was talk of people being burnt out, or shot, or chased out, a sense of harassment and menace. It brought back memories of the fear of Daddy's train being stoned on the way to the Eucharistic Congress, or of attacks on Catholics, but it seemed to have nothing to do with village life, where many of the visitors we played with, who came every year, were Protestants, and where our Protestant neighbours, although they went down the street to church rather than up to chapel, and carried Bibles and prayer books under their arms instead of rosary beads in their pockets, were friendly and generous and never scary or threatening.

Some of the Belfast folk stayed on into the winter, presumably after the riots, and some went to school – children from Cromac Street and Joy Street and Eliza Street who introduced us to the joys of Belfast street songs and games and skipping rhymes. They also, between the desks, and entirely unofficially, produced a version of Irish history and an analysis of events on the basis of sectarian strife that was entirely new to us. In this, Catholics were a hunted species and Protestants the chasers, the victors, the temporary holders of the spoils. [. . .]

11.3 BEING PART OF A PSYCHIATRIC COMMUNITY

Keith Shires

Source: interview by Premilla Trevedi for the Mental Health Testimony Archive, now held by the British Library National Sound Archive (ref. C905/01/01–02).

[. . .] I was taken in hospital and, and I . . . I . . . I went to the reception ward in Shenley and I was mixing with people who were quite a lot older than me and I didn't feel very happy there, so I ran away, with my clothes, so I was transferred to the adolescents unit near . . . in the same hospital, Villa Twenty Four, which is quite well known I think, and they were going to give me insulin treatment, which I was ... and my parents agreed to have that for me, but I was so terrified about it that I ran away in my pyjamas from the unit, and ... I, I got about a hundred yards and a nurse followed me ... was chasing me ... but what must have been fate, he dropped the keys to the ward when he was chasing me, so I got away, and I suppose I felt in a way like a fugitive. I felt very strange because I was still in my dressing gown and ... nightclothes and I felt like a fox. I kept to one side, close the hedge, so I could only be seen from one side and it reminded me of *Great Expectations* with ... Magwitch who bloody escapes from the wooden hulks where he was a prisoner. Unfortunately for me I got about five miles from the hospital and ... I went ... I went to this farm, and some farmer ... farm ... farm woman ... farmer's wife was there and she was a bit taken aback at first, naturally, as if she thought I was some candid camera or something, you know ... but she was ... her husband had mental health problems so she was very understanding, so she rang my parents up and they took me back to Shenley, but while I was there with her, this woman, and she said ... she made a cup of tea and said, you know, listen to a record, LP, which it was then, not CD then, and ... I listen to Mozart's Prague Symphony and that was very pleasant so ... my parents came and picked me up and took me back to the hospital and I was put in a secure ward, but before I went back ... this woman said she'd come and visit me, the farmer's wife, and she did, and she gave me two books, which ... which she came in and saw ... one was *Aku-Aku* by Thor Heyerdahl about the civilisation of Easter Island, and the other one was Alan Paton's *Cry the Beloved Country*. So I read the book and I was very appreciative, though I've never seen her since. But, to the hospital's credit, they never rang the police when I ran away which I think was very good of them, but I did experience a harsh regime where you were shut in, you were locked in. And ... though they ... though the psychiatrist who I transferred to, Dr Cooper, who was quite well known for his work with R.D. Laing in the sixties, I transferred to his care and I was in this ... at this particular locked ward for about a month, and they were all a lot older than me, than me. I was only seventeen, but some of the men were in their mid ... mid-fifties or even older, and ... so I couldn't relate to a lot of the people ... I did to some, and ... when I ran away from ... the other year ... 'cause of the insulin treatment. I'm digressing on now, but I think it's important that they abandoned that treatment because one of the patients went into a coma and somebody rang the *Evening Standard*, there was quite a hue and cry about it, so they abandoned the treatment, so after a month in this ward [...] they transferred me back to the original unit I was supposed to go in, but it was now the adolescent unit without the particular treatment which frightened me, and that ... Then I was with David Cooper who wrote the book *Psychiatry and Anti-psychiatry*, and I was there for about six or seven months, and ... you went home and you got ... you had to sign a form ... but you could go on home leave, go Friday evening ... and I would come back Sunday evening, you had to sign a form, and if they thought you weren't well enough then they would ... they would cancel your home visit, but most of the time it was OK. After a period of several months I got quite friendly with everybody there, 'cause many of the young people ... it ... it wasn't mixed, it was an all-male ward, at the time ... many of them were university people that had broken up under pressures, and so it was quite an intellectual atmosphere there, and David Cooper encouraged us all because he allowed us into his consulting room every Saturday morning and we used to discuss things, a lot of different things, and it was very encouraging ... for ... he was quite open, there was no sort of professional status ... you know ... which was distancing ... would distance a lot of professionals, 'cause they feel they've got to be ... they've got to be detached to get the job ... objective opinion of you, but some of them carry it too far and they often go into the field of prejudice and ... negativism, but he was quite open and we used to discuss things with him and it was quite impressive really to be there with him and the other people, and often the chief male nurse would come in as well ... join in, so it was quite a civilised atmosphere ... and there was no problems of professional detachment, which I believe is necessary to a degree, but it was quite a friendly, open, equal environment and it helped me a great deal. Well I was there for about six months, and then I decided ... they decided that I could go home, so I came home, but I did after that ... for two or three years, go and visit them on Saturdays sometimes to see Dr Cooper ... I wasn't under him at the time, I was transferred to my GP, and I ... I ... I left, left him, but went on the Saturdays often to see him and the other people I knew there and that went on for two or three years, then I sort of grew away from it. [...]

11.4 THEY ALL HELP EACH OTHER ON THE ISLAND

Janet Foster

Source: *Docklands*, UCL Press, London, 1999, pp. 190–1.

I was shocked when I first come here.... I s'ppose I'd been here about nine months to a year, one day someone said to me 'My car's broke down, are you doin' anythink this morning?' and I said 'No not really.' So she said 'You wouldn't mind running me down to Stratford, would yer?' I thought bloody cheek, all the way to Stratford, so I said 'No alright then.' I thought bloody cheek, but I'll take her anyway.

I went down to Stratford, did her a bit of shopping and she said to me 'You wouldn't, on the way back, pull into the garage to see if my car's done?' and I said 'Yeah OK', thinking I'm gonna be bloody out all day with 'er, I'm not gonna get anythink done indoors, you know. Called round her car was done so she said to me 'I don't know my way 'ome from here' . . . so she said 'You wouldn't wait for me and show me the way home?' I said 'Yeah OK', brought her all the way back and she said 'I really appreciate that, thanks very much.'. . . I didn't realise that they all did this for each other . . . she didn't feel she had a cheek asking me . . . the Islanders will all 'elp each other out. If I said to 'er 'Would you run me to East Ham, I haven't got a car', she'd say 'Yeah' and we've become quite close friends. . .

When I was pregnant . . . I was really ill, I was just so ill I couldn't get out of the bed. It was just the worst experience of my life. Barby picked Emily up probably for the nine months, took her to school, picked up of a night brought her home. I bought her a big bunch of flowers and I kept sayin' to her 'I'm sorry.' She said 'Please don't keep sayin' sorry for goodness sake. Don't worry about it. I'll come every morning I'll pick her up, you don't wanna worry about it, really.'. . . I've got into the habit meself now of doin' it like if someone says 'Oh I've got a hospital appointment', I say 'Well is it early cos I'll take the kids to school for yer if you want' and I go and pick 'em up and we drop each other's kids round to dance classes and 'Oh well if you can't make it I'll pick her up and take her home, give her a bit of tea and drop her off later.' But when I first came here I'd never had that experience before . . . I didn't realise the whole of the island was doin' it for each other.

They don't mind what they do for each other. It's just such a tight close-knit thing with them. . . . They don't mind, they'll do it . . . because there'll always be a time when that person can help you back anyway . . . All the Islanders are like it, their mums were like it, their dads were like it and their grandparents were like it. . . .

11.5 COMMUNITIES ON THE MOVE

Kevin Hetherington

Source: *New Age Traveller: Vanloads of Uproarious Humanity*, Cassell, London, 2000, pp. 80–6.

[. . .] It is important to recognize that New Age travellers do not always move around the country in convoys, nor are they always on the road. For many, there is often a distinctive seasonal pattern to the way they travel and to the choice of particular sites where a group might stay for some months.

In the past, festivals have usually been held between the months of May and September, mainly because in Britain the weather's better. During the winter, it is more common for Travellers to park up in some remote or out-of-the-way upland or rural area, or return to live with friends or relatives in towns and cities, or perhaps to move into squats.

As well as sites that have a symbolic importance, practical considerations just as much as the romance of a life on the open road will influence where Travellers live. There is no contradiction here. While considerations of an imaginary and idealized landscape in which to live are important, this is often more a utopian dream than reality. Pragmatic decisions in a land where many people are hostile to your presence will lead to ordinary and mundane solutions. Sites where there is less chance of eviction, the need for local sources of water and wood and opportunities to work will also be important considerations in where Travellers choose to live. [...]

When asked the direct question, 'what would you consider home?' most Travellers are equivocal in their answers. That equivocation perhaps comes from the idea, common in Western societies, that associates the home with rootedness in a settlement and a dwelling that are seen as part of mainstream lifestyles. In answering the question they generally mention first what they call their 'tribe', their families, or sometimes the localities in which they travel rather than their vehicle. Yet when talking about the hostility they often encounter when on the road or parked up, it is often their vehicles which come to be seen as home in the sense of being a personal and intimate space that has been violated by intruders such as bailiffs or the police. Indeed, a number of Travellers I have spoken to have suggested that it was the freedom of having their own personal space in the form of their vehicle that was an important reason for leaving urban housing, usually of a low-grade rented kind. To travel, one also has to live, but giving up on the idea of a settled life in a house does not mean giving up the idea of home. This idea of home is expressed, therefore, through a mixture of sentiments about families, possessions and extended communal units (*Bund*):

> *Everybody wants to be part of something ... people want to feel they have a place where they belong. I don't mean a physical place ... the analogy I would use is that people are very much like leaves on a tree ... what gives the leaf its meaning is the tree. People want to know that they are part of something larger like that they also want to know where it is that they fit in. They want to be loved basically.*

As another long-term Traveller and festival-goer suggested about her life amongst people on the road,

It really is a family, with Travellers that I know. When I meet them, that's home, that's my family ... it's very supportive, very caring, it doesn't matter that elements of the family have changed, there's usually a core group that haven't changed and that for me, it really is like coming back to my family ... I can be myself [with them]. There's a common bond [amongst] persecuted minority groups, that is always a strong common bond.

[...]

Travellers have numerous sources of income which range across the spectrum of types of work from paid employment to illegal activities. The image of Travellers as work-shy dole scroungers persists amongst those who oppose Travellers and their way of life. There are some, typically town-based crusties who have never been on the road, who do indeed come close to fitting this stereotype, but for many Travellers, work is an important part of living on the road and it is within the varied sources of the informal economy where that work is found. This is not to say that they do not sign on at the same time. Seasonal labour, such as fruit picking, hop picking and farm work, is generally one significant source of income, especially in the autumn. Festivals, as suggested above, have always been of major importance to Travellers' livelihoods in the past. Many Travellers attend festivals to sell goods they have either made or acquired. These range from selling, bartering or exchanging vehicle parts and rebuilt wood-burning stoves, through to frying potato chips on site to sell to other festival-goers. A large number of Travellers also place considerable emphasis on traditional craft skills and folk or circus forms of entertainment, many of which they learn and use as a source of income. Again, entertaining at festivals as clowns, jugglers, fire-eaters and folk musicians can be a source of income, as can busking or begging in towns. Selling hand-made ornaments, tools, New Age artefacts and clothing at festivals, or in some cases on the streets in cities, is another source of income. It is notable that for what is a predominantly rural lifestyle such articles are generally intended to convey an aura of organic, rural authenticity, as they are often made out of wood, leather or hand-dyed natural fibres.

Drugs are a source of income, although most Travellers whom I interviewed emphasized that drugs such as marijuana, LSD and Ecstasy were the mainstay of the Traveller lifestyle rather than the so-called 'hard drugs' such as heroin, crack and cocaine. Even then, these are mainly used for personal consumption and not generally as the main source of income for the majority. It would be wrong to see all Travellers as drug dealers, just as it would be wrong not to recognize that this does go on. In that respect, Travellers are no different from any other group within society, as drug consumption, despite long-standing prohibition, is an endemic feature of British life.

Social security payments are also a major source of income for many Travellers, but again, not the sole source. Other sources include scrapping, skipping (scavenging from builders' skips), poaching, dog breeding and a variety of forms of casual labour. In other words, think of any activity that might find a niche within the informal or 'black economy' and there will no doubt be a group of Travellers somewhere who derive an income from it.

Such a way of life, where there are few external support systems, makes skills and the communal networks in which they can be exchanged important. Developing skills is positively encouraged amongst most Travellers, especially skills that can be used to provide some kind of income. Craft, musical and entertaining skills are particularly popular, usually learned after people have become Travellers and have to adapt to living on the road. There is a good deal of skill sharing and mutual aid amongst Travellers, not only in learning these sorts of skills, but also others that are necessary for being able to get by on the road, such as providing an education for their children. The ability to carry out vehicle maintenance, especially given that many have old vehicles, is an important set of skills that often needs to be learned. Constructing temporary dwellings known as 'benders', or even tepees for some Travellers, are other skills that can be learned. [. . .]

In all, this is a communal way of life that exists on the fringes of society but one that has economic and cultural relationships with that society. It is about making an alternative space for oneself to live as nomads together with family, friends or partners. The hardships associated with poverty and exposure to the elements are doubled by the hostility that most people feel towards Travellers and the almost constant threat of eviction that hovers over almost every Traveller site. But that hardship and the conflicts surrounding it only seems to add to the sense of being part of an elect, a special community that has come together because of its ideals and has shared all the problems posed by society. The utopian vision of the freedom of the open road in a beautiful land on the one hand and, on the other, the everyday experience of living on a muddy site with an eviction notice nailed to the gatepost, do not stand in contradiction but are fused together in this idea of a communal space and the solidarity that it provides for its inhabitants. [. . .]

11.6 THE SPIRIT OF COMMUNITY

Amitai Etzioni

Source: *The Spirit of Community*, Fontana, London, 1995, pp. 30–6.

[...] *No society can function well unless most of its members 'behave' most of the time because they voluntarily heed their moral commitments and social responsibilities.* There can never be enough police ... inspectors and accountants to monitor the billions of transactions that occur every day. And who will guard the guardians? Even if half the society were to police the other half, who would police this vast police to ensure that *it* obeyed the law? The only way the moral integrity of a society can be preserved is for most of the people, most of the time, to abide by their commitments voluntarily. The police powers of the government should be called upon only as a last resort to deal with the small number of sociopaths and hard-core recalcitrants, those who do not have moral commitments or sufficient impulse control to heed those commitments.

Unfortunately the record shows, even after only a cursory examination of our world, that from drug abuse to corporate crime, illegal and immoral behaviors have broken through this important line of voluntary self-restraint. Large segments of the population do not voluntarily do what they are supposed to do. It follows that we must shore up our moral foundations to allow the markets, government, and society to function properly again.

How do we shore up morality? How can we encourage millions of individuals to develop a stronger sense of right and wrong? [...] We gain our initial moral commitments as new members of a community into which we are born. Later, as we mature, we hone our individualized versions out of the social values that have been transmitted to us. As a rule, though, these are variations on community-formed themes.

[...] When the term *community* is used, the first notion that typically comes to mind is a place in which people know and care for one another – the kind of place in which people do not merely ask 'How are you?' as a formality but care about the answer. This we-ness (which cynics have belittled as a 'warm, fuzzy' sense of community) is indeed part of its essence. Our focus here, though, is on another element of community, crucial for the issues at hand: *Communities speak to us in moral voices. They lay claims on their members.* Indeed, they are the most important sustaining source of moral voices other than the inner self.

Communitarians, who make the restoration of community their core mission, are often asked which community they mean. The local community? The national community? The sociologically correct answer is that communities are best viewed as if they were Chinese nesting boxes, in which less encompassing communities (families, neighborhoods) are nestled within more encompassing ones (local villages and towns), which in turn are situated within still more encompassing communities, the national and cross-national ones (such as the budding European Community). Moreover, there is room for nongeographic communities that crisscross the others, such as professional or work-based communities. When they are intact, they are all relevant, and all lay moral claims on us by appealing to and reinforcing our values.

But, we are asked, given the multiple communities to which people belong (the places where they live and work, their ethnic and professional associations, and so on), can't a person simply choose at will which moral voice to heed? Aren't people using the values of one community to free themselves from obligations that others may press on them – leaving them free to do what they fancy? It is true that you can to some extent play these multiple affiliations against one another, say spend more time with friends at work when people in the neighborhood became too demanding. However, societies in which different communities pull in incompatible directions on basic matters are societies that experience moral confusion; have moral voices that do not carry. We need – on all levels, local, national – to agree on some basics.

How can the moral voice of the community function when it is well articulated and clearly raised?

[. . .] When I discuss the value of moral voices, people tell me they are very concerned that if they lay moral claims, they will be perceived as self-righteous. If they mean by 'self-righteous' a person who comes across as without flaw, who sees himself as entitled to dictate what is right (and wrong), who lays moral claims in a sanctimonious or pompous way – there is good reason to refrain from such ways of expressing moral voices. But these are secondary issues that involve questions of proper expressions and manner of speech.

At the same time we should note that given our circumstances, our society would be much better off if some of its members sometimes erred on the side of self-righteousness (on which they are sure to be called) than be full of people who are morally immobilized by a fear of being considered prudish or members of a 'thought police.' . . . I realize that when I speak of the value of the two-parent family, many of my single-parent friends frown. I do not mean to put them down, but their displeasure should not stop me or anybody else from reporting what we see as truthful observations and from drawing morally appropriate conclusions. It is my contention that *if we care about attaining a higher level of moral conduct than we now experience, we must be ready to express our moral sense,* raise our moral voice a decibel or two. In the silence that prevails, it may seem as if we are shouting; actually we are merely speaking up.

As more and more of us respond to the claims that we ought to assume more responsibilities for our children, elderly, neighbors, environment, and communities, moral values will find more support. Although it may be true that markets work best if everybody goes out and tries to maximize his or her own self-interest (although that is by no means a well-proven proposition), moral behavior and communities most assuredly do not. They require people who care for one another and for shared spaces, causes, and future. Here, clearly, it is better to give than to take, and the best way to help sustain a world in which people care for one another – is to care for some. The best way to ensure that common needs are attended to is to take some responsibility for attending to some of them.

To object to the moral voice of the community, and to the moral encouragement it provides, is to oppose the social glue that helps hold the moral order together. It is unrealistic to rely on individuals' inner voices and to expect that people will invariably do what is right completely on their own. Such a radical individualistic view disregards our social moorings and the important role that communities play in sustaining moral commitments. Those who oppose statism must recognize that communities require some ways of making their needs felt. They should welcome the gentle, informal, and – in contemporary America – generally tolerant voices of the community, especially given that the alternative is typically state coercion or social and moral anarchy. [. . .]

CHAPTER 12

THE REGENERATION OF COMMUNITIES

Steve Clarke

Introduction

The regeneration of communities may appear to be a rather abstract idea, open to a wide variety of interpretations. Do we intend to knock down large areas of our towns? Can we arrange for intensive investment to bring economic prosperity to areas in decline? Alternatively, could we aim at something more social – arranging for the rebirth of community spirit and neighbourhood institutions? Surely it would be beneficial if we could achieve all of these (National Assembly for Wales 2000a)?

Since 1997, in the flurry of social policies that seem to be the hallmark of the New Labour agenda, the words 'community', 'partnership' and 'stakeholder' have been attached to as many social and economic initiatives as possible (Oppenheim 1999; Social Exclusion Unit 1998; Welsh Office 1998). In Wales, which is to be the focus of this chapter, the whole image of the new Assembly reflects this theme (National Assembly for Wales 2000b; 2000c). Whereas this might appear to be mere political froth to disguise the tougher edges of public administration, its impact will be far more significant. The government is actually introducing, with a certain degree of stealth, a far-reaching initiative that amounts to social engineering on a grand scale.

We will consider the implementation of the policy of community regeneration in Wales. The policy covers a broad canvass and attempts to achieve its objectives through integrating economic and social policies. Some influential politicians and senior officials are seeking radical change in the nation's political agenda because they are convinced that government has grown too far away from its electorate. Their views might be summed up as 'Devolved government in Wales has something to prove. It must demonstrate that it is seeking new paths to prosperity through responsiveness to local needs and innovation at the point of delivery.'

Crisis in the Welfare State

The economy of the Welfare State is at a crossroads. There are deep-rooted public expectations, born of fifty years of striving towards the provision of universal services, linked to rising levels of general economic prosperity. Surely, our standard of living is underwritten in some way, and the achievements of civilisation as we know are not reversible phenomena? The facts show a grimmer picture. This notional prosperity is failing to reach into many deprived parts of society, and the phenomenon of poverty is growing (Barclay 1995; Drakeford 1997; Howarth *et al.* 1998; National Assembly for Wales 2000d). Must we view as inevitable the emergence of an 'underclass' of over one million, made up of permanently or semi-permanently unemployed, aged, disabled and other people (Hills 1995; Murray 1990; Stepney *et al.* 1999)? Won't the rationing of services within the non-medical welfare and care sectors produce a reservoir of unmet need (Clarke 2000)?

It seems that we live in a society given over to values that are remarkably different from those that prevailed at the time when the Welfare State was established in the immediate post-Second World War period. Attitudes towards a social contract, class inter-dependence, and social awareness, have given way to the values of laissez-faire in the free market economy. Margaret Thatcher's denial that there is such a thing as 'society' (Thatcher 1988) has taken root through the major economic forces that were released over the past thirty years. In some way, this process has now to be reversed, if aspirations to live, as far as is possible, as one society, are to be realised. Failure will bring about communities which are isolated and divided by unbridgeable barriers of stigma, poverty and exclusion.

Communitarianism

An essentially conservative attitude towards community which emerged from the USA in recent years has been publicly endorsed by Tony Blair and New Labour (Etzioni 1993; 1995a; Lund 1999; MacKian 1998). This approach is best described as Communitarianism, and combines social fears about the disintegration of society through the lack of socialisation and control over young males (from single-parent families), the decline of the traditional family, and the need to rebuild the 'traditional village society' that may have once flourished (MacKian 1998). 'Community' must be re-built based upon the nuclear family and the neighbourhood school (Etzioni 1995b). In addition, there is a perception that the tax-paying public will not stand for higher levels of taxation, especially when there are perceptions of wastage in the services (subsidising the 'feckless poor'), and also funding the detached and expensive bureaucracy of government itself.

Since 1990 new policies have produced new relationships between the state and the voluntary sector. The role of voluntary organisations in the sphere of health and welfare is now ever more commonly provided through contracted, specialised organisations. These are now more like businesses but are formally accountable through contracts with the service planning authorities which decide on priorities. The result is that there is little surplus in contracts for preventive work, or support for those not in the greatest need. This is where the reservoir of unmet need originates.

The problem can be stated quite starkly. Whereas there is a greater understanding of social need in the realms of work, health, welfare and well-being, there is a breakdown of a sense of social cooperation, and the desire to share the burden of care. More people are falling through the welfare safety net if they do not immediately qualify as high priority. Outside of the priority areas, the shortage of resources means that the state cannot generate the necessary infrastructure for the economy to re-absorb its victims. Division, hardship and detachment follow, and the 'Two Britains' divide out into an 'underclass' and those who are economically and socially secure.

This is the difficulty that confronts the National Assembly for Wales. In a small economy beset by contractions and under-investment, with large rural areas to service, and diverse ethnic and cultural needs to accommodate, there is just not enough in the public kitty. Thus, the Assembly has tried to create alternative resources to promote a sense of public responsibility, social inclusion as well as mechanisms for overcoming economic detachment. Every effort is now directed towards exploiting the one resource that has not yet been formally targeted in any systematic way – the community at large. To achieve this, policies are framed to ensure that funding (and auditing/evaluation frameworks) reflect a community regeneration approach. Local agencies of government must now engage in stakeholder-inclusive planning, decision-making and activities.

Community development

If community regeneration is the planned and positive change of the physical, economic and social fabric of a defined area of society, then community development is the process that puts ordinary people, as active and valued participants, into planning and delivering these changes. Thus, community development is the vehicle for delivering community regeneration. Formally, community development can be defined as the mobilisation and integration of the maximum amount of social, economic and political resources for the achievement of planned, sustainable social change. It is a deliberately structured activity. The aims of community development are normally quite far-reaching in relation to the physical, social and/or economic environment. As such, it makes an impact on the culture of any particular community, and also on the relationships between communities. For the purposes of community development, *community* can be defined as any geographical area, or any group of people who may share common identity, needs, or other characteristic(s) that identifies them as subjects of a planned change process (Clarke 2000). This definition enables the identification and inclusion of groups who have many diverse needs, even without the same geographical boundaries (such as ethnic, religious, generation or gender characteristics). There may be many sub-divisions of social identity within any geographical area, or within a seemingly homogeneous population. Defining the 'community' is a crucial step in regeneration. Thus, organising collective or composite responses to the need for change is one of the most complex ingredients of the community development process.

Typically, the involvement of people requires a great deal of preparation and direction. Citizens must identify their priorities, and put them in some sort of order. This tends to be done through the medium of representative organisations which may or may not exist in advance of a community development initiative. These may be assessed in advance (by agents of the strategic agency seeking community change), and new organisations may have to be formed to cater for specific interests or characteristics in the community. Initially, these organisations may be generated around the community's interests prior to their being involved in any larger-scale strategy. Any outside agency seeking the active and positive cooperation of a community will need to invest in this local development process. A community will need to be aware of its capabilities in terms of its ability to speak for itself and exercise its civic power. Without this ingredient, the momentum of active participation and inclusion will drain away (Barr *et al.* 1996; Clarke 2000; Hawtin *et al.* 1994; Henderson and Thomas 1987). In this way, organised communities can then be oriented towards the agenda of the state and the need to engage in change-directed activities in cooperation with the state. Historically, the significance of community development as a model for intervention is that communities do take the lead from the state, and that this model works (Clarke *et al.* 2001).

The model we have described above might appear to be somewhat cynical, authoritarian and bereft of sympathetic principles. It has deliberately been described in stark terms with its underlying assumption that people will just not go where you want them unless they are actually coerced. This is not really an option for community development approaches in our society. Alternatively, they may be offered compensation that is in keeping with their contribution, or offered something much better than the status quo. This approach is the basis of most successful community development programmes. Simply put, it is a model which is based on self-interest.

In contrast to the idea of manipulation, the promising of fraudulent rewards, or the creation of unrealistic expectations, there is a highly developed body of ethics, and methodological theory that defines the range of acceptable behaviour for professionals and public officials in these matters (Midgley 1995). Basically, these state that the greater the level of involvement by members of communities in all the process of planning, decision-making and judging the success of change, the more beneficial and authentic is the community development method involved (Barr *et al.* 1996; Burns 1991; Carmen and Sobrado 2000; Chambers 1997; Cracknell 2000; Goulet 1995; Patton 1997). This represents the reference point for those concerned with community regeneration. Their work will be measured against it. Certainly, this is the framework against which the initiatives of the National Assembly for Wales will be judged (National Assembly for Wales 2000c).

We live in a society where there is a great deal of centralised control over the decisions surrounding social policies, such as public investment, social programmes and planning the environment. The state is the largest player in these activities, and its agents have traditionally had expectations of remaining in control, after due process of deferment to the democratic process. New policies from central government have now suggested that the structure of decision-making should change somewhat. Nevertheless, the state is still to be the final arbiter of the shape, direction and nature of change and progress in these areas. Therefore, for the state to remain in charge of a regeneration process, it must adopt a model of social intervention that allows it to exercise control without coercion.

In Wales, community development is the preferred method across a wide range of strategies, namely: social exclusion – *Communities First*; health – *Healthy Living Centres, Investment for Health*; childcare – *Sure Start*; economic regeneration – *Objective 1, Sustainable Wales*; interagency cooperation – *Voluntary Sector Compact*. All of these strategies require local and health authorities as well as voluntary agencies to establish the appropriate mechanisms for local partnerships. These must be responsive to local needs and aspirations and build the sustainable engagement of stakeholders into the processes of change. These are not inconsequential requirements, and they represent a challenge to the power of the traditional authorities in the way that they shape policies and the direction of development. It is with this mechanism that central government has begun to address the perceived problem of local democracy being too distant from the electorate. There is one consolation for the local authority, however. This is the way in which community development initiatives are designed. Managing the apparent conflict between interests and power blocs in a joint exercise for change is where the expertise of the community development worker is brought in.

In strategically designed community development initiatives it is usual to presuppose that the state will lead the enterprise (National Assembly for Wales 2000e). This ensures that the shape and direction of what happens on the ground are directed towards the state's own desired outcomes. Social planning is the term applied to the over-arching process. This is an initiative that combines overall strategic planning with a focused approach to locality development initiatives (Rothman 1995). The social planning process creates the framework within which experts, funders and lead field agencies prioritise their overall objectives. They then lay out a pattern for localised investment, change and development for intensive intervention and social change. Locality development, the building of organisations and networks to target local objectives, follows in keeping with the strategic plan. These become the delivery systems for the realisation of the centrally-developed strategic plan. They are developed from community resources, acting either separately or in concert with resources from the planning agencies (Barr 1996; Clarke 2000; Miller and Steele 2000).

Communities First

Launched after intensive consultations over most of 2000, *Communities First* represents a concerted approach to 'establish cross-sectoral and multi-agency methods of designing policy and local service delivery and will involve the direct participation of the community in planning and developing the services delivered to that community' (National Assembly for Wales 2000d, p. 4). It is a 'new concept in regeneration' (2000b, p. 5). This approach was introduced to draw in the bulk of the community in addressing the 'long, slow social and economic decline' of their communities which left them 'severely deprived by comparison to the rest of Wales' (2000d, p. 3).

All sectors (statutory, non-statutory, private and independent) in the social and economic field were to be drawn into the process of partnership to target the most deprived communities in Wales. Frictions and loss of focus were to be dramatically reduced by insisting on 'joined-up' government, and the specific difficulties of local communities in taking a lead in such initiatives would be addressed through the design of the local programmes. It was recognised from the start that 'community based development groups are fulfilling an essential function and are often best placed to deliver locally sensitive programmes which raise capacity and participation' (2000d, p. 7). To achieve this, 'a wide-ranging and cross-cutting agenda of community development will be pursued in the communities needing support' (2000d, p. 7).

Local authorities launched pilot projects. They identified their own priority areas, using social planning community development techniques within partnerships, and tested these assumptions on the ground using locality development methods. The National Assembly then ratified bids for further projects with reference to an Index of Multi-deprivation (National Assembly 2000e). A rolling programme of funding (£81 million of 'extra' money, plus linkages to other mainstream funding) followed. In this way, communities across Wales have been targeted for social change through local development in full cooperation with the local authorities. The Assembly recognises that communities of interest have just as much right to public resources as do geographical areas, and so funding decisions will be based upon a broad range of criteria. After many years of neglect, the terms of 'bottom-up government' and community development can now be heard at corporate planning meetings.

Conclusion

In adopting a strategy of community regeneration, government in Wales has demonstrated a commitment to policies and direct action that will address prevention as well as social support for the most needy. If communities become more aware and inclusive in supporting their own members, high-intensity services can be targeted on the most critical problems. This will allow for specific savings to be made, and the inclusion of others, for example homeless people, within the sphere of central services rather than being peripheral as at present. Wales does not have tax-raising powers, and so the budget is more or less fixed. The adoption of bottom-up community regeneration principles by government will realise the cumulative and sustainable potential of community development, and enhance the state of engagement and well-being in society at large. In so doing, Wales is demonstrating a commitment to an international movement (Mittelmark 1999; Tsouros 1992) that, since 1987, has been moving government closer to its citizens. It is widely recognised that traditional methods have not delivered the goods as far as the social benefits of economic progress are concerned. Community regeneration through community development places the community firmly in the frame, and sets out the basis for negotiating a fresh social contract for a more democratic and less bureaucratic society.

REFERENCES

Barclay, Sir P. (1995) *Joseph Rowntree Foundation Inquiry into Income and Wealth*, Volume 1. York, Joseph Rowntree Foundation.
Barr, A. (1996) *Practising Community Development*, Revised Edition. London, Community Development Foundation.
Barr, A., S. Hashagen and R. Purcell (1996) *Monitoring and Evaluation of*

Community Development in Northern Ireland. Belfast, Voluntary Activity Unit/Dept. of Health and Social Services.

Burns, D. (1991) 'Ladders of Participation', *Going Local*, 18, 14–15.

Carmen, R. and M. Sobrado (eds) (2000) *A Future for the Excluded: Job Creation and Income Generation by the Poor*. London, Zed Books.

Chambers, R. (1997) *Whose Reality Counts? Putting the Last First*. London, Intermediate Technology.

Clarke, S. (2000) *Social Work as Community Development: a Management Model for Social Change*, Second Edition. Aldershot, Ashgate.

Clarke, S., A. Byatt, M. Hoban and D. Powell (eds) (2001) *The History of Community Development in South Wales*. Cardiff, University of Wales Press.

Cracknell, B.E. (2000) *Evaluating Development Aid: Issues, Problems and Solutions*. New Delhi, Sage.

Drakeford, M. (1997) 'The Poverty of Privatization: Poorest Customers of Privatized Gas, Water and Electricity Industries', *Critical Social Policy*, 17, 2, 115–32.

Etzioni, A. (1993) *The Spirit of Community: the Reinvention of American Society*. New York, Simon Schuster.

Etzioni, A. (1995a) 'Nation in Need of Community Values', *The Times*, London, p. 9.

Etzioni, A. (1995b) 'Responsibility', in Atkinson, D. (ed.) *Cities of Pride: Rebuilding Community, Refocusing Government*. London, Cassell, pp. 33–6.

Goulet, D. (1995) *Development Ethics: a Guide to Theory and Practice*. London, Zed Books.

Hawtin, M., G. Hughes and J. Percy-Smith (1994) *Community Profiling: Auditing Social Needs*. Buckingham, Open University Press.

Henderson P. and D.N. Thomas (1987) *Skills in Neighbourhood Work*, Second Edition. London, Allen & Unwin.

Hills, J. (1995) *The Joseph Rowntree Inquiry into Income & Wealth*, Volume 2. York, Joseph Rowntree Foundation.

Howarth, C., P. Kenway, G. Palmer and C. Street (1998) *Monitoring Poverty and Social Exclusion: Labour's Inheritance*. York, New Policy Institute/Joseph Rowntree Foundation.

Lund, B. (1999) 'Ask Not What Your Country Can Do For You': Obligations, New Labour and Welfare Reform', *Critical Social Policy*, 19, 4, 447–62.

MacKian, S. (1998) 'The Citizen's New Clothes: Care in a Welsh Community', *Critical Social Policy*, 18, 1, 27–50.

Midgley J. (1995) *Social Development: The Developmental Perspective in Social Welfare*. London, Sage.

Miller, S. and A. Steele (2000) 'Regeneration and Community Partnership: a Contradiction in Terms?' *The Scottish Journal of Community Work & Development*, 6, Autumn, 5–14.

Mittelmark, M.B. (1999) 'Health Promotion at a Community-wide Level', in Bracht, N. (ed.) *Health Promotion at the Community Level*, Second Edition. Thousand Oaks CA, Sage.

Murray, C. (1990) *The Emerging British Underclass*. London, IEA Health & Welfare Unit.

National Assembly for Wales (2000a) *A Sustainable Wales – Learning to Live Differently*. Cardiff, National Assembly for Wales.

National Assembly for Wales (2000b) *Better Wales*. Cardiff, National Assembly for Wales.

National Assembly for Wales (2000c) *Communities First* (2nd Consultation Document). Cardiff, National Assembly for Wales.

National Assembly for Wales (2000d) *'Communities First': Regenerating our Most Disadvantaged Communities – A Consultation Paper*. Cardiff, National Assembly for Wales.

National Assembly for Wales (2000e) *The Welsh Index of Multiple Deprivation*. Cardiff, National Assembly for Wales.

Oppenheim, C. (1999) 'Poverty and Social Exclusion: an Assessment', *Local Work*, CLES, 15, July.

Patton, M.Q. (1997) *Utilization-Focused Evaluation: the New Century Text*, Third Edition. Thousand Oaks, CA, Sage.

Rothman, J. (1995) 'Approaches to Community Intervention', in Rothman, J., Erlich, J. and Tropman, J.E. (1995) *Strategies of Community Intervention*, Third Edition. Itasca, Illinois, F.E. Peacock, 26–63.

Social Exclusion Unit (1998) *Bringing Britain Together: a National Strategy for Neighbourhood Renewal*. London, Cabinet Office, Cm 4045.

Stepney, P., R. Lynch and B. Jordan (1999) 'Poverty, Social Exclusion and New Labour', *Critical Social Policy*, 19, 1, 109–28.

Thatcher, M. (1988) Interview with *Woman's Own*. London, 17.06.1988.

Tsouros, A.D. (1992) *World Health Organization Project: a Project Becomes a Movement*. Milan, WHO Healthy Cities Project/SOGESS.

Welsh Office (1998) *Better Health Better Wales*. London, Stationery Office, Cm 3922.

WHO (1986) *Ottawa Charter for Health Promotion*. Ottawa, World Health Organization.

CHAPTER 13

SOCIAL CHANGE, NETWORKS AND FAMILY LIFE

Chris Phillipson, Miriam Bernard, Judith Phillips and Jim Ogg

Family relationships have traditionally been viewed as a major part of the everyday life of older people. Older people are seen as being supported through such ties, as well as through friendships and contacts with neighbours. But important questions might be asked about these relationships: how is the family life of older people changing? To what extent do kinship relations still operate as the mainstay of life in old age?

To answer these questions, this chapter draws on a research project which returned to three areas, the locations for some classic studies of family life of England completed in the 1940s and 1950s. These were Wolverhampton (Sheldon 1948); Bethnal Green (Townsend 1957 and Young and Willmott 1957); and Woodford in Essex (Willmott and Young 1960). Hereafter these are referred to as 'the baseline studies'. This chapter reviews the methods we used to study family change, highlights relevant findings from the research, and concludes with a summary of the main changes that have affected these three communities.

In the 1940s and 1950s, research focused upon people living within what Frankenberg termed 'an environment of kin' (1966: 187). Subsequently, under the influence of modernisation theory, the focus turned to the break-up of the extended family (Cowgill and Holmes 1972). Research in the 1980s and 1990s, however, has presented a more complex picture: on the one hand emphasising the importance of family-based care, set in the context of a gendered division of labour; on the other, highlighting the move towards a more individualised family, with relationships based on

Source: S. McRae (ed.) *Changing Britain: Families and Households in the 1990s*, Oxford University Press, Oxford, 1999.

individual 'commitments' rather than 'fixed obligations' (Finch 1989; 1995: 61).

Our approach was to identify the central conclusions of the baseline studies, and to consider the extent to which these still apply to older people living at the end of the twentieth century. Our research provides a test of these different views by asking:

- How has family life changed in the three communities over the past fifty years?
- How different are relationships in old age now, in contrast with the period following the Second World War?

Fieldwork

As a way of documenting the range of relationships that affect the lives of older people, the research draws on the idea of them being part of a 'social network' (Wenger 1992). Measurements of social networks typically build upon three types of questions:

- the *exchange* question: this identifies those who might have performed some kind of service for the older person (McCallister and Fischer 1978; Wenger 1984);
- the *role relation* question: this focuses on people who are related to the individual in some formalised or prescribed way (Cochran *et al.* 1990);
- the *subjective* question: this identifies those 'close to' or on 'intimate terms' with the older person (Kahn and Antonucci 1980).

We were interested in examining changes in those whom older people might list as important in their life, and so we took the subjective question as the key measure. We asked older people to make their own assessment regarding who was most important in their life and what roles these people played in the provision of support. We presented the respondent with a diagram of three concentric circles, with the smaller circle in the centre in which the word 'you' was written. Respondents were asked to place in the inner circle the names of those persons who are 'so close and important' that they 'could not imagine life without them'. They were then asked to place those they considered less close but still important in the middle and outer circles. In each case, having named the individual with whom they were close, respondents were asked about their relationship with that person (e.g. sibling, friend, spouse). Having done this, respondents were then asked about the different types of help and support that these network members provided or received.

This technique was originally devised by Kahn and Antonucci (1980; see also Antonucci 1995). It makes no *a priori* assumptions about the nature of the network in which people are involved. Family ties may be important, but other relationships may also be shown to be significant.

Data collection was carried out in two main phases: the first comprised a questionnaire survey of around 200 people of pensionable age in each of the three areas. This was designed to explore social and family change since the time of the baseline studies, as well as details about personal networks. The second phase had a number of elements, the main part of which comprised a series of qualitative interviews with sixty-two white people drawn from the social survey, who were over the age of seventy-five. An additional group of interviews was also undertaken with Asian respondents in Bethnal Green and Wolverhampton (Phillipson *et al.* 2000). Possibly these are two of the more vulnerable groups of older people and the purpose of both sets of interviews was to examine the issue of social change from their standpoints.

Experiences of family life

Drawing on the social network approach, our research demonstrates a mixture of continuities and discontinuities. Household structure has been one important change since the 1950s (Table 13.1). Then, notably in Bethnal Green and Wolverhampton, older people defined their lives in the context of family groups. In Bethnal Green, for example, as many as 46 per cent shared a dwelling with relatives and in Wolverhampton just 10 per cent were living alone. Some fifty years later, 72 per cent of our respondents in Bethnal Green were living either with a spouse or on their own. In Wolverhampton, the figure was 78 per cent; and in middle-class Woodford as high as 83 per cent.

Thus the contrast over the two periods is between an old age spent with others and one where it is experienced initially with one other person and then alone (mostly by women). Middle-class Woodford in fact represents what may become the norm, with nearly 50 per cent of pensioner households comprising the older couple. Bethnal Green however demonstrates the continuing importance of multigenerational households within the inner city: 26 per cent of households being of two generations or more. These were drawn predominantly from the Bangladeshi families in our sample. The comparable figure in Townsend's study was 41 per cent, so

Table 13.1 Household composition

| | Bethnal Green | | Wolverhampton | | Woodford |
	1954–5	1995	1945	1995	1995
Lives alone	25	34	10	37	35
Lives with spouse or partner only	29	38	16	41	48
Lives with others	46	28	74	22	17
N (=100%)	203	195	477	228	204

the change is considerable, but not as great as might be expected. In contrast, just 13 per cent of pensioner households in suburban Woodford comprise two or more generations.

From this evidence, Frankenberg's 'environment of kin' has undergone significant alteration. Older people are certainly much less likely to share the lives of children and grandchildren on a daily basis under the same roof. But kinship and family ties still matter, a point that may be illustrated in at least two ways. Using the measure described earlier, the 627 people interviewed named an average of 9.3 members of their networks (standard deviation: 5.4). All but seven of those interviewed could identify someone 'close' and important in their life. Few older people, therefore, would appear to be 'isolated' in the sense of lacking close relationships – a finding which held for all three areas. This may be taken as representing at least some degree of continuity with the baseline studies. Leaving aside partners or spouses, it is clear that friends and children are the dominant groups. Other groups such as other relatives and neighbours appear to be much less important on the type of measure we have used. Overall, the personal networks of older people are dominated by kin, who form 73 per cent of those named. Children make up 20 per cent of network members. They are, however, relatively few in number within each network: the average number of children per network was 1.9 overall, with 2.1 in the case of Wolverhampton, and 1.8 in Bethnal Green and Woodford.

The numerical importance of kin – children especially – is matched by the way in which they also provide the emotional core within the network. They comprise the bulk of those listed in the inner circle. The following extract from one of the qualitative interviews, illustrates this point. Mr Green is aged 75 and lives with his wife in Bethnal Green. They have one son who now lives in an adjoining borough. Mr Green acknowledges the security provided by his immediate family:

> *Oh, I think that family life is 100 per cent important. In every way because I mean for myself now this, I have only got one son right, there is peace of mind, I am under the weather, the wife had a very bad spell and so family life then was ... it showed family life you know what I mean, it showed family life, everybody was prepared to, I mean at the drop of a hat they would be there ... anything on the phone, I mean my son has got a car ... and we have got their home phone numbers, posted up down there and that to us is. It doesn't matter what time of the day or night, if there is a problem, pick the phone up ... so you know family life is very, very important.*

A second illustration of the importance of kin concerns the proximity of children. Of those listing children in their personal network (including those living with one of their children), a majority in each of the areas had access to a child within a distance of four miles or less (64 per cent in Bethnal Green; 71 per cent in Wolverhampton; and 60 per cent in Woodford). Here are some extracts from our qualitative interviews of older people talking about the contact that they have with their children.

Mrs Harris is 81 and, following a serious illness, the family decided that she should move to the home of one of her three children (a daughter also living in Woodford):

> *I thought I wasn't quite ready to look for a retirement home, depending on how my cancer was going to progress. So it was decided that I come here to my daughter's. Well my other daughter lives very near as well so I mean she will take me to the shops sometimes, she will take me to the Post Office to collect my pension and I will go and spend a day with her now and again.*

Mr Cole is 77 and was born in Bethnal Green. He lives with his wife and has four of his five children living around the East End:

> *One lives ... locally, that is my daughter. My other daughter lives in Bow. My other son lives in Stratford. And my other son lives at Enfield ... My youngest daughter works [locally] so consequently we can see her anytime we want to. But normally we go out once or twice a week with her.*

Mr Ellis is 91 and lives in Wolverhampton. He was widowed thirty years ago. He has lived in his present house for fifty years. He has two children.

> *Ken, the elder one ... he still lives at Codsall, where he's lived for twenty years. Jill has just recently moved house but it's only about half a mile away from where she was before. She's come a tiny bit nearer to me. Codsall is about seven miles from here, and where Gillian lived before was Fairgate, about five miles from here. And now it's about four or something like that. So I, she always comes as she has done for ages to take me up to the Post Office on pension day and do what shopping I need while she is here you see.*

Changes

But, in addition to household structures, the relationships of older people have also changed a great deal since the 1940s and 1950s. In the first place, elderly people living together as couples has more prominence now than was evident in the baseline studies. As Lynn Jamieson (1998: 136) has argued:

> *the historical shift from 'the family' to 'the good relationship' as the site of intimacy is the story of the growing emphasis on the couple relationship.*

Older people (men especially) see their partner both as a confidant and a source of support in times of crisis, whether through illness or financial hardship. This reflects a more general point about changing relationships between generations: no longer living side-by-side in the same street or house, and with a less dominant 'mum' at the centre of the family, couples have moved to centre stage. This has also produced a significant change in the relationship between parents and children, one highlighted in the desire to live in 'independent' households and for there to be 'intimacy at a distance' (Rosenmayr and Kockeis 1963).

Second, friends are also more prominent now in older people's social networks. The significance of friendship has been a major theme in the work of researchers such as Jerrome (1992), Adams and Allan (1998) and Pahl (2000). In our survey we found that friends are the largest single group listed in respect of intimate ties, and they may play a substantial role in providing emotional support. For the never-married, friends were listed as important sources of help (one in three would draw upon a friend for help with most areas of support). For those who were married, friends appeared to have a complementary role to partners and children.

The role played by friends may be especially important in middle-class areas such as Woodford where relatives may be geographically more dispersed. This was a central finding in the earlier study of Woodford, where local networks of friends (largely organised by women) were viewed as having functions somewhat similar to the extended family of the East End (Willmott and Young 1960). Our findings suggest that the cohort of people who moved from the East End to suburbs such as Woodford has maintained active links with friends in the immediate area. Such ties are important in sustaining leisure and social activities in retirement, although in many cases (again as the Willmott and Young study suggests), this represents a continuation of a pattern established much earlier in life.

A third change is that whilst some children may live near, older people still face the challenge of managing relations within more dispersed networks. In some respects, this is aided by the growth of new forms of communication. In the early 1950s, only one fifth of *all* households had access to a telephone (Obelkevich 1994: 145), with a lower proportion still in pensioner households. By the 1990s, telephone ownership had become near universal (although it should be noted that 13 per cent of respondents in Bethnal Green did not have use of a telephone, compared with 9 per cent in Wolverhampton, and 3 per cent in Woodford). More importantly, the telephone has come to symbolise the contact which can still be maintained with distant children and siblings. We found, for example that, overall, one in three of our respondents had last been in touch with someone in their network, not face-to-face, but via the telephone. Growth in the use of mobile phones and e-mail has also served to accelerate trends towards electronic rather than face-to-face communication. These developments may create pressures, especially for working-class pensioners.

Mr Pinner is an 81-year-old widower living on the thirteenth floor of a tower block in Bethnal Green. He has four children.

> *The son in Bracknell rings up every night. Bill, in Wales, he rings up once a week, something like that. Jerry, the one over in Ireland, as I say, I can't speak to him until he speaks to me because he is not on the phone. He was on the phone, but his wife kept ringing up home from over there all the time and he run up a bill of over £400. So if he wants to make a call he goes to a call box. Then after a while, I got the number of the call box like, and when the pips go I say put the phone down and then I ring him back.*

Finally, social networks have themselves been subject to more general changes, affecting the communities in different ways. Comparing the three areas, it is Wolverhampton which in 1995 best approximates to the idea of the 'local extended family'. Strong local networks still flourish within the locality, notwithstanding significant social and demographic changes since the 1940s.

In the case of Bethnal Green, economic and social changes have affected kinship networks in complex ways. The situation of the Bangladeshi families could be described as reminiscent of the 'family groups' described by Sheldon (1948) and Young and Willmott (1957). Mr Hussein provides an example here:

> *Mr Hussein is aged 70 and lives in a four bedroomed flat on the third floor of a council block in Bethnal Green. He came to Britain from Bangladesh in the late 1950s ... There are ten people in the flat: Mr Hussein (who rents the flat), his wife, his mother-in-law, four sons, two daughters, and a grandchild. He also has a nephew living in the same block. Three sisters and one brother also live in East London.*

Many white respondents had contrasting experiences, with kin often spread over considerable distances, as in the example above of Mr Pinner. This dispersal of the network had most obviously affected pensioner households in Woodford, although here geographical mobility was viewed as a normal part of family development. Mrs Lewin, for example, had two children: a son living in Colchester and a daughter in Stansted, Essex. She also had three grandchildren now living in different parts of the Midlands and Southern England. Asked about their moving away, she commented: 'They should branch out on their own. Otherwise you don't get anywhere do you?.' This illustrates how nuclear families within a middle-class kinship network tend to maintain greater distance between themselves (Jerrome 1996). Jerrome concluded that middle-class parents may be less intensively involved with their adult children on a day-to-day basis, and that everyday contact is as likely to occur with peers as with children.

Conclusion

This chapter has reviewed some ways in which family life is experienced by older people. Overall, the findings confirm that the family has retained its influential role. It is, though, a different type of family compared with that of the 1950s. Indeed, an important conclusion from this research is that talking about *the* family life of older people has become a more complex task. There are many more different 'types' of older people than was the case just after the Second World War, and many more different types of families (not least through Britain being a multicultural society). But the family in some form is still central to support in later life, even if this is often focused around a small number of network members. And other relationships certainly do matter, especially for those without children, those who are single, or those who are estranged from their family (and the last may be an increasingly significant group in the caseloads of health and social services workers).

Locality also seems to matter. Not because locality produces some kinds of relations rather than others; rather, we can use ideas about locality and community to illustrate the important social and economic differences that exist among older people.

Overall, the message from the research is that family relationships continue to be a major part of growing old, but there are constraints as well: some operating through choice, others through the pressures which arise through particular life histories and particular environments. Either way, the experience of diversity and variety in the family and community life of older people is an important theme and conclusion to this investigation into family relationships and social networks.

NOTE

1   The work on which this chapter is based was supported by a grant from the Economic and Social Research Council, reference number L315253021. A full discussion about the research methodology, along with the research findings, is contained in Phillipson *et al.* (2001).

REFERENCES

Antonucci, T. (1995) 'Convoys of social relations: family and friendships within a life span context'. In Blieszner, R. and Bedford, V.H. (eds) *Handbook of Ageing and the Family*. New York: Greenwood Press.

Adams, R. and Allan, G. (1998) *Placing Friendship in Context*. Cambridge: Cambridge University Press.

Cochran, M. *et al.* (1990) *Extending Families*. Cambridge: Cambridge University Press.

Cowgill, D. and Holmes, D. (eds) (1972) *Ageing and Modernisation*. New York: Appleton-Century-Crofts.

Finch, J. (1989) *Kinship Obligations and Family Change*. Cambridge: Polity Press.

Finch, J. (1995) 'Responsibilities, obligations and commitments'. In Allen, I. and Perkins, E. (eds) *The Future of Family Care for Older People*. London: HMSO.

Frankenberg, R. (1966) *Communities in Britain*. Harmondsworth: Penguin Books.

Jamieson, L. (1998) *Intimacy: Personal Relationships in Modern Societies*. Cambridge: Polity Press.

Jerrome, D. (1992) *Good Company: an Anthropological Study of Older People in Groups*. Edinburgh: Edinburgh University Press.

Jerrome, D. (1996) 'Ties that bind'. In Walker, A. (ed) *The New Generational Contract: Intergenerational Relations, Old Age and Welfare*. London: UCL Press.

Kahn, R. and Antonucci, T. (1980) 'Convoys over the life course: attachment, roles and social support'. In Baltes, P.B. and Brim, O. (eds) *Life-Span Development and Behaviour* (Vol. 3). New York: Academic Press.

McCallister, L. and Fischer, C. (1978) 'A procedure for surveying personal networks', *Sociological Methods and Research*, 7: 131–147.

Obelkevich, J. (1994) 'Consumption'. In Obelkevich, J. and Catterall, P. (eds) *Understanding Post-War British Society*. London: Routledge.

Pahl, R. (2000) *Friends*. Cambridge: Polity Press.

Phillipson, C., Alhaq, E., Ullah, S. and Ogg, J. (2000) 'Bangladeshi families in Bethnal Green: older people, ethnicity and social exclusion'. In Warnes, T., Warren, L. and Nolan, M. (eds) *Care Services for Later Life*. London: Jessica Kingsley Publishers.

Phillipson, C., Bernard, M., Phillips, J. and Ogg, J. (2001) *The Family and Community Life of Older People: Social Networks and Social Support in Three Urban Areas*. London: Routledge.

Rosenmayr, L. and Kockeis, E. (1963) 'Propositions for a sociological theory of ageing and the family', *International Social Service Journal*, 15, 3, 410–426.

Sheldon, S. (1948) *The Social Medicine of Old Age*. Oxford: Oxford University Press.

Townsend, P. (1957) *The Family Life of Old People*. London: Routledge and Kegan Paul.

Wenger, G.C (1984) *The Supportive Network*. London: Allen and Unwin.

Wenger, G.C. (1992) *Help in Old Age – Facing up to Change*. Liverpool: Liverpool University Press.

Willmott, M. and Young, P. (1960) *Family and Class in a London Suburb*. London: Routledge and Kegan Paul.

Young, M. and Willmott, P. (1957) *Family and Kinship in East London*. London: Routledge and Kegan Paul.

CHAPTER 14

PROBLEMATIZING SOCIAL CARE NEEDS IN MINORITY COMMUNITIES

Ken Blakemore

Much of the discussion about minority ethnic and 'racial' communities and community care in Britain (the author's included) has, to date, stressed the problematic nature of health and social care in the community for black and Asian people. The sharpest needs have been given attention while less urgent needs and examples of relative success in community care have hardly been mentioned. [...]

There has been a negative bias in research on ageing and community care in minority communities. In other words, researchers have looked for problems. But they have not necessarily looked for examples of ways in which minority communities or older people themselves have grappled with these problems.

Equally, there has been little or no awareness of the ways in which the reform of community care might have affected black and South Asian people (NISW 1990, Patel 1990, Ahmad and Atkin 1996). Changes in community care policy during the 1990s brought to a head the leading question of how much community exists 'out there' in the form of available carers, and resources such as time, money and facilities. The reality is that, as with the white majority, black and South Asian minority families and communities are often thrown back on their own resources when faced with the needs of their dependants. In addition, stereotypes of extended family life in minority communities feed the assumption among service

Source: 'Health and social care needs in minority communities: an over-problematized issue?' *Health and Social Care in the Community*, 2000, 8.1, pp. 22–30.

planners and providers that black and South Asian people are more willing to 'look after their own' than people in the white majority (Blakemore and Boneham 1994). This in turn raises questions about the extent of need for community care in minority communities and how the resources available in those communities compare with the position for the majority.

Three kinds of 'resources' in South Asian and African-Caribbean communities can be identified:

a. The size and proportions of ageing cohorts in different communities;
b. Family change and residence patterns;
c. Economic assets: employment and housing.
[. . .]

Ageing cohorts

The minority communities taken as a whole are, on face value, in a much better position than the majority. In Britain, almost one-fifth of the white population is over retirement age compared to only 6 per cent of the African-Caribbean, 4 per cent of the Indian and 1 or 2 per cent of the Pakistani and Bangladeshi communities (OPCS 1991). Looked at in this basic way, most minority families in Britain still have very few aged relatives. Most of the 'grandparent generation' is still under 60 years of age. [. . .] As immigration from the Caribbean peaked in the 1950s there is a disproportionately large group of African-Caribbeans now in their late fifties and early sixties. A quarter of all the people in Britain who define themselves as African-Caribbean (including those born in the UK) are aged between 45 and 60/65 years (see OPCS 1991 p. 25). This is a significantly larger proportion than in the white majority population (22 per cent), larger than in Indian communities (16 per cent), and much larger than in the Pakistani and Bangladeshi minorities (12 and 14 per cent, respectively).

As far as 'care resources' are concerned, the 'late middle-age bulge' among African-Caribbeans appears to offer, on the one hand, considerable resources for cohort self-sufficiency and a pool of potential support for those who suffer from chronic illnesses and other problems.

On the other hand, though, three factors detract from this optimistic estimate: firstly, there is evidence from earlier community surveys (Bhalla and Blakemore 1981, Fenton 1985) of poor health among late middle age/early old age cohorts of African-Caribbean people.

Secondly, there is already a considerable proportion of African-Caribbean people (under pensionable age) living alone – for example, the 1991 Census recorded that in Birmingham over one-quarter of the 'Black Caribbean' households were composed of a lone adult with no children (OPCS 1992 p. 327). While living alone need not be problematic, observation of individual cases and survey results (Berry et al. 1981, Blakemore and Boneham 1994) show that there is a substantial and growing number, among those living alone, of rather isolated older women (often widowed) in the African-Caribbean community. It is among this group of relatively disengaged individuals or formerly 'self-reliant pioneers' that one finds cases of sudden change to a dependent or chronically ill status and it is such people who have relatively few potential carers to call upon.

Thirdly, the demographic bulge of the migrant generation of the 1950s and 1960s is quite tightly compressed in time terms (Peach 1991). Many African-Caribbean migrants of this period are therefore now crossing the threshold of sixty years of age together. Rather quickly, and in the space of five to ten years, the balance is likely to shift from this being a cohort group with an excess of potential carers to a cohort group with rapidly increasing care needs.

The African-Caribbean community is distinctive in being the most tightly bunched cohort group reaching retirement age. Of the South Asian communities, those of Indian origin or descent (chiefly Sikh and Gujerati communities) come closest to the Caribbean pattern, but even so have a significantly lower percentage of people in the pre-retirement group than either the Caribbean or the majority white population. The Pakistani and Bangladeshi communities are even younger in age structure. [. . .]

Worryingly high rates of illness in the older African-Caribbean population have already been mentioned. As pointed out above, community surveys in Birmingham and Bristol identified a considerable number of rather vulnerable older black people who have to cope with long-term illnesses of various kinds. They often have to do so either on their own or without the support of large families or networks of relatives (Bhalla and Blakemore 1981, Fenton 1985). The findings of these earlier community surveys of older black people have been supported by other studies of mortality rates in minority ethnic communities. Balarajan (1995), for instance, discusses an excess of deaths from stroke among African-Caribbeans aged between sixty-five and seventy-four years (approximately 50 per cent higher than the norm in England and Wales). Balarajan also points out that mortality rates from stroke are even higher in the Bangladeshi community (twice the rate in England and Wales), slightly above the England and Wales rate in the Pakistani community and well above in the Indian community. [. . .]

Data from the 1991 Census on incidence of limiting long-term illness show that while the percentage of ill people is higher in the white majority (reflecting the age structure of the majority population), the relative illness rate (adjusted for age) is higher in the minority communities. Relative illness rates are particularly high among Pakistani and Bangladeshi men and women and among African-Caribbean women.

The data also show that, from a household point of view, minority households (which tend to be larger than in majority) are – in the case of African-Caribbean and Indian communities – about as likely to have a member with a limiting long-term illness as do households in the white majority; in the Pakistani and Bangladeshi communities, the percentage of households with a member who is chronically ill is significantly greater than in the majority.

Family change and residence patterns

How resilient are family ties in minority communities? How far will ideals of care for older people continue to be translated into practical support and action? [. . .] It is important to be aware of signs of change and to consider their significance in relation to changing patterns of residence and household size.

Firstly, there is evidence from the voluntary organizations which provide services to older African-Caribbean and Asian people that families are not as supportive to older people as they were. In 1985, I reported on two surveys of forty Asian and African-Caribbean voluntary organizations (Blakemore 1985). In 1993, a number of these organizations were contacted again. Only twelve responded – some organizations had been closed down and colleagues had moved to unknown addresses.

It was significant that eleven of the twelve responses from voluntary organizations included statements which in one way or another pointed to losses of family support in the past five years. Respondents were anxious to avoid either moralistic or culturalist explanations of a 'decline of family values' nature, and some sought to explain increasing need for community support as one of the inevitable outcomes of social change.

For example, an Age Concern organization in Leicester identified moves to smaller houses and job mobility as key reasons for 'fast growing' needs for community services in the older population. A Gujerati Indian association in London had identified 'more and more people feeling lonely without receiving enough response from the family' and added, 'the family system is slowly but steadily disintegrating with the young generation seeking more freedom'.

African-Caribbean organizations responded in much the same way. For example, a Caribbean association in London which provided services to over 250 older people every week reported that 'family support over the past five years has declined steadily', and another – a day centre for older African-Caribbeans – had found that 'the extended family seems to be breaking down . . . people are becoming more introspective'.
[. . .]

A third sign of change which will affect the position of older people can be found in changing attitudes to extended family living. Stopes-Roe and Cochrane's (1990) survey revealed that in terms of values and attitudes among younger Asians there is still a great deal of support for the extended family. But the authors also detected signs of change. Not only did two-thirds of young Asian women express a preference for nuclear family living but, more unexpectedly, so did one-third of the fathers and 40 per cent of the mothers.

In view of these normative changes in attitudes to family life and the position of older people, it is interesting to note the differences in actual patterns of family residence and household structure among South Asian communities. The 1991 Population Census provides evidence of the proportions of households which are 'three or more adults with one or more dependent children' (a rough and ready indicator of joint family living and/or multigenerational households). In all the 'Asian' groups the proportions of such larger households are much higher than in the white and 'African-Caribbean' populations, which have only a few per cent.

But there are also some significant differences among the South Asian groups identified by the census. In Birmingham, for example, significantly fewer Indian households were of the larger kind (26 per cent) than either Pakistani or Bangladeshi households (32 and 36 per cent, respectively).

There are yet further inter- and intra-ethnic differences in percentages of families living in larger-sized households, according to geographical area and the nature of the housing stock in each town or city.

For example, our comparison of South Asian communities in Birmingham and Coventry showed that large households (of six or more people) are much more common in the former city than the latter (Blakemore and Boneham 1994 p. 82). [...] These differences in domestic residence patterns are reflections not only of differences between two distinctively different 'ethnic' communities but also of the ways in which other factors – housing stock in the two cities, for instance – affect household size. The trend towards smaller households and separate living arrangements for the older generation will not necessarily entail less actual support of older people, though a shift in expectations has undeniably taken place in some minority communities and a proportion of families. In the future, when a rising proportion of older South Asian people become frail, the extended family may be able to provide some daily care but, when this has to be done at a distance, risks of neglect and isolation increase.

Also, older South Asian people are vulnerable to two additional sources of stress and disadvantage: firstly, they are international migrants and have to deal with the psychological aspects of growing old in a 'foreign' country; secondly, they are in 'racial' and ethnic minorities. If they are unsupported by a family or wider group of kin they are particularly vulnerable to direct racism (abuse, hostility and attack), indirect racism (as shown in the non-provision of appropriate services), or simple isolation in a society they are not readily able to communicate with.

Residence patterns among older African-Caribbean people seem to indicate even greater risk of isolation. Again, one has to beware of problematizing living alone when most older people who do so are successfully independent and are often connected to some kind of social network. [...]

Increasing numbers of African-Caribbean people on the verge of retirement age are seriously considering whether to leave Britain. This is a controversial issue and the evidence of migration statistics reveals some inexplicable falls in numbers of older African-Caribbeans (Peach 1991). However, significant drops in the totals of older black people in Britain are occurring and only a small proportion is accounted for by mortality.

Even if a considerable proportion do leave, however, it is likely to be the older people who are already relatively well-connected socially and those who have accumulated savings and other assets who will return, rather than 'the marooned', or those who are rather isolated, relatively poor, and increasingly in need of care.

Employment and housing

[. . .] Earlier community surveys (for example, Bhalla and Blakemore 1981) discovered substantially lower pensioner incomes among the minorities than white older people in the same neighbourhoods. Opportunities to build up occupational pensions, and to acquire houses which have appreciated or retained their value, have been limited, historically, in black and Asian communities.

However there are clearly discernible differences between the various minority communities in terms of economic well-being despite 'the persistence of inequality . . . [and] . . . strong elements of continuity in racial disadvantage' (Jones 1993 p. 151). Jones's report on Britain's Asian and African-Caribbean minorities reveals elements of both continuity and divergence, with 'African Asian, Indian and Chinese groups . . . making progress in terms of education and employment' (1993 p. 152) but continuing sharp disadvantage among African-Caribbeans and especially Pakistanis and Bangladeshis. The latter groups 'remain concentrated in the lower job levels, and are subject to much higher rates of unemployment than other ethnic groups' (Jones 1993 p. 156).

What do these trends mean for health and social care? One way to consider this question is to examine what has been happening among some of the better-off Asian communities, such as African Asians and Indians in south London and the east Midlands.

As discussed above in relation to family change, there are some signs of loss of contact with the older generation as sons and daughters set up homes on their own and are more likely than before to become geographically and socially mobile. On the other hand, the assets of such families and their communities can do much to offset these losses. Though community and voluntary sector-run services in South Asian communities as a whole tend to be rather limited and to cater for men rather than women (Blakemore 1985), this is not the case among the Indian and African Asian communities in Leicester, for instance. Here, a range of services are used by women as well as men and these include day centre and leisure facilities, 'drop-in' visits to frail older people, a varied meals service to Hindus, Sikhs and Muslims, welfare rights advice and counselling, hospital visiting services, and local and foreign holidays. This range of services, when combined with the development of sheltered and residential accommodation, can be compared with the growth of a parallel welfare system in Jewish communities. Ambitious developments of this kind are dependent not only on concern in the community and the willingness of volunteers to help run services, but just as importantly on the economic resources a community can muster: cash donations, transport, accommodation. [...]

By 1995, the white male unemployment rate in Britain stood at 8 per cent while the rate among the Indian community was 12 per cent. In the Pakistani and Bangladeshi (27 per cent) and Black communities (24 per cent), unemployment was at a strikingly higher level (ONS 1996 p. 46). Unemployment, and related problems of economic deprivation and poverty, are concentrated in the Pakistani, Bangladeshi and black communities.

Rates of unemployment among economically-active Pakistani and Bangladeshi women are even higher than among their male counterparts. Is it fair, then, to conclude that despite problems of poverty, the presence of a majority of Pakistani and Bangladeshi women in the home (whether resulting from high unemployment or from traditional expectations) implies a plentiful supply of potential carers?

There are several objections to this argument. One is that we cannot assume that traditional expectations of unconditional support for older people will or should be maintained indefinitely. Another is that such assumptions can be sexist. It is the women who are expected to shoulder the larger share of domestic and caring tasks, much as they do in the majority community (Qureshi and Walker 1989), though patterns of domestic work vary between ethnic communities – in Pakistani communities, for instance, it is often the men who do the shopping. There is also the question of whether women in minority ethnic communities receive enough help in the form of support, advice and training from social services. The 'plentiful supply of care' assumption also implies that older women will be cared for as well as older men, but given the ambivalent or uncertain position that some older women occupy in their husbands' families (for instance, widows who have no sons to protect their interests), age in itself is not always the guarantee of devoted care that it might appear to be.

Family care in most Pakistani or Bangladeshi homes is warm and supportive but the point is that it is not inevitably so. As in any community, severe tension and conflict is bound to arise in some families. If the family is already struggling with problems of racism, poverty, high rates of unemployment, inadequate housing and overcrowding (OPCS 1992 p. 326), such tensions are likely to be difficult to resolve.

The housing occupied by Pakistani and Bangladeshi families is more likely to lack the amenities and improvements which make it easier to care for frail older people. For instance, while under one-third of white and 'African-Caribbean' residents in the West Midlands live in households with no central heating and under one-quarter of Indians do so, 58 per cent of Pakistanis and just over half of Bangladeshis lack this amenity (OPCS 1992, p. 326).

Ratcliffe (1997) summarizes selected housing characteristics by 'ethnic' group. Looking at the key facilities that help families to provide care – for instance ownership of a car, accommodation that is not overcrowded, central heating – by and large it is African-Caribbean, Pakistani and Bangladeshi households which again appear to be at a distinct disadvantage compared with both the white majority and the Indian communities. Significantly, the latter (Indian) community has a lower proportion of households with no car or central heating than the white majority.

Conclusion

All black and South Asian communities face common problems of 'racial' discrimination and social disadvantage to a greater or lesser extent. These structural problems of disadvantage are bound to be reflected in (a) the resources available to different communities and their ability to meet social and care needs themselves, and (b) the planning, appropriateness and delivery of health and care services. However, within this broad conclusion it is clear that some communities, or subgroups within communities, are likely to fare better than others in meeting community care needs and gaining access to social and health services. [. . .]

The evidence shows that some older South Asian and African-Caribbean people have considerably greater needs than older people in the majority population. Need is evident in relation to higher rates of serious illness, poverty and inadequate housing. There are also questions to be asked about whether health and social services adequately meet the needs of older black and South Asian people. This subject has not been the focus of the discussion here. However, it should not be forgotten that neither mainstream social and health services nor informal community networks of support can be relied upon to step in where family support is found wanting. Also, a significant number of older people in minority ethnic groups are reliant on a rather narrow base of family support or, especially in the case of the African-Caribbean community, might not have any close relatives to rely upon.

Finally, though, the point that some older people in black and Asian communities have greater needs than the majority and suffer neglect should not be allowed to define the situation as one which is wholly problematic for community care. Some older people in minority communities are in greater need of care than older people in the majority but by and large have their care needs met (and may even be in a better position, in terms of family support and social contact, than some older people in majority communities). Yet others have fewer needs and problems than the people in the majority community who are very old and frail.

Also, at the level of the community rather than the individual, the evidence shows that both the resources available to Britain's diverse ethnic minority population and care needs (as expressed, for instance, by dependency ratios) vary widely from one group to another. The position of minority ethnic communities has often been portrayed as one of common disadvantage compared with the position facing the white majority. In this way existing research has tended to racialize the debate about minority needs, focusing on problems in community care as if they affect all black people equally. In fact, some minority communities are in a much better position than others to lessen the impact of 'race' discrimination, inadequate care services and social disadvantage. All the signs point to increasing inequalities in community care among Britain's minority black and South Asian communities, while the black/white divide becomes less distinct than it was.

REFERENCES

Ahmad W.I. and Atkin K. (eds) (1996) *'Race' and Community Care*. Open University Press, Buckingham.

Balarajan R. (1995) Ethnicity and variations in the nation's health. *Health Trends* 27 (4), 114–119.

Berry S., Lee M. and Griffiths S. (1981) *Report on a Survey of West Indian Pensioners in Nottingham*. Nottingham Social Services, Nottingham.

Bhalla A. and Blakemore K. (1981) *Elders of the Minority Ethnic Groups*. AFFOR, Birmingham.

Blakemore K. (1985) The state, the voluntary sector and new developments in provision for the old of minority racial groups. *Ageing and Society* 5 (2), 175–190.

Blakemore K. and Boneham M. (1994) *Age, Race and Ethnicity*. Open University Press, Milton Keynes.

Fenton S. (1985) *Race, Health and Welfare: Afro-Caribbean and South Asian People in Central Bristol*. Department of Sociology, University of Bristol, Bristol.

Jones T. (1993) *Britain's Ethnic Minorities*. Policy Studies Institute, London.

NISW (National Institute for Social Work) (1990) *Black Community and Community Care*. NISW, London.

ONS (1996) *Social Trends 26*. HMSO, London.

OPCS (1991) *Labour Force Survey 1988 and 1989*. HMSO, London.

OPCS (1992) *1991 Census, County Report, West Midlands (Part 1)*. HMSO, London.

Patel N. (1990) *A 'Race' Against Time?* The Runnymede Trust, London.

Peach C. (1991) *The Caribbean in Europe. Research Paper no. 15*, Centre for Research in Ethnic Relations, University of Warwick, Warwick.

Qureshi H. and Walker A. (1989) *The Caring Relationship – Elderly People and their Families*. Macmillan, Basingstoke.

Ratcliffe P. (1997) Race, ethnicity and housing differentials in Britain. In: V. Karn (ed.) *Ethnicity in the 1991 Census*, Vol. 4. The Stationery Office, London.

Stopes-Roe M. and Cochrane R. (1990) *Citizens of this Country, the Asian–British*. Multilingual Matters, Clevedon.

CHAPTER 15

A CHILD'S VIEW OF CARE IN THE COMMUNITY

Meera Syal

Mama was rummaging about in what we called the Bike Shed, one of two small outhouses at the end of our backyard, the other outhouse being our toilet. We'd never had a bike between us, unless you counted my three-wheeler tricycle which was one of a number of play items discarded amongst the old newspapers, gardening tools, and bulk-bought tins of tomatoes and Cresta fizzy drinks. Of course, this shed should have really been called the bathroom, because it was where we filled an old yellow plastic tub with pans of hot water from the kitchen and had a hurried scrub before frostbite set in, but my mother would have cut out her tongue rather than give it its real, shameful name.

'Found it, Mrs Worrall!' she shouted from inside the shed. Mrs Worrall, with whom she shared adjoining, undivided backyards, stood in her uniform of flowery dress and pinny on her step. She had a face like a friendly potato with a sparse tuft of grey hair on top, and round John Lennon glasses, way before they became fashionable, obviously. She moved like she was underwater, slow, deliberate yet curiously graceful steps, and frightened most of the neighbours off with her rasping voice and deadpan, unimpressed face. She did not smile often, and when she did you wished she hadn't bothered as she revealed tombstone teeth stained bright yellow with nicotine. But she loved me, I knew it; she'd only have to hear my voice and she'd lumber out into the yard to catch me, often not speaking, but would just nod, satisfied I was alive and functioning, her eyes impassive behind her thick lenses.

Source: *Anita and Me*, Flamingo, London, 1997, pp. 57–68.

She would listen, apparently enthralled, to my mother's occasional reports on my progress at school, take my homework books carefully in her huge slabs of hands and turn the pages slowly, nodding wisely at the cack-handed drawings and uneven writing. Every evening, when she came to pick up our copy of the *Express and Star* once my papa had finished reading it (an arrangement devised by my mother, 'Why should the poor lady have to spend her pension when she can read ours?'), she'd always check up on me, what I was doing, whether I was in my pyjamas yet, whether I was mentally and physically prepared to retire for the night. At least, that's what I read in her eyes, for she never spoke. Just that quick glance up and down, a slight incline of the head, a satisfied exhalation.

I wondered if she was like Mrs Christmas, childless, and maybe that was why she was so protective of me. But mama told me, with a snort of disgust, that she had three grown-up sons and a few grandchildren also. 'But I've never seen them! Do they live far away?' I persisted.

'Oh yes, very far. Wolverhampton!' she quipped back.

It had seemed quite a long way to me when we had driven there for my birthday treat, but I guessed by my mother's flaring nostrils and exaggerated eyebrow movements that she was being ironic, the way Indians are ironic, signposting the joke with a map and compass to the punchline.

'But why don't they come and see her then?'

My mother sighed and ruffled my hair. 'I will never understand this about the English, all this puffing up about being civilised with their cucumber sandwiches and cradle of democracy big talk, and then they turn round and kick their elders in the backside, all this It's My Life, I Want My Space stupidness, You Can't Tell Me What To Do cheekiness, I Have To Go To Bingo selfishness and You Kids Eat Crisps Instead Of Hot Food nonsense. What is this My Life business, anyway? We all have obligations, no one is born on their own, are they?'

She was into one of her Capital Letter speeches, the subtext of which was listen, learn and don't you dare do any of this when you grow up, missy. I quite enjoyed them. They made me feel special, as if our destiny, our legacy, was a much more interesting journey than the apparent dead ends facing our neighbours. I just wished whatever my destiny was would hurry up and introduce itself to me so I could take it by its jewelled hand and fly.

She paused for oxygen. 'I mean, Mrs Worrall is their mother, the woman who gave them life. And she on her own with Mr Worrall, too. I tell you, if my mother was so close, I would walk in my bare feet to see her every day. Every day.'

She turned away then, not trusting herself to say anything more. There was still something else I wanted to ask but I knew it would have to wait. I had grown up with Mrs Worrall, I had seen her every day of my life, but I had never seen or heard Mr Worrall. Ever.

My mother emerged from the shed holding aloft an old dusty glass vase which she blew on, and then scuffed with the sleeve of her shirt before handing it to Mrs Worrall who took it with a pleased grunt. 'Please, Mrs Worrall, have it. We never use it.'

Mrs Worrall nodded again and cleared her throat. 'He knocked mine over. I was in the way, in front of the telly. *Crossroads*. He likes that Amy Turtle. So he got a bit upset, see.'

Mama nodded sympathetically. 'How is he nowadays?'

Mrs Worrall shrugged, she did not need to say, same as always, and went back inside her kitchen.

'Mum, I'm starved, I am,' I wheedled. 'Give me something now.'

She busied herself with shutting the shed door, not looking at me, her face drawn tight like a cat's arse. 'There's rice and daal inside. Go and wash your hands.'

'I don't want that . . . that stuff! I want fishfingers! Fried! And chips! Why can't I eat what I want to eat?'

Mama turned to me, she had her teacher's face on, long suffering, beseeching, but still immovable. She said gently, 'Why did you take money for sweets? Why did you lie to papa?'

'I didn't,' I said automatically, blind to logic, to the inevitable fact that my crime had already been fretfully discussed while I'd been having the best day of my life being Anita Rutter's new friend.

'So now you are saying papa is a liar also? Is that it?'

I pretended to take a great interest in a mossy crack in the yard concrete, running my sandal along it, deliberately scuffing the leather. I knew how I looked, pouting, defiant in the face of defeat, sad and silly, but I could not apologise. I have still never been able to say sorry without wanting to swallow the words as they sit on my tongue.

Mama knelt down on the hard floor and cupped my face in her hands, forcing me to look into her eyes. Those eyes, those endless mud brown pools of sticky, bottomless love. I shook with how powerful I suddenly felt; I knew that with a few simple words I could wipe away every trace of guilt and concern ebbing across her face, that if I could admit what I had done, I could banish my parents' looming unspoken fear that their only child was turning out to be a social deviant. 'I did not lie,' I said evenly, embracing my newly-born status as a deeply disturbed fantasist with a frisson that felt like pride.

After my mother had retreated back into the kitchen, Mrs Worrall came out and stood in her doorway, wiping her large floury hands on her front, watching me kick mossy scabs across the yard. 'Come and give us a hand, Meena,' she said finally. I hesitated at the back door; I'd seen glimpses of her kitchen practically every day, I knew the cupboards on the wall were faded yellow, the lino was blue with black squares on it and the sink was under the window, like in our house. But I'd never actually been inside, and as I stepped in, I had a weird feeling that I was entering Dr Who's Tardis. It was much bigger than I had imagined, or it seemed so because there was none of the clutter that took up every available inch of space in our kitchen.

My mother would right now be standing in a haze of spicy steam, crowded by huge bubbling saucepans where onions and tomatoes simmered and spat, molehills of chopped vegetables and fresh herbs jostling for space with bitter, bright heaps of turmeric, masala, cumin and coarse black pepper whilst a softly breathing mound of dough would be waiting in a china bowl, ready to be divided and flattened into round, grainy chapatti. And she, sweaty and absorbed, would move from one chaotic work surface to another, preparing the fresh, home-made meal that my father expected, needed like air, after a day at the office about which he never talked.

From the moment mama stepped in from her teaching job, swapping saris for M & S separates, she was in that kitchen; it would never occur to her, at least not for many years, to suggest instant or take-away food which would give her a precious few hours to sit, think, smell the roses – that would be tantamount to spouse abuse. This food was not just something to fill a hole, it was soul food, it was the food their far-away mothers made and came seasoned with memory and longing, this was the nearest they would get for many years, to home.

So far, I had resisted all my mother's attempts to teach me the rudiments of Indian cuisine; she'd often pull me in from the yard and ask me to stand with her while she prepared a simple *sabzi* or rolled out a chapatti before making it dance and blow out over a naked gas flame. 'Just watch, it is so easy, beti,' she'd say encouragingly. I did not see what was easy about peeling, grinding, kneading and burning your fingers in this culinary Turkish bath, only to present your masterpiece and have my father wolf it down in ten minutes flat in front of the nine o'clock news whilst sitting cross-legged on the floor surrounded by spread sheets from yesterday's *Daily Telegraph*.

Once, she made the fatal mistake of saying, 'You are going to have to learn to cook if you want to get married, aren't you?'

I reeled back, horrified, and vowed if I ended up with someone who made me go through all that, I would poison the bastard immediately. My mother must have cottoned on; she would not mention marriage again for another fifteen years.

'Shut the door then,' said Mrs Worrall, who swayed over to the only bit of work surface that was occupied, where a lump of pastry dough sat in a small well of white flour. Otherwise, all was bare and neat, no visible evidence of food activity here save a half-packet of lemon puffs sitting on the window sill.

'What you making?' I asked, peering under her massive arm.

'Jam tarts. Mr Worrall loves a good tart. Mind out.'

She bent down with difficulty and opened the oven door, a blast of warm air hit my legs and I jumped back.

'What's that?'

'What yow on about? It's the oven.'

I'd never seen my mother use our oven, I thought it was a storage space for pans and her griddle on which she made chapatti. Punjabis and baking don't go together, I've since discovered. It's too easy, I suppose, not enough angst and sweat in putting a cake in the oven and taking it out half an hour later.

'Yow ever made pastry?' I shook my head. I'd always wondered what the crispy stuff on the bottom of jam tarts was, and here was Mrs Worrall making it in her own home. I was well impressed. 'Hee-y'aar,' said Mrs Worrall, putting a small bowl in front of me in which she poured a little flour and placed a knob of lemony butter. 'Always keep your fingers cold. That's the secret. Now rub your fingers together ... slowly. You wanna end up with breadcrumbs...' I squeezed the butter, feeling it squash then break against my fingers, and started to press and pummel it into the flour like I'd seen mama do with the chapatti dough.

'No! Too hard! It'll stick! Gently, dead gentle...' I slowed down, tried to concentrate on feeling each grain of flour, made my fingers move like clouds, and saw a tiny pile of breadcrumbs begin forming at the bottom of the bowl.

'I'm doing it! Look! Pastry!'

Mrs Worrall grunted. 'Not yet, it ain't...'

She left me to it whilst she quickly rolled out the large lump of pastry into an oval and pressed a cutter over its surface, slipping the tart cases into a large tin tray. Her fingers moved swiftly and lightly, as if they did not belong to those flapping meaty arms. She then took my bowl off me and stared at the contents critically. 'Not bad. Now binding. Use warm water, not cold. But the fork has to be like ice, see...'

She poured in a little liquid from a steel, flame-blackened kettle and handed me a fork from a pan of cold water in the sink. I pressed the crumbs together, watching them swell and cling to each other, until they gradually became a doughy mass.

'It's like magic, innit?'

'No. Your mum does that,' she said. 'This is your one. Alright?'

I nodded, and she quickly rolled out my dough, which I noticed stuck to the rolling pin much more than hers, cut out a small shape and placed it onto the tray before shoving the whole thing in the oven.

[...]

'Can I have lemon curd in my one, Mrs Worrall?' I jabbered, eager to distract her. She did not answer but wiped her hands on her pinafore and said, 'Come and say hello to Mr Worrall.' She opened the door leading into the sitting room and I blinked rapidly, trying to adjust my eyes to the gloom. The curtains were drawn, split by a bar of red sunset light where they did not quite meet, and the small black and white television set sitting on the dining table was on full volume. *Opportunity Knocks* was on, one of my very favourite programmes where ordinary people who felt they had a great untapped talent could try their luck at singing, impressions, unicycling whilst juggling hatchets, whatever, and if the great British public voted them the best of the acts, could return again and again every week, gathering more acclaim, accolades and possibly bookings at dizzying venues like the Wolverhampton Grand until they were finally knocked off first place by the new young pretender to the variety throne. The unicyclist is dead, long live the fat man from Barnet doing Harold Wilson impressions!

From the first time I watched that show, I knew that this could be my most realistic escape route from Tollington, from ordinary girl to major personality in one easy step. But I'd never seen anyone who wasn't white on the show, not so far, and was worried that might count against me. Hughie Green was doing his famous one-eye-open, one-eyebrow-cocked look right down the camera and he announced, 'Let's see how our musical muscle man, Tony Holland, does on our clapometer!' An oiled, bulging bloke in micro swimming trunks appeared briefly and rippled his belly muscles into animal shapes as the audience whooped and hollered and the clapometer began at fifty and rose and rose, climbing slowly along until it nudged ninety and there were beads of sweat forming on Tony's undulating diaphragm.

Mrs Worrall suddenly switched the TV off and another wail of protest came from a far dark corner. 'Later. Say hello to Mrs K's littl'un first, eh?' She pushed me forward and I suddenly became aware of the smell of the room which seemed to be at one with the gloom, the smell of a sick room, unaired and lonely, of damp pyjamas steaming, sticky-sided medicine bottles, spilled tinned soup and disinfectant under which there hovered the clinging tang of old, dried-in pee. A shape took form before me, thin useless legs in clean striped pyjamas, the toes curled and turned inwards, passive hands with fingers rigid and frozen as claws, a sunken chest making a bowed tent of the pyjama top, and finally Mr Worrall's face, wide blue-blue staring eyes and a mouth permanently open, asking for something, wanting to talk, with the bewildered, demanding expression of an unjustly punished child.

Mr Worrall moaned loudly again, nodding his head vigorously, a few drops of spit fell onto his chin which Mrs Worrall expertly wiped away with her pinafore hem. She took up his hand and placed it on mine, his fingers seemed to rustle like dry twigs but, amazingly, I could feel the pump and surge of his heartbeat throbbing through his palm. I wanted to pull my hand away but I looked up to see Mrs Worrall's eyes glittering behind their bottle bottom frames. 'Hello Mr Worrall,' I said faintly. Mr Worrall jerked his head back violently and gave a yelp. 'He likes you,' Mrs Worrall said, the glimmer of a smile playing round her mouth. 'It was the shells. In the war. He got too close. He was always a nosey bugger.'

I felt it was maybe alright to pull my hand away now, and I carefully replaced his back onto his lap, like replacing a brittle ornament after dusting. Mr Worrall jerked forward, I felt his breath on my face, it was surprisingly sweet-smelling, like aniseed, like Misty's warm steamy mouth used to smell. 'That's enough now,' said Mrs Worrall, pushing him back into his chair and gathering his blanket around his knees. 'It's nearly time for your wash. You want a wash, eh?' Mr Worrall seemed tall, even sitting down. He must have been over six foot before the shells got him. Now I knew two war veterans, him and Anita's dad. I felt annoyed that my papa had not done anything as remotely exciting or dangerous in his youth, or if he had he'd kept it quiet.

'How do you get Mr Worrall upstairs? Have you got a lift or something?' I asked as she busied herself with removing his socks. 'Ooh, we never use the upstairs, do we? No. Not been up there for twenty-two years.' My gaze travelled to the small door leading onto the stairs, the same as in our house, which fooled people into thinking there was another bigger room leading off from the lounge. It was padlocked from the outside, its hinges rusted.

All this time when I had run up and down our landing and imagined the Worralls ambling about on the other side of the wall, tutting about the noise, our adjoining bookends, I had never realised that next door were empty rooms, cobweb-filled, echoing, unused rooms. I felt queasy, my hunger had become nausea; Mrs Worrall was attempting to kneel, her fat knees cracking, and I suddenly saw what the last twenty-two years of her life must have been, this endless uncomplaining attendance of a broken, unresponsive body, the wiping of spittle and shit, the back-breaking tugging and loading and pulling and carrying, all the nights in front of the television whilst the Deirdre Rutters and the Glenys Lowbridges were putting on lipstick and waltzing off to pubs and bingo and dances and Mrs Worrall's big treat was an extra lemon puff in front of *Crossroads*, whilst her husband dozed off.

Not all the English were selfish, like mama sometimes said, but then again, I did not think of Mrs Worrall as English. She was a symbol of something I'd noticed in some of the Tollington women, a stoic muscular resistance which made them ask for nothing and expect less, the same resignation I heard in the voices of my Aunties when they spoke of back home or their children's bad manners or the wearying monotony of their jobs. My Aunties did not rage against fate or England when they swapped misery tales, they put everything down to the will of Bhagwan, their karma, their just desserts inherited from their last reincarnation which they had to live through and solve with grace and dignity. In the end, they knew God was on their side; I got the feeling that most of the Tollington women assumed that He had simply forgotten them.

'I've got to go,' I mumbled, backing away on Bambi legs, 'Mum's waiting...'

Mrs Worrall wordlessly helped me into the kitchen which now smelt like a bakery, yeasty and welcoming and warm. She retrieved the metal tray from the oven on which stood ten perfect tartlets and one which resembled a relief map of Africa. Nevertheless, she filled it with lemon curd from a twist-top jar, and threw in another two tarts for mama and papa, warning me, 'Wait a minute, or that curd'll tek the skin off yer tongue.'

I carried the three trophies on a napkin carefully to the door, and then paused to call out, 'Bye Mr Worrall!' as cheerily as I could manage. I did not expect an answer but I felt Mrs Worrall's eyes gently guide me to my back door.

CHAPTER 16

COMMUNITY AND STIGMA

16.1 THE PRINCIPLE OF NORMALIZATION

Wolf Wolfensberger and Stephen Tullman

Source: *Rehabilitation Psychology*, 27.3, 1982; reprinted in A. Brechin and J. Walmsley (eds) *Making Connections*, Hodder and Stoughton, London, 1989, pp. 211–19.

The principle of normalization first appeared in North America in the late 1960s (Wolfensberger 1980). Since then, it has evolved into a systematic theory that can be used as a universal guiding principle in the design and conduct of human services, but which is especially powerful when applied to services to people who are devalued by the larger society. [...]

In discussing the normalization principle..., we use the following simple definition: 'Normalization implies, as much as possible, the use of culturally valued means in order to enable, establish, and/or maintain valued social roles for people.' Though very brief, this definition has a vast number of implications for human services, ranging from the most global to the most minute. The definition reflects the almost paradigm-breaking assumption that the goal of human services with the most impact is social role enhancement or role defense.

Obviously, this definition reflects the assumption that if a person's social role were a societally valued one, other desirable things would be accorded that person within the resources and norms of his or her society.

In order to perceive the crucial function of role enhancement, it is necessary to understand the dynamics of deviancy making. A person can be considered 'deviant' or devalued when a significant characteristic is negatively valued by that segment of society that constitutes the majority or holds norm-defining power. [...]

Obviously, how a person is perceived affects how that person will be treated and has the following implications:

1   Devalued people will be badly treated. Others will usually accord them less esteem and status than non-devalued citizens. Devaluated people are apt to be rejected, even persecuted, and treated in ways that tend to diminish their dignity, adjustment, growth, competence, health, wealth, life span and so on. [. . .]

2   The negative treatment accorded devalued persons takes on certain forms that express the way society conceptualizes the roles of a devalued person or group. For example, if a group of children is (unconsciously) viewed as animals, then they may be segregated in a special class that is given an animal name – often even the name of animals that are seen as expressive of a devalued children's identity. Thus a class for retarded children may be called 'The Turtles'. [. . .]

In the habilitation area it is very common for the sick role and perception to be attributed to clients who certainly are no sicker than most of the population, and who really need a developmental approach, adult education, industrial apprenticeship training and the like. Instead, they are interpreted as sick by association with medically trained staff. [. . .]

3   How a person is perceived and treated by others will, in turn, strongly determine how that person subsequently behaves. The more consistently a person is perceived as deviant, therefore, the more likely it will be that he or she will conform to that expectation and emit the kinds of behaviour that are socially expected, often behaviours that are not valued by society. [. . .]

The fact that deviancy is culturally defined opens the door for psychologists to effect a two-pronged strategy of enabling devalued persons to attain a more valued membership in society by (1) reducing or preventing the differentness or stigmata that may make a person devalued in the eyes of observers and (2) changing perceptions and values regarding devalued persons so that a given characteristic is no longer seen as devalued.

Social role enhancement is the ultimate goal, but both stigma reduction/prevention and societal attitude changing can be pursued through two major subgoals: (*a*) the enhancement of the social image of a person or group and (*b*) the enhancement of the competence of the person or group, including bodily, sensory, intellectual and social performance, and the practice of valued skills and habits.

Image enhancement and competency enhancement are believed to be reciprocally reinforcing, both positively and negatively. A person who is competency impaired is at high risk of being seen and interpreted as being of low value and of suffering from image impairment; a person who is impaired in image and social value is apt to be responded to in ways that reduce his or her competency. Both processes work equally in the reverse direction.

The definition of normalization used here places emphasis on 'the use of culturally valued means.' Service structures, programs, methods, technologies, and tools are all means toward the normalization goal, and their value in the eyes of society is determined largely by the degree to which these means are used within the larger culture with and for *valued* persons of the same age, sex, and so on. For example, the culturally valued analogue for the schedules of an educational program for handicapped children would be the daily, weekly, and yearly schedules of a school for nonhandicapped children of the same age. Culturally valued analogues for a vocational program for young adults might include apprenticeship, vocational school, night classes in vocational subjects, on-the-job training, and adult education. It would not include 'job therapy', make-believe work (valued people who perform fake work are at high risk of getting devalued), or playing games.

It is possible to schematicize the normalization principle in a number of ways that can help one to understand it better, and that can form a basis for the formulation of a variety of specific implementive measures. One way to schematicize the principle is to classify its implications into different levels of social systems as follows:

1   Actions on the level of the person concerned, usually a client.
2   Actions on the level of the person's relevant *primary* social systems (e.g., family) and *secondary* social systems (e.g. neighborhood, community, service agency).
3   Actions on the level of society as a whole; that is, society's values, language usage, laws, customs, and so on.

Thus combining the second and third levels, all action implications could be represented by the schema in Table 16.1.

Normalization is concerned with the identification of the unconscious, and usually negative, dynamics within human services that contribute to the devaluation and oppression of certain groups of people in a society, and with providing conscious strategies for remediating the devalued social status of such people. Furthermore, such normalization-based service evaluation instruments as Program Analysis of Service Systems (PASS) and especially Program Analysis of Service Systems Implementation of Normalization Goals (PASSING) have been deliberately structured so as to reward consciousness of human service issues on the part of human service personnel.

Thus, a human service for devalued people must do everything within its power to break the negative roles into which its devalued clients have been cast, and to establish such clients in as many positive social roles as possible.

Table 16.1 Implications of the two major goals of the normalization principle on three levels of social organization.

Levels of action	Major action goals	
	Enhancement of personal competencies	Enhancement of social images
The Individual	Eliciting, shaping, and maintaining useful bodily, mental, and social competencies in persons by means of direct physical and social interactions with them	Presenting, managing, addressing, labeling, and interpreting persons in a manner that creates positive roles for them and that emphasizes their similarities to, rather than their differences from, other (valued) persons
Primary and Secondary Social Systems	Eliciting, shaping, and maintaining useful bodily, mental, and social competencies in persons by adaptive shaping of such primary and secondary social systems as family, classroom, school, work setting, service agency, and neighborhood	Presenting, managing, labeling, and interpreting the primary and secondary social systems that surround a person or that consist of persons at risk so that these systems, as well as the persons in them, are perceived in a valued-fashion
Societal Systems	Eliciting, shaping, and maintaining useful bodily, mental, and social competencies in persons by appropriate shaping of such societal systems and structures as entire school systems, laws, and government	Shaping cultural values, attitudes, and stereotypes so as to elicit maximum feasible acceptance of individual differences

Conservatism

Many people have negatively valued characteristics, but these are usually so few or minor that they do not place a person into a deviant role or hinder his or her functioning. Unlike other citizens, however, devalued people exist in a state of heightened vulnerability to further devaluations and negative experiences.

[...]

The conservatism corollary of normalization posits that the greater the number, severity, and/or variety of deviancies or stigmata of an individual *or* the greater the number of deviant people there are in a group or setting, the greater the impact of (1) the reduction of one or a few of the individual stigmata, (2) the reduction of the number of deviant people in the group, or (3) the balancing off (compensation) of the stigmata or deviancies by the presence or addition of positively valued manifestations. [...]

It is not enough for a human service to be merely neutral in either diminishing or enhancing the status of devalued persons in the eyes of others; it must seek to effect the most positive status possible for its clients. For example, on occasions where either a suit and tie or a sports jacket and sports shirt are equally appropriate attire, the man at value-risk in society would fare better wearing the suit-and-tie combination.

Societal integration

[...] Because segregation tends to make people more devalued and more dependent, society pays a high price for it in many complex and deeply hidden ways.

Normalization requires that a devalued person or group has the opportunity to be personally integrated into the valued social life of society. Devalued people would be enabled to live in normative housing within the valued community and with valued people; be educated with their non-devalued peers; work in the same facilities as other people; and be involved in a positive fashion in worship, recreation, shopping, and all the other activities in which members of a society engage.
[...]

It must be emphasized that the type of integration implied by normalization theory is very specific: personal social integration and valued social participation. 'Physical integration,' which merely consists of the physical presence of devalued people in the community, is only a potential *facilitator* of actual individual valued social participation. Also, social integration is not the same as 'mainstreaming' and 'deinstitutionalization,' which often are not truly integrative.

Additional perspectives on the normalization principle

In respect to the goal of normalization, one can say that a person is normalized if he or she has that culturally normative degree of personal autonomy and choice that society extends to its non-devalued members, has access to the valued experiences and resources of open society much as would be the case for a typical citizen, and is free to and capable of choosing and leading a life style that is accessible to at least the majority of other people of the same age. These goals are not attainable for every person, so it is important to keep in mind the qualifying phrase 'as much as possible' in the normalization definition. Normalization strategies must take into account the particular individual concerned, the limits of our current know-how, and the individual's own choice of his or her personal goals and means. Low expectations, inappropriate pessimism, stereotyping, and the like, can have a very destructive effect on the person involved. Consequently, an adaptive human management approach is to maintain a healthy skepticism when confronted with the assertion that a specific normative human service measure or interpretation is unattainable or unrealistic.

The normalization principle has sometimes been criticized as imposing cultural uniformity. In truth, it (1) promotes social tolerance and bridge building, (2) opens up an enormous range of valued options that are commonly denied to almost a third of our population, and (3) enables (not coerces) many people who have been devalued and excluded *against their will* to participate more fully. Only a few people or groups can be said to truly and deliberately choose social marginalization and devaluation of their own free will. Even when they say they do, they often do so only reactively in response to *prior* rejection by society. [...]

REFERENCE

Wolfensberger, W. The definition of normalization: Update, problems, disagreements, and misunderstandings. In R. J. Flynn and K. E. Nitsch (Eds), *Normalization, social integration, and community services*. Baltimore: University Park Press, 1980.

16.2 STIGMA AND SOCIAL IDENTITY

Erving Goffman

Source: Reprinted with the permission of Simon and Schuster, Inc., from Stigma: Notes On the Management of Spoiled Identity by Erving Goffman. Copyright © 1963 by Prentice Hall: copyright renewed 1991 by Simon & Schuster, Inc., pp. 11–15, 17–18.

The Greeks, who were apparently strong on visual aids, originated the term *stigma* to refer to bodily signs designed to expose something unusual and bad about the moral status of the signifier. The signs were cut or burnt into the body and advertised that the bearer was a slave, a criminal, or a traitor – a blemished person, ritually polluted, to be avoided, especially in public places. Later, in Christian times, two layers of metaphor were added to the term: the first referred to bodily signs of holy grace that took the form of eruptive blossoms on the skin; the second, a medical allusion to this religious allusion, referred to bodily signs of physical disorder. Today the term is widely used in something like the original literal sense, but is applied more to the disgrace itself than to the bodily evidence of it. Furthermore, shifts have occurred in the kinds of disgrace that arouse concern. Students, however, have made little effort to describe the structural preconditions of stigma, or even to provide a definition of the concept itself. It seems necessary, therefore, to try at the beginning to sketch in some very general assumptions and definitions.

Society establishes the means of categorizing persons and the complement of attributes felt to be ordinary and natural for members of each of these categories. Social settings establish the categories of persons likely to be encountered there. The routines of social intercourse in established settings allow us to deal with anticipated others without special attention or thought. When a stranger comes into our presence, then, first appearances are likely to enable us to anticipate his category and attributes, his 'social identity' – to use a term that is better than 'social status' because personal attributes such as 'honesty' are involved, as well as structural ones, like 'occupation'.

We lean on these anticipations that we have, transforming them into normative expectations, into righteously presented demands.

Typically, we do not become aware that we have made these demands or aware of what they are until an active question arises as to whether or not they will be fulfilled. It is then that we are likely to realize that all along we had been making certain assumptions as to what the individual before us ought to be. Thus, the demands we make might better be called demands made 'in effect', and the character we impute to the individual might better be seen as an imputation made in potential retrospect – a characterization 'in effect', a *virtual social identity*. The category and attributes he could in fact be proved to possess will be called his *actual social identity*.

While the stranger is present before us, evidence can arise of his possessing an attribute that makes him different from others in the category of persons available for him to be, and of a less desirable kind – in the extreme, a person who is quite thoroughly bad, or dangerous, or weak. He is thus reduced in our minds from a whole and usual person to a tainted, discounted one. Such an attribute is a stigma, especially when its discrediting effect is very extensive; sometimes it is also called a failing, a shortcoming, a handicap. It constitutes a special discrepancy between virtual and actual social identity. Note that there are other types of discrepancy between virtual and actual social identity, for example the kind that causes us to reclassify an individual from one socially anticipated category to a different but equally well-anticipated one, and the kind that causes us to alter our estimation of the individual upward. Note, too, that not all undesirable attributes are at issue, but only those which are incongruous with our stereotype of what a given type of individual should be.
[. . .]

Three grossly different types of stigma may be mentioned. First there are abominations of the body – the various physical deformities. Next there are blemishes of individual character perceived as weak will, domineering or unnatural passions, treacherous and rigid beliefs, and dishonesty, these being inferred from a known record of, for example, mental disorder, imprisonment, addiction, alcoholism, homosexuality, unemployment, suicidal attempts, and radical political behaviour. Finally there are the tribal stigma of race, nation, and religion, these being stigma that can be transmitted through lineages and equally contaminate all members of a family. In all of these various instances of stigma, however, including those the Greeks had in mind, the same sociological features are found: an individual who might have been received easily in ordinary social intercourse possesses a trait that can obtrude itself upon attention and turn those of us whom he meets away from him, breaking the claim that his other attributes have on us. He possesses a stigma, an undesired differentness from what we had anticipated. We and those who do not depart negatively from the particular expectations at issue I shall call the *normals*.

[. . .] The stigmatized individual tends to hold the same beliefs about identity that we do; this is a pivotal fact. His deepest feelings about what he is may be his sense of being a 'normal person', a human being like anyone else, a person, therefore, who deserves a fair chance and a fair break. (Actually, however phrased, he bases his claims not on what he thinks is due *everyone*, but only everyone of a selected social category into which he unquestionably fits, for example, anyone of his age, sex, profession, and so forth.) Yet he may perceive, usually quite correctly, that whatever others profess, they do not really 'accept' him and are not ready to make contact with him on 'equal grounds'. Further, the standards he has incorporated from the wider society equip him to be intimately alive to what others see as his failing, inevitably causing him, if only for moments, to agree that he does indeed fall short of what he really ought to be. Shame becomes a central possibility, arising from the individual's perception of one of his own attributes as being a defiling thing to possess, and one he can readily see himself as not possessing.

[. . .]

16.3 LIBERATION AND SCHIZOPHRENIA

David Cooper

Source: *The Dialectics of Liberation*, Penguin, Harmondsworth, 1968, pp. 7–8.

The Congress on the Dialectics of Liberation was held in London at the Roundhouse in Chalk Farm from 15 July to 30 July 1967. . . . I would like to outline . . . how the Congress came about and in particular why we, the organizers, arranged this meeting between these particular people, why we generated this curious pastiche of eminent scholars and political activists.

The organizing group consisted of four psychiatrists who were very much concerned with radical innovation in their own field – to the extent of their counter-labelling their discipline as anti-psychiatry. The four were Dr R.D. Laing and myself, also Dr Joseph Berke and Dr Leon Redler. Our experience originated in studies into that predominant form of socially stigmatized madness that is called schizophrenia. Most people who are called mad and who are socially victimized by virtue of that attribution (by being 'put away', being subjected to electric shocks, tranquillizing drugs, and brain-slicing operations, and so on) come from family situations in which there is a desperate need to find some scapegoat, someone who will consent at a certain point of intensity in the whole transaction of the family group to take on the disturbance of each of the others and, in some sense, suffer for them. In this way the scapegoated person would become a diseased object in the family system and the family system would involve medical accomplices in its machinations. The doctors would be used to attach the label 'schizophrenia' to the diseased object and then systematically set about the destruction of that object by the physical and social processes that are termed 'psychiatric treatment'.

16.4 CRITICAL PSYCHIATRY

Phil Thomas and Joanna Moncrieff

Source: http://www.critpsynet.freeuk.com

New Labour's 'new' look at mental health policy has some nasty surprises for those who believed that 1 May 1997 heralded a new dawn of tolerance, understanding and social inclusion for those suffering from mental health problems. The government is proposing changes that have serious implications for the human rights of people who use psychiatric services. Although the National Service Frameworks contain positive developments like home treatment, the government's priority appears to be increasing coercion and control for those using mental health services. The Green Paper reforming the 1983 Mental Health Act includes proposals for compulsory treatment in the community, and is accompanied by a Joint Home Office and Department of Health initiative on the management of people with so-called dangerously severe personality disorders (DSPD). If enacted, this would enable psychiatrists to detain such people indefinitely, even though they had committed no offence. We would be the only democracy in the world in which you could be locked up for life without having committed an offence. Compulsory treatment in the community and reviewable detention represent serious challenges to human rights, and this has fuelled concern inside the profession. In January 1999 the Critical Psychiatry Network first met in Bradford to discuss these concerns, and has since made clear its opposition to compulsory treatment in the community and reviewable detention for people with DSPD. To understand critical psychiatry we must consider the recent context in which medicine and psychiatry have been practised.

[. . .] Psychiatry has always been deeply split between care and healing on the one hand, and coercion and social control on the other. Government legislation, in shifting the balance away from care towards control, is making this split even clearer. No other medical speciality has the equivalent of the psychiatric survivors' movement, confirmation of the coercive nature of psychiatry.

Critical psychiatry is part academic, part practical. Theoretically it is influenced by critical philosophical and political theories, and it has three elements. It challenges the dominance of clinical neuroscience in psychiatry (but does not exclude it); it introduces a strong ethical perspective on psychiatric knowledge and practice; it politicizes mental health issues. Critical psychiatry is deeply sceptical about the reductionist claims of neuroscience to explain psychosis and other forms of emotional distress. It follows that we are sceptical about the claims of the pharmaceutical industry for the role of psychotropic drugs in the 'treatment' of psychiatric conditions. Like other psychiatrists we use drugs, but we see them as having a minor role in the resolution of psychosis or depression. We attach greater importance to dealing with social factors, such as unemployment, bad housing, poverty, stigma and social isolation. Most people who use psychiatric services regard these factors as more important than drugs. We reject the medical model in psychiatry and prefer a social model, which we find more appropriate in a multicultural society characterized by deep inequalities.

The practice of critical psychiatry has important ethical implications. It is often difficult to work in the biomedical model in a way that really respects and engages with the patient's beliefs and preferences. What point is there in respecting the patient's view if you believe that the main objective is to rectify a neurochemical imbalance in someone's brain? The social model, on the other hand, recognizes that the meaning of distress is culturally contingent, and so engaging with the person's belief systems and values is of paramount importance. This can only be achieved by listening carefully and respecting the person's beliefs. Critical psychiatry also brings a political perspective on mental health issues. The biomedical model locates distress in the disordered function of the individual's mind/brain, which relegates social contexts to a secondary role. This is problematic because it completely overlooks the role of poverty and social exclusion in psychosis. One of critical psychiatry's most important tasks is the creation of a new dialogue between survivors, mental health service users and psychiatrists, a dialogue that recognizes the value of different types of expertise. Psychiatrists are experts by profession, but service users are experts by experience. The best outcomes will only be achieved when these two types of expertise can work in alliance, something that critical psychiatry argues must happen now. The government already recognizes the importance of alliance between patient experts and health professionals in the area of chronic physical illness, by establishing an Expert Patients' Task Force to consider how professionals can work in partnership with expert patients. We believe that this model must be applied to the field of mental health, and we hope the government will not waste an excellent opportunity to act on this.

16.5 THE SANATORIUM AT VIRGINIA WATER

Bill Bryson

Source: *Notes from a Small Island*, Doubleday, London, 1995, pp. 80–4.

Virginia Water is an interesting place. It was built mostly in the Twenties and Thirties with two small parades of shops and, surrounding them, a dense network of private roads winding through and around the famous Wentworth Golf Course. Scattered among the trees are rambling houses, often occupied by celebrities [... and] when I first saw it, [it felt] rather like walking into the pages of a 1937 *House and Garden*.

But what lent Virginia Water a particular charm back then, and I mean this quite seriously, was that it was full of wandering lunatics. Because most of the patients had been resident at the sanatorium for years, and often decades, no matter how addled their thoughts or hesitant their gait, no matter how much they mumbled and muttered, adopted sudden postures of submission or demonstrated any of a hundred other indications of someone comfortably out to lunch, most of them could be trusted to wander down to the village and find their way back again. Each day you could count on finding a refreshing sprinkling of lunatics buying fags or sweets, having a cup of tea or just quietly remonstrating with thin air. The result was one of the most extraordinary communities in England, one in which wealthy people and lunatics mingled on equal terms. The shopkeepers and locals were quite wonderful about it, and didn't act as if anything was odd because a man with wild hair wearing a pyjama jacket was standing in a corner of the baker's declaiming to a spot on the wall or sitting at a corner table of the Tudor Rose with swivelling eyes and the makings of a smile, dropping sugar cubes into his minestrone. It was, and I'm still serious, a thoroughly heart warming sight.

Among the five hundred or so patients at the sanatorium was a remarkable idiot savant named Harry. Harry had the mind of a small, preoccupied child, but you could name any date, present or future, and he would instantly tell you what day of the week it was. We used to test him with a perpetual calendar and he was never wrong. You could ask him the date of the third Saturday of December 1935 or the second Wednesday of July 2017 and he would tell you faster than any computer could. Even more extraordinary, though it merely seemed tiresome at the time, was that several times a day he would approach members of the staff and ask them in a strange, bleating voice if the hospital was going to close in 1980. According to his copious medical notes, he had been obsessed with this question since his arrival as a young man in about 1950. The thing is, Holloway was a big, important institution, and there were never any plans to close it. Indeed there were none right up until the stormy night in early 1980 when Harry was put to bed in a state of uncharacteristic agitation – he had been asking his question with increasing persistence for several weeks – and a bolt of lightning struck a back gable, causing a devastating fire that swept through the attics and several of the wards, rendering the entire structure suddenly uninhabitable.

It would make an even better story if poor Harry had been strapped to his bed and perished in the blaze. Unfortunately for purposes of exciting narrative all the patients were safely evacuated into the stormy night, though I like to imagine Harry with his lips contorted in a rapturous smile as he stood on the lawn, a blanket round his shoulders, his face lit by dancing flames, and watched the conflagration that he had so patiently awaited for thirty years.

The inmates were transferred to a special wing of a general hospital down the road at Chertsey, where they were soon deprived of their liberty on account of their unfortunate inclination to cause havoc in the wards and alarm the sane. In the meantime, the sanatorium had quietly mouldered away, its windows boarded or broken, its grand entrance from Stroude Road blocked by a heavy-duty metal gate topped with razor wire. I lived in Virginia Water for five years in the early Eighties when I was working in London and occasionally stopped to peer over the wall at the neglected grounds and general desolation. [. . .] For well over a decade this fine old hospital, probably one of the dozen finest Victorian structures still standing, had just sat, crumbling and forlorn, and I had expected it to be much the same – indeed, was rehearsing an obsequious request to the watchman to be allowed to go up the drive for a quick peek since the building itself couldn't much be seen from the road.

So imagine my surprise when I crested a gentle slope and found a spanking new entrance knocked into the perimeter wall, a big sign welcoming me to Virginia Park and, flanking a previously unknown vista of a sanatorium building, a generous clutch of smart new executive homes behind. With mouth agape, I stumbled up a freshly asphalted road lined with houses so new that there were still stickers on the windows and the yards were seas of mud. One of the houses had been done up as a show home and, as it was a Sunday, it was busy with people having a look. Inside, I found a glossy brochure full of architects' drawings of happy, slender people strolling around among handsome houses, listening to a chamber orchestra in the room where I formerly watched movies in the company of twitching lunatics, or swimming in an indoor pool sunk into the floor of the great Gothic hall where I had once played badminton and falteringly asked the young nurse from Florence Nightingale for a date, with a distant view, if she could possibly spare the time, of marrying me. According to the rather sumptuous accompanying prose, residents of Virginia Park could choose between several dozen detached executive homes, a scattering of townhouses and flats, or one of twenty-three grand apartments carved out of the restored sani, now mysteriously renamed Crosland House. The map of the site was dotted with strange names – Connolly Mews, Chapel Square, The Piazza – that owed little to its previous existence. How much more appropriate, I thought, if they had given them names like Lobotomy Square and Electro-convulsive Court. Prices started at £350,000.

I went back outside to see what I could get for my £350,000. The answer was a smallish but ornate home on a modest plot with an interesting view of a nineteenth-century mental hospital. I can't say that it was what I had always dreamed of. All the houses were built of red brick, with old-fashioned chimney pots, gingerbread trim and other small nods to the Victorian age. One model, rather mundanely known as House Type D, even had a decorative tower. The result was that they looked as if they had somehow been pupped by the sanatorium. You could almost imagine them, given sufficient time, growing into sanitoria themselves. Insofar as such a thing can work at all, it worked surprisingly well. The new houses didn't jar against the backdrop of the sanatorium and at least – something that surely wouldn't have happened a dozen years ago – that great old heap of a building, with all its happy memories for me and generations of the interestingly insane, had been saved. I doffed my hat to the developers and took my leave.

AGEING, LEARNING DIFFICULTIES AND MAINTAINING INDEPENDENCE

Alan Walker and Carol Walker

The application of normalisation to service provision has been criticised for neglecting gender, class and race (Brown and Smith 1992). The same criticism may be levelled with regard to age, though it has not been hitherto. Although normalisation hinges on the position of the individual, its operationalisation through the medium of service delivery inevitably concentrates attention on group needs, interests and expectations and, if it is inappropriately applied, this can lead to group stereotyping. Thus normalisation may force people with learning difficulties into narrowly defined patterns of conformity which do not reflect their individuality (Dalley 1992).

It is reasonable to ask what is 'normal' for any particular group in society. Is what is regarded as 'normal' or widely accepted as such, a desirable optimum or the result of historical development or just a matter of resource constraints? What is 'normal' is not necessarily ideal or even appropriate. This sort of dilemma is familiar to social gerontologists who have, for example, questioned the official denial of poverty (Walker 1980) or disability (Townsend 1981) in old age on the grounds that these are 'normal' features of ageing. Our research has revealed that care workers treat older people with learning difficulties differently to younger people and have different expectations of their abilities and appropriate lifestyles (Walker *et al.* 1993). This has important implications for the nature of the support or care that is provided and, in particular, whether the care of older people with learning difficulties is structured on the expectation of dependence rather than the goals of increasing independence or inter-dependence.

One of the major criticisms made of normalisation, particularly from within the liberation movement of disabled people, is that rather than demanding that wider society unconditionally accepts and integrates those members who are in any respects 'different', it requires the individual to adapt to the norms of society, to 'compete in the world of the able-bodied and the able-minded' (Walmsley 1991, p. 227). Furthermore, it is assumed that 'the values and norms of behaviour and appearance in society are worth striving for' (Hattersley 1991, p. 3). Lawson (1991), as a user of mental health services, shares the doubts of other critics of normalisation (Chappell 1994) when its attainment implies 'conformity to an unjust world', and questions its usefulness when the predominant value system itself is unacceptable. [. . .]

All of these criticisms have particular resonance if they are applied to the situation of older people with learning difficulties. The ageing of the learning disabled population has important implications for the concept of normalisation, which is based on the premise that people with learning dif-ficulties should share similar life experiences to their peers in the wider community. However, the limitations of the normalisation concept are clearly demonstrated with regard to older people with learning difficulties because the experiences of their reference group – in this case older people – are themselves often limited and restricted by society's attitudes. Thus, the goals set for older people with learning difficulties and the service responses offered to them will, in turn, be restricted by the socially con-structed stereotype of old age as a period of dependency (Walker 1980).

Care or support?

We can illustrate the practical implications of this from findings of our study of older people with learning difficulties living in the community. Those in formal care usually lived in small-scale, shared, supported housing, the most popular model of community care currently being adopted in Britain for this group. Our research found that, in many important respects, a bifurcation was occurring in the treatment of older and younger people within service provision for people with learning dif-ficulties, similar to that which exists between older people and learning disability services.

People with learning difficulties are not a homogeneous group. They vary widely in their levels of physical and developmental abilities and disabilities. The problems they face in their everyday lives are compounded by the stigma that they have suffered and, for large numbers, by their enforced social exclusion from the wider community. The kind of help and assistance which people with learning difficulties require therefore varies widely. Some people with learning difficulties need care, i.e. the need for others to undertake tasks on their behalf, including personal care needs or cooking and preparation for meals (Qureshi and Walker 1989). In this sense care is something done *to* the recipient both in terms of 'tending' with physical needs and, especially but not only by informal carers, with emotional needs. Other people with learning difficulties may not need assistance with physical tasks, but either because of their level of competence or because of restricted opportunities in the past, may require only support, i.e. the help of others to assist them to do things for themselves. This may involve helping them to gain confidence and then giving them the opportunity to do things for themselves, from routine self-care or household tasks, to making decisions and participating in activities in the community. Support, in this sense, should be a process of empowerment.

If individuals are to achieve the highest level of independence and integration possible, maintaining the correct balance between care and support is crucial. Insufficient care can undermine the individual's quality of life and can restrict activities for which he or she needs only support. Care when given unnecessarily can create dependency (Walker 1981, 1982). If insufficient or inappropriate support is available then the individual will not be able to obtain and/or maintain control over important aspects of daily living. Conversely, too much or the wrong type of support may limit the individual's self-determination by being over-protective, thus fostering dependence rather than independence.

We found that service providers tended to concentrate on the need to *care* for older people and, therefore, to over-state their levels of dependency, rather than to support them in independent living as they did with younger people. Care workers frequently espoused a view of older people that was remarkably similar to Cumming and Henry's (1961) disengagement thesis which portrayed old age as a period of mutual disengagement between the individual and society. For example, many care workers assumed that because older people in general tended to lead more sedentary lives, to go out less than younger people, and to have fewer friends, they needed to expend less effort in developing activities and fostering the social integration of this section of the learning disabled population. This age discriminatory assumption became, thereby, a self-fulfilling prophecy.

The assumption of dependence among older people

Care staff felt that it was less important to help older people to develop new skills or to try to maintain existing skills than was the case for younger people. For example, 30 per cent of care workers of the older group in our study did not think that providing or organising personal skills training was an important part of their job; no-one working with the younger group held this view. Consequently, only three out of ten people aged sixty or over were currently receiving any personal skills training or had received any in the previous twelve months, compared to eight out of ten of those under sixty. Care workers of the older group were half as likely to think that the person with learning difficulty they were working with was capable of learning a new skill – even though, as discussed earlier, overall, this group was more able than the younger group.

[. . .] In the care workers' own words:

> *He's growing old gracefully. We can't be so hard now, he can relax. (It's) easier with younger (people, they're) not as set in their ways. Anthea's old keyworker would say she shouldn't be set goals because she is too old. I don't agree. I think everybody should have the chance. I'm hoping that he will become more independent but I'm worried that because of his age he may not.*

And the familiar stereotype:

> *Younger people need new things. They need to get out more. Older people are more content.*

[. . .]

If people are over-protected then increasing dependence is inevitable, so it is not surprising that care workers were less likely to report that people over fifty had become more competent in recent years. In examining this finding it is difficult to disentangle how far this difference can be explained by the ability levels of the service users or by the lower expectations of care workers and the reduced opportunities consequently given to the older group, both of which were illustrated in comments from the care workers:

> *I feel that younger people should learn more, whereas older people may not need training.*

> *There aren't so many options for older people. There are less activities for someone who is old and disabled.*

[. . .]

This age discriminatory assumption by service providers of decline and increasing dependency has implications for the continued presence of older people with learning difficulties in the community. In our work we have found that residential care is now considered as an appropriate option for an older person with learning difficulties where it would definitely *not* be deemed so for younger people (Walker *et al.* 1996a). One district social care purchaser in the North West reported that although special permission had to be sought from the Regional Health Authority to resettle people from hospital (though not from a community setting) to a residential care home (contrary to regional policy guidelines), it was now generally accepted that nursing home provision could be used.

> *There is a small number of people who are going into nursing home settings ... (They) tend to be very elderly, who if they were in the main population ... would be accommodated in that type of resource.*

The danger with this view is that, as resources are squeezed increasingly, residential homes will be seen as a less expensive alternative to providing the enhanced support necessary to enable someone to stay in their own home – just as they are for the wider population of older people. In both cases community care is not a cheap option if it is to genuinely improve the quality of life of both those in need of care and their families.

[. . .]

The older people with learning difficulties in our study benefited less from services provided for and used by people with learning difficulties generally. However, few had much contact with services for older people either. This is partly explained by their age. As a result of severe resource constraints these services now tend to cater for the very elderly and, consequently, the younger elderly, fifty to seventy-year-olds, are often deemed too young or not frail enough for such services. However, there is also a reluctance on the part of the older person's service sector to take on people with learning difficulties. As a result they fall between the two services – a clear case of double jeopardy.

> *I think they are a bit patronised ... They are people with learning disabilities first rather than older people. Therefore, if you try to get them into an old people's service the learning disability precludes them. Community care and day centres provided for the elderly don't cater for those with learning difficulties – they are expected to muck in.*

> *...she's too old to go to a day centre but at the over 60s club they don't want her because of her disability. Nothing there for them. You get the normal older people centres but they don't welcome people with learning difficulties ... (and) the Gateway Clubs, for instance, are not appropriate for older people.*

[. . .]

The limits of normalisation

There has been very considerable progress over the past thirty years in ideas and policies towards the care and support given to people with learning difficulties. This has been influenced positively by the debate on normalisation which has stressed the importance of enabling this group to live ordinary lives within communities and to be involved in the decisions which affect them. The practical application of this philosophy to service provision for older people with learning difficulties reveals both some of the limitations of the philosophy itself, and the dilemmas which result from the very different traditions underpinning services for people with learning difficulties and those for older people.

One of the main problems with the philosophy itself is that 'normal' provision itself may not be adequate or appropriate. Policy makers and service providers have been slow to respond to the specific needs of some groups, such as ethnic minorities. Or, as with older groups, they have created or enhanced dependency among older people by not providing sufficient or appropriate support to enable them to maintain independent lives in their own homes. This is particularly significant for people with learning difficulties as they get older, because, in contrast to services for older people, learning disability services over recent years have concentrated not on the containment and care of this group, but on supporting them towards a realisation of greater choice and independence. Thus, the ageist assumptions and stereotypes that are built into the traditional pattern of care offered to older people mean that people with learning difficulties face much more restrictive, and possibly segregated, lives when they get older.

The research findings show that many of these stereotypes are now creeping into learning disability services. In other words there is a failure to learn lessons from gerontology about the adverse impact of age stereotypes on the quality of older people's lives. Age itself was often used by service providers as an explanation for older people not leading more active lives or being trained to do more themselves – despite the fact that, as a whole, the older people in our sample had a wider range of competencies than their younger peers. Perhaps most indicative of the insidious effect of age stereotyping was the fact that reinstitutionalisation into older persons' homes was accepted as a viable option, although similar residential type settings definitely would not even be considered for younger people. Activities outside the home and social networks were deemed to be less important for older people because this was associated by formal carers with the natural process of ageing. To the extent that older people are inactive and are socially isolated, it is clear that this is usually not a result of choice but is one of the aspects of their lives that they would most wish to change.

[...]

Despite the professional definitions of normality implicit within them [. . .], goals of normalisation appear very positive compared to the tradition of service provision for older people which, as outlined above, has been based on a model of growing dependence rather than independence. Notwithstanding the valid criticisms made of normalisation, its application to services for the wider population of older people could have as dramatic an impact on services for them as it has had on the development of learning disability services in the last two decades and, moreover, its implementation could serve to confront the now dominant age discriminatory construction of services and attitudes towards older people. [. . .]

REFERENCES

Brown, H. and Smith, H. (1992) *Normalisation: a reader for the nineties* (London, Tavistock/Routledge).

Chappell, A.L. (1994) A question of friendship: community care and the relationships of people with learning difficulties, *Disability, Handicap and Society*, 9, 419–434.

Cumming, E. and Henry, W. (1961) *Growing Old: the process of disengagement* (New York, Basic Books).

Dalley, G. (1992) Social welfare ideologies and normalisation: links and conflicts, in H. Brown and H. Smith (eds) *Normalisation: a reader for the nineties*, pp. 100–111 (London: Tavistock/Routledge).

Hattersley, J. (1991) The future of normalisation, in S. Baldwin and J. Hattersley (eds), *Mental Handicap: social science perspectives* (London: Tavistock/Routledge).

Lawson, M. (1991) A recipient's view, in S. Ramon (ed.), *Beyond Community Care: normalisation and integration work* (Basingstoke, Macmillan/MIND).

Qureshi, H. and Walker, A. (1989) *The Caring Relationship* (London, Macmillan).

Townsend, P. (1981) Elderly people with disabilities, in A. Walker and P. Townsend (eds), *Disability in Britain*, pp. 91–118 (Oxford, Martin Robertson).

Walker, A. (1980) The social creation of poverty and dependency in old age, *Journal of Social Policy*, 9, 49–75.

Walker, A. (1981) Community care and the elderly in Great Britain: theory and practice, *International Journal of Health Services*, II, 541–557.

Walker, A. (1982) Dependency and old age, *Social Policy and Administration*, 16, 116–137.

Walker, C., Ryan, T. and Walker, A. (1993) *Quality of Life after Resettlement for People with Learning Difficulties* (Manchester, North Western Regional Health Authority).

Walker, A., Walker, C. and Ryan, T. (1996a) Older people with learning difficulties leaving institutional care – a case of double jeopardy, *Ageing and Society*, 16, 1–26.

Walmsley, J. (1991) 'Talking to Top People': some issues relating to the citizenship of people with learning difficulties, *Disability, Handicap and Society*, 6, 219–232.

CHAPTER 18

WHITENESS AND EMOTIONS IN SOCIAL CARE

Yasmin Gunaratnam

Race equality received increased attention in the health and social care fields at the turn of the century, particularly following the Stephen Lawrence Inquiry Report (Macpherson 1999). Within social care, strategic policy and service development initiatives have highlighted institutional structures and practices that need to be changed both in mainstreaming and achieving race equality in service provision and in 'workforce development'.

In this chapter I argue that these formal developments are based upon a somewhat partial, abstract and rationalist understanding of race equality that is far removed from the complex, difficult and emotional aspects of day-to-day work in social care. Policies on race equality perform the vital function of defining a framework within which the concepts, meanings, knowledge and skills relating to race equality can be made explicit. They have, however, neglected to address the complex ways in which power relations can produce, and be produced by, the tiny detail of 'everyday' practices, identifications and interactions. As Ann Phoenix has pointed out there is value to be gained in analysis of issues at the microsocial level, since:

> [...] it is generally easier to see how policy definitions construct not only specific ways of understanding social problems, but also their associated subject positions and solutions. In doing so, those policies frequently claim to be addressing the needs of particular subjects while taking little account of the subjects' constructions of self and their social positioning.
>
> (Phoenix 2000: 95)

Although this is certainly true for race equality policies, I will argue that there has also been insufficient recognition given to the subjectivity and experiences of workers who have ultimate responsibility for translating policy intentions into 'reality' (Gunaratnam *et al.* 1998). In fact there are a number of contradictions in approaches to 'race' that serve to position staff in different ways according to which differences are being addressed and how. For example, attention has been given to monitoring characteristics of the social care workforce in terms of gender, age, ethnicity, community identity and illness and disability (Balloch *et al.* 1999). Yet, we know little about how these factors shape and are shaped by the ways in which staff see, feel about, and position themselves, their work and their relationships with colleagues, service users and carers.

More specifically, black and 'minority ethnic' staff have been the focus of particular attention. Human resource strategies have aimed to increase the numbers of minoritised staff recruited to and promoted within the workforce (Alexander 1999). In addition, the cultural knowledge and/or language skills that they are seen as possessing have been valued by service managers in the delivery of multicultural services (Lewis 2000). Yet, what is most striking in current policy and service developments on race equality is that few attempts have been made to examine qualitatively the ways in which white workers contribute towards the construction of 'racialised' practices in social care. By racialisation, I am referring to a dynamic process that both generates and is produced by its reliance upon (either explicitly or implicitly) biological or cultural categorisations of difference.

This chapter will address this gap, by using data generated in group discussions with white hospice social workers.[1] I will focus upon the value for both policy and service development of addressing, and engaging with, the social, occupational and subjective experiences of white social care workers not only in working with issues of racialised difference, but also in how they give meaning to 'being white'. In the last decade or so there has been increased attention given to the analysis of 'whiteness' as an essential part of the study of 'race', ethnicity and difference (Frankenberg 1993; Roediger 1990; Ware 1992). This work has begun to make explicit the ways in which 'whiteness' is a part of everyday practices and discourses, yet is also naturalised as 'non-racial'. Rather than understanding whiteness as a biological category, it has been seen as a social construction that has different histories accompanied by different forms of maintenance and resistance.

By drawing upon key concepts from this work, I aim to show how an interrogation of the links between professional identifications and whiteness can deepen our understanding of the challenges of race equality in the sector.

Uneasy representations

The data upon which this chapter is based were generated during five group discussions over a twelve month period with essentially the same group of white, female hospice social workers. The first group consisted of four women and the remaining groups were held with three of the women. Unlike one-off group interviews, the longitudinal nature of this part of the study meant that trust and rapport were built up over time. I believe that this had a significant impact in reducing levels of threat in discussions as they might have been constituted by both my identity as an interviewer of colour and the discussion of matters of 'race' and difference. Unlike other researchers (Lewis and Ramazanoglu 1999), I did not find that the women always distanced themselves from racist practices and identifications through the use of impersonal accounts. Rather, I see these women as being 'race cognizant' (Frankenberg 1993), in so far as they acknowledged race differences and power relations whilst also often making visible their own whiteness. This positioning was not, of course, stable and I have tried to chart the complex ways in which they grappled and negotiated with varying levels of awareness and experience within the discussions.

It is also important to point out that the analysis and representation of the data from these discussions raises ethical issues. As Lewis and Ramazanoglu have pointed out, there are potential political tensions in any research on racialised power relations, particularly the 'political tensions between both respecting people's accounts of their identities, and also identifying white privilege as unmerited' (1999: 29). In re-presenting the accounts in the following sections, my aim is not to make moral evaluations about the individual women, but rather to examine how they, as white, female social workers, produce, manage and negotiate the interrelations between their whiteness and their professional identities, and the implications of this for race equality in social care.

Culturally competent practitioners

In the group discussions, issues relating to 'cultural competence' were a recurring theme, serving to draw attention to the 'dilemmas' of intercultural work.

Alexander (1999) has highlighted cultural competence as an area of practice that is of 'strategic importance' in the achievement of race equality in health and social care. In a report commissioned by the Department of Health into race equality across 'all aspects of its work', cultural competence was defined as denoting 'a set of skills and knowledge that have at their base the acceptance of the legitimate values, beliefs and behaviour patterns of people who are from another ethnic group' (Alexander 1999: 21). The emphasis upon the unproblematic 'acceptance' of the values, beliefs and behaviours of people from different ethnic groups informs practitioners in very broad terms of what approach they should take. However, without acknowledging any of the complexities or difficulties of inter-cultural work, this definition is both too 'neat' and too abstract to be of real value in everyday practice. Little recognition is given to the dynamic and often contradictory nature of cultural systems, categorisations and identifications and how these might relate to professional values and practices. Diversity within ethnic groups is also obscured (Pinkney 2000; Williams 1999).

The social workers talked about these issues primarily in terms of the pressures of 'getting it right' and 'getting it wrong'. They were concerned about their ability to 'read' and respond to what were seen as specific 'cultural' needs. They also expressed difficulties in addressing and evaluating differences of perspective between carers and service users. In the following extract, 'Jo' describes some of the difficulties that she encountered in responding to what she constructs as differences between individual choice and cultural prescription. In this particular case there were differences in opinion between an Ethiopian service user and his friends about what should happen to his body after death.

JO: I really struggled with what to do about that, er, because I found that I didn't know the cultural prescriptions or the religious prescriptions which he had been brought up . . . and I felt . . .

JANE: Quite sort of . . . hesitant . . . and not clear about how to work?

JO: Yes . . . who should I listen to? and (was) unclear about, and conflicted about the, you know, individual patient choice versus cultural prescriptions or religious prescriptions and I would always go with patient choice, but I mean, it was partly difficult because sometimes he wasn't conscious to say it. But also feeling . . . that it was quite hard to disagree with these people (the friends) who perceived themselves as being extremely helpful and knowing something that I didn't know . . . I mean I didn't know about their cultural issues . . .

Drawing upon notions of cultural competence, Jo cites her own ignorance of Ethiopian cultural and religious customs as shaping her personal 'struggle' with the case. This ignorance is represented as dulling and confusing her professional judgement, distancing her from the frames of reference of the service user, whilst also lending authority to the opinions of the young man's friends. The implication within the narrative is that knowledge of Ethiopian culture would have lessened the intensity of Jo's dilemma. We also get a sense that Jo's 'usual' practice ('I always go with personal choice') is undermined through encounters with racialised difference. Moreover, both white and professional authority to interpret, arbitrate and then define the legitimacy and extents of need, remain unchallenged: neither Jo nor Jane doubted that Jo had 'work' to do.

However, in exploring this issue with her further, it became apparent that cultural knowledge was not as central to the dilemma as first suggested. Indeed, as Jo continued, the emphasis upon her lack of cultural knowledge moved into a more complex commentary. This problematised and situated her commitment to 'individual rights' within constructions of whiteness, Western cultural contexts and within the social work tradition.

YASMIN: . . .I was just interested . . . in what you were saying in terms of the conflict between individual choice and then cultural prescription and, or religious prescription, and how do you deal with that in terms of white families?

JO: Again you go with individual choice.

YASMIN: Right. . .

JO: But that again, that's my cultural heritage to go with individual choice. But that's where I am and that's how it is for me and I guess I accept that that's how it is for me and I'm not going to (. . .) be, I'm not going to be different to how I am, though (. . .), but I am very aware that that is a particular view that we have . . . But you see, again that, it's, it's difficult, only because that is my, our, you know what's important is individual choice, and I think that's very much a social work tradition.

The implication is that issues of individual choice are less problematic in work with white (non-migrant) service users because of Jo's 'cultural competence' and professional and racialised identities as a white (non-migrant) social worker. Here the tensions between identity as constituted through the individual and through cultural collectivities are recast along lines of 'race'. Through this positioning white people can be addressed as individuals, whereas people racialised as 'minorities' are seen primarily as cultural beings, with group identity overwhelming the possibility of any individuality or agency (Joppke 1996). This way of reading and responding to cultural difference can thus reinforce and make natural racialised systems of dominance ('I'm not going to be different to how I am'), whilst also making these systems seem inevitable and unchangeable.

At a broader level, it can also be seen how the rhetoric of cultural competence can serve to inhibit or restrict the practice of white staff (Gunaratnam 1997) through the production of racialised barriers of 'experience'. To quote Gail Lewis, exclusions can be set up through the categories of 'sameness' and 'otherness' so that:

There are fixed 'black' and 'white' experiences, understandings and perceptions of 'self', and no room is allowed for the possibility of shared understandings, correspondences of experience or fluidity of identity across group boundaries, nor indeed of heterogeneity within groups.
(Lewis 2000: 127)

There were occasions, however, where the women talked about being able to 'cross' such racialised boundaries. One of the ways in which they did this was by using gendered identifications to produce commonalities of experience or need. In a broadly similar account to Jo's, Anna talked about difficulties that arose with an African woman who wanted her body to remain in the UK after her death, so that the money could be used to support her children:

ANNA: But the culture says that her body must go back and so there's a huge wrangle going on within the family now, and the men will win because the men in the family always get their say. Um, but I was thinking how it touches me as a worker ... And I was thinking that's often a conflict ... you know, is it that I only respect ... other cultures' attitudes so ... long as it doesn't impinge on my own values? Which are that, you know, that the kids are more important and they should benefit...

What is significant in this example is that gender identifications are used to mediate the construction of racialised and culturalised differences in a way in which connections are also made with professional values. Most significantly, in doing so, Anna does not use the gendered identifications to evade completely racialised difference. Rather, the links are problematised in that the simultaneous strain between closeness and distance in Anna's identifications is used to highlight and question the conditional nature of her 'respect' for cultural differences.

Emotions and inter-cultural practice

While dilemmas about how to conceptualise and place 'cultural' experiences can serve to create dilemmas for inter-cultural practice, it is also the case that such dilemmas are produced through emotions. The group discussions with the social workers all produced accounts in which the emotional components of inter-cultural and anti-oppressive practice were often described and deliberated about.

It would be overly simplistic to argue that emotions have been completely excluded from discussions and initiatives on race equality, since they formed a critical part of Race Awareness Training in the 1980s. However, I would argue that such initiatives failed to fully integrate a concern with emotions with both policy development and wider social power relations. Moreover, I would also argue that the backlash against such training (see Sivanandan 1985), led to conceptions of the 'rational actor' being reasserted in approaches to race equality in contemporary social care. Indeed, the mounting critique of the dominance of such conceptions (Hoggett 2000; Twigg 2000) has led to calls that:

> *social policy needs a subject in which mind and body, reason and*
> *passion, self and other, agent and object are held simultaneously in*
> *mind without splitting one from the other.*
>
> *(Hoggett 2000: 143)*

Attention to what has been called 'emotional labour' (Hochschild 1983; James 1989) provides such an area of analysis. Here it is possible to explore forms of subjectivity and how they might relate to racialised differences in social care. In examining representations of emotional labour in talk about inter-cultural and anti-oppressive practice, I want to concentrate upon one particular area: the management and negotiation of fear about 'race'.

A particular source of fear that the hospice social workers talked about was the fear of being racist, or being seen to be racist. As Lewis and Ramazanoglu found in their study of identifications amongst white women, fears about racism, particularly in work roles could give women a 'forced awareness' of their whiteness as it 'implicated them in responsibility for potentially racist practices' (1999: 50). Jane talked about such fears within the specific context of social work practice:

JANE: I think for me there's a sense of double jeopardy about if I'm racist, I think, because you know, professionally, I make mistakes all the time. I could have done things better. I, I shouldn't have done that, that was a mistake, and I process it and I'm not thrilled with it. I process it and OK hopefully next time it will be better, um but for me the devastation is sort of both professional and personal, you know that I as a white social worker have got it wrong, haven't got it right yet, but also I as a white person who, who carry the, you know, tradition of persecution, have, have, hurt and done it wrong. And I think for me, it's, it's that combination which happens almost uniquely I think around racism, particularly for me with black people. . . in a way that doesn't happen around anything else professionally.

In this extract, Jane makes explicit a series of links between current practices, professional and white privilege and traditions of race oppression. She ties these into fears of inflicting further 'hurt' upon people of colour. In this context, the threat of being racist is identified as being unique in its potential to 'devastate' and make vulnerable professional and personal identifications and is brought into being primarily through the presence or actions of racialised 'others'. In Jane's account, the emotional labour involved in the routine reflexive monitoring of practice is inadequate in evaluating the nature and quality of practice in 'race' work. Racism becomes 'something inescapable' (Frye 1992: 150), placing onerous burdens upon white social workers to 'get it right' and not be racist.

For Jo, these fears were also more than personal:

JO: I don't actually think it is just a literal fear of being accused of being racist, I actually think it is a fear of triggering the rage and fury … about white people's history of treatment of black people … I don't know, how much… does that immobilise us? Does that stop … me taking risks with families?

Here, accusations of racism, while painful personally, are seen as less threatening than the 'triggering' of the historically built-up 'rage and fury' that can be embodied in racialised others. A sense of vulnerability but also vigilance is constructed in whiteness, a sense that is justified implicitly by the simultaneous positioning of 'black people' as dangerous and volatile. What is particularly interesting is the connections that Jo makes between her management of this fear and how this might result in the inhibition of the risk-taking elements of her practice. As I have argued elsewhere (Gunaratnam *et al.* 1998), racism in service provision is not simply produced through direct and intentional actions. It can also be produced when service users do not get the best or more creative forms of practice that are often generated through professional risk-taking. In this way, emotional labour around fears of racism can intertwine with practice to produce the very inequalities that race-cognizant workers are most fearful of. The critical paradox being that race awareness can itself serve to reinforce racist systems and practices.

In exploring the emotional nature of 'race' work in social care, the contradictions of the gaps between policy and practice can become even more apparent. One such contradiction lies in the way training in social care has emphasised the need for white workers to be race aware, yet has not recognised the two main implications of such awareness. First, the encouragement of race awareness is 'troublesome' and 'troubling' for professionals, and can lead in complex ways to further inequalities in practice. For example, from the above accounts it can be seen that varying levels of 'race' consciousness can produce dilemmas, complications and restrictions for practice when links are made between whiteness, power, professional identity and racism. Second, awareness of such connections, or indeed the repression of such awareness, entails 'work' that has effects upon the performance of professional roles and the achievement of race equality objectives in service provision. At the same time this work is largely invisible within social care agencies and is not accounted for by them.

Conclusion

This chapter has examined the links between whiteness, subjectivity and emotions in 'race work' in social care, through the re-presented accounts of white, female social workers. However, it is important to recognise that such re-presentations are also framed at two further levels. First, social work theory and training has long been concerned with challenging forms of oppression (Pinkney 2000), and the need to work sensitively with ethnic diversity has been emphasised by processes of globalisation and the development of transnational perspectives in teaching and practice (Razack 1999). Second, policy developments in social care have led to the pursuit of equal opportunities and anti-racism within organisations, leading to particular public expectations of professional practice. In short, there are specific social, professional and organisational pressures upon white workers in social care to be anti-racist. Moreover, these pressures, together with the contradictions and confusions in anti-racist approaches (Gilroy 1990), have meant that, whilst there are considerable anxieties about 'race' and racism at both individual and institutional levels, many current race equality initiatives fail to fully address and engage with such anxieties or their implications. Thus, although many social care workers may be aware of the challenges and complexities that the emotional components of 'race' present in their work, the bureaucratic emphasis in the current outcome-related focus upon 'institutional racism' appears to have left little legitimate space for equally important issues of process.

Recognising and engaging with the social, occupational and subjective experiences of white workers in social care has significant implications for how we understand and approach race equality in service provision and in employment. While some progress has been made towards answering quantitative questions about the social care workforce in terms of 'who they are' and 'where they are', we know very little about the qualitative question of '*how* they *are*'. Thus whole areas of experience and practice have often remained hidden from both analytic and political attention. As this discussion has illustrated, the complex and varying ways in which whiteness is produced amongst social care workers is central to understanding and challenging different forms of racialised power and practices. If dismantling institutional racism is to be taken seriously then we cannot continue to ignore the challenges of engaging with both subjectivity and whiteness.

NOTE

1   The research that this chapter is based on was funded by the Economic and Social Research Council (R00429534133). The group discussions with social workers were part of a larger research project that included interviews with service users, group interviews with a range of hospice professionals, and forms of service observation and participant observation.

REFERENCES

Alexander, Z. (1999) *Study of Black, Asian and Ethnic Minority Issues.* London: Department of Health.

Balloch, S., McLean, J. and Fisher, M. (eds) (1999) *Social Services: Working under Pressure*. Bristol: The Polity Press.

Frankenberg, R. (1993) *White Women, Race Matters: The Social Construction of Whiteness*. London: Routledge.

Frye, M. (1992) White Woman Feminist. In *Wilful Virgin: Essays in Feminism*. Freedom, California: Crossing.

Gilroy, P. (1990) The End of Anti-Racism. In W. Ball and S. Solomos (eds) *Race and Local Politics*. London: Macmillan.

Gunaratnam, Y. (1997) Culture is Not Enough: a Critique of Multiculturalism in Palliative Care. In D. Field, J. Hockey and N. Small (eds) *Death, Gender and Ethnicity*. London: Routledge.

Gunaratnam, Y., Bremner, I., Pollock, L. and Weir, C. (1998) Anti-discrimination, Emotions and Professional Practice, *European Journal of Palliative Care*, 5 (4): 122–124.

Hochschild, A. (1983) *The Managed Heart: Commercialisation of Human Feeling*. Berkeley: University of California Press.

Hoggett, P. (2000) Social Policy and the Emotions. In G. Lewis, S. Gewirtz and J. Clarke (eds) *Rethinking Social Policy*. London: The Open University in association with Sage Publications.

James, N. (1989) Emotional Labour: Skill and Work in the Social Regulation of Feelings, *Sociological Review*, 37, 15–47.

Joppke, C. (1996) Multiculturalism and Immigration: A comparison of the United States, Germany and Great Britain. *Theory and Society*, 25(4), 449–500.

Lewis, B. and Ramazanoglu, C. (1999) Not Guilty, Not Proud, Just White: Women's Accounts of Their Whiteness. In H. Brown, M. Gilkes and A. Kaloski-Naylor (eds) *White? Women: Critical Perspectives on Race and Gender*. York: Raw Nerve Books.

Lewis, G. (2000) *'Race', Gender, Social Welfare: Encounters in a Postcolonial Society*. London: Polity Press.

Macpherson, W. (1999) *The Stephen Lawrence Inquiry: Report of an Inquiry*. London: Home Office.

Phoenix, A. (2000) Constructing Gendered and Racialised Identities: Young Men, Masculinities and Educational Policy. In G. Lewis, S. Gewirtz and J. Clarke (eds) *Rethinking Social Policy*. London: The Open University in association with Sage Publications.

Pinkney, S. (2000) Anti-Oppressive Theory and Practice in Social Work. In C. Davis, L. Finlay, and A. Bullman (eds) *Changing Practice in Health and Social Care*. Buckingham: The Open University.

Razack, N. (1999) Anti-Discriminatory Practice: Pedagogical Struggles and Challenges, *British Journal of Social Work*, 29: 231–250.

Roediger, D.R. (1990) *Towards the Abolition of Whiteness: Essays on Race, Politics, and Working Class History*. London: Verso.

Sivanandan, A. (1985) RAT and the Degradation of Black Struggle, *Race and Class*, 25(2): 1–33.

Twigg, J. (2000) Social Policy and the Body. In G. Lewis, S. Gewirtz and J. Clarke (eds) *Rethinking Social Policy*. London: The Open University in association with Sage Publications.

Ware, V. (1992) *Beyond the Pale: White Women, Racism and History*. London: Verso.

Williams, C. (1999) Connecting Anti-racist and Anti-oppressive Theory and Practice: Retrenchment or Reappraisal? *British Journal of Social Work*, 29: 211–230.

CHAPTER 19

ON BECOMING A DISABLED PERSON

Andrew Hubbard

I was in the final year of my degree course. I'd already been having problems with my eyes because of diabetes – diabetic retinopathy – and had had one or two minor haemorrhages and quite a lot of laser treatment to try to prevent this. Anyway, I was having a shower just before dinner in my hall of residence and I had these two really large haemorrhages. I quite literally went blind within about thirty seconds. So you can imagine. Next thing, I found myself in hospital. Unfortunately, in my right eye, the blood blocked the drainage system. The pressure got so high that it destroyed the whole of that eye – retina, all the nerves, the lot. So that was gone. But I suppose I was lucky it didn't happen in the left. Actually it took about three or four years before most of that haemorrhage drained away and, interestingly, that did restore some degree of partial sight, although it was all peripheral. I was twenty-two when it happened and I'm now forty-five. So I have had almost exactly half my life with near perfect vision and half first, with virtually no sight and then a very little sight. So I've been a non-disabled person and a disabled person.

I did complete the degree, which was amazing. In fact, looking back, I wish I'd left it or come back. But it was very much expected at that time and I responded to what was expected of me. It was a challenge. Then that was finished and there was absolutely nothing, no job prospects. In fact I didn't even know where I was going to live. I didn't want to go back to my family because I was afraid of losing my independence.

So a year passed. I had some rehabilitation. I went away on a residential course and learned some basic mobility. I did learn typing skills, which was useful. And they taught me braille, which was useful in part but I couldn't read it very well because I'd got some peripheral neuropathy and I couldn't feel that sensitively with my finger tips. But most of it was what these people thought I should do and learn. They never asked how you felt. It was woodwork, making baskets, making clay animals. The message was clear: 'You are blind and the world is sighted. It's your problem. The responsibility is yours.' So I was stuck there for three months, with about fifty other adults, being drilled. We were all jammed into little attic rooms. We had to go to bed at half past nine, weren't allowed to go out, couldn't have drink or cigarettes, lights out at ten o'clock. Although it was a fantastic gothic stately home, it was a horrible place. I remember a friend who came to visit saying: 'The least of people's problems here is that they can't see!'

About a year later I got in touch with a career adviser from the RNIB and he suggested speech therapy. Part of my degree had been in linguistics and it seemed ideal for me. I got onto a highly regarded course in London, which lasted three years. It was a post-graduate option in 'Speech and language pathology' as it was called then. I thoroughly enjoyed it. It was quite liberating. But, looking back, I was already, unconsciously I suppose, developing the idea that the only way I would succeed in life would be through complete denial of my disability. This was a strategy that had been shaped during my rehabilitation period and by everything else that was happening around me. I wanted to be normal. I wanted other people to treat me as normal. And I thought I was actually capable, strong enough certainly, and clever enough to cope as though I didn't have any problems. That worked great in college and everything was going fine. There was quite good learning support even then, although most support came from other students. I qualified, I got a very good MSc and I got a one-year contract working in the college's clinic for aphasic adults.

I thoroughly enjoyed working in the clinic. The group I really got on with was a mixed group of aphasic language-impaired patients. It was not about teaching skills but about allowing people to discover their own strengths and needs. Working in this way, as a group facilitator, was wonderful. But it only lasted a year. So that came to an end and, after six months, I still hadn't got another job. I'd applied but been turned down. And the reason was always the same, basically: 'We don't think you'd be capable of carrying out speech therapy work if you can't see.' They never actually said that, of course. They said there would be too many steps in this building, or 'We think transport might be a problem – how are you going to get here?' All sorts of obstacles and barriers were being put up which, at that my point in my life, I didn't realise was a form of oppression that I needed to challenge. I just went along with it, kidding myself I suppose that 'Well you know they're only thinking of my best interests really.'

So six months went past and I was living in this flat in south London with my partner Jon and things were getting really difficult. We had rent arrears. The housing conditions were awful, just terrible, and Glenda, my guide dog, didn't even have a garden. You had to walk into a recreation area with the dog at night, a dangerous area and all that. And I thought, 'This is no good, we're not getting anywhere'. So I applied for a job as a speech therapist in the town where I was at University. I applied because I knew the area. To my amazement I was asked to come for an interview. I think I got the job because they were desperate to fill lots of empty posts. For the interview, I was driven to a clinic on a housing estate where they'd obviously decided to put me. They opened a filing cabinet and said, 'Can you read the name at the top of this set of notes?' and I squinted and thought I had to do my best to see it or otherwise I wouldn't get the job. And I said, 'Yes' and they said, 'That's OK then'. Actually the woman in charge was just crazy about dogs. I think it was the dog that got the job. She used to say at staff meetings, 'This is my best therapist', patting Glenda.

At the beginning everything seemed fine. Actually I think I was feeling really pleased with myself. I'd done an extra training course. I'd gone to London. I'd coped with all that and I'd got a permanent job. I didn't see a lot of the problems immediately. It never occurred to me to say 'This isn't working for me' or 'I need more support with this'. I received very little, if any support. I didn't have an assistant. In fact, at that time, there were no assistants. So I struggled on and was moved around a couple of places and eventually ended up at a hideous clinic in the centre of town. After a while I started to feel that things were going wrong. I felt isolated. I had no support. And then, three years ago, my eyesight started to deteriorate again, ironically due to the laser surgery I'd had twenty years before. I knew things were deteriorating. And, looking back, I did cope quite well, but I had become so depressed that I didn't notice how bad things were. I was on automatic pilot – in and out to work. Things got worse, health, social, personal life, to such a degree that it came to the point that I couldn't cope any longer. No one appeared to have noticed how bad things had got for me and I went off sick. By now I had worked in this job for fourteen years.

At this point I reconnected with my brother who I hadn't really been in touch with for ten years. He had had a complete life change himself, divorce, new partner, a really impressive change actually – and we spoke about things. I was ambivalent about my situation because I thought it was all my fault. But he pointed out the lack of support and said that I had not been recognised as a disabled person. My reaction to that was 'No' because I had never wanted to play that role. And now I realise that if you deny disability you start to develop a sense of isolation. Your life becomes a performance and gradually you don't value yourself at all because everything you do is pretend.

When I went off sick, I really was at the lowest point I'd ever been. I think there were a number of reasons but the most important was having had some extremely bad news about my eyesight – they couldn't do any surgery to halt the process of deterioration. I didn't have to make a choice about surgery – it wasn't going to happen. There was a 90 per cent certainty of total blindness. When that news was reported back to my employers, their first reaction was that they were very, very sorry of course. But then they asked me to consider the option of taking early retirement on ill-health grounds. I was in the paralysis of depression. I didn't know what to say. Eventually I decided that I couldn't afford to take early retirement and said, 'No'. I was getting advice from the Union by now and I asked if my job could be restructured. They didn't respond for a further ten weeks, during which time I was plagued by personal anxiety and blame. When they did respond it became clear that they weren't keen on me returning to work. We had more meetings. They asked me, 'Why haven't you explored the benefits available to you? We're sure you'll find you'll be pleasantly surprised.' They tried to persuade me that if I couldn't see people's faces then I couldn't assess their communication needs. They accused me of not filling in my forms and daily returns properly. Eventually it came to the end of the line. I'd been off sick for twelve months and my contract was terminated. They said I could not return to my post on grounds of incapacity. I knew I wasn't incapable. They'd made no assessments or adjustments. They didn't have grounds to say that.

My first response was a feeling of relief that it had finally come to a head. But then I felt lost. It was like some kind of familiar pattern was happening all over again, like in London. I felt a strong sense of personal responsibility, blame, guilt and failure. But I contacted the RNIB and was put in touch with the local Disability Initiative. They interviewed me and I was asked to join a new Disability Equality Training course for trainers. So only a month after my contract of employment had been terminated, I started the course and it has absolutely and completely turned my life around and therefore the way ahead.

The course was twelve weeks, one day a week. It wasn't a fast track but more like a motorway with a lot of hairpin bends. It was totally liberating. It was contrary to all my background, all my experience of education and virtually all my experience as a working professional. It was designed not to teach people, or even to train them, but to create the conditions for learning. And what we did was learn about ourselves through active participation with each other. We were guided obviously, but it soon became clear that this was about personal development. Much more powerfully though, it was about challenging my identity. The core aim of the whole thing was to identify myself as a disabled person and value my difference. So we were taken on an incredible emotional rollercoaster – I found it fantastic. But this was only the beginning of a process, which is by no means finished.

I had great difficulties in the first week and I thought 'I'm not coming back.' The course leaders seemed rather radical: 'You're all disabled people', they said. Looking back, they were playing devil's advocate and intended to challenge us. But I was faced with a great dilemma because I had repressed my disabled identity for the last twenty-four years. Suddenly that was being challenged. In quite a sensitive way, but challenged it was. I started having big problems. I didn't think I could change to see myself as a disabled person. I had absorbed all of society's standards, beliefs, images, everything – this was the image of disability that I'd grown up with and that still exists. For me, embracing disability would be to lose all power and control over my own life, to lose my identity and my status altogether. I struggled because the concepts of the medical and social models of disability are terribly difficult and we had to try to deal with that in one day. Obviously we were meant to take away those thoughts and feelings and then start trying to see things differently.

As the course progressed, I became more and more passionate and actually at one point angry. Some kind of crusade was developing. I started to experience difficulties with friends. I was getting a lot of interesting reactions. One friend said, 'I don't like you being empowered like this, it changes everything.' And I realised then that in changing myself, I was upsetting other people, upsetting the status quo and the nice way that we all seemed to be with each other. That was yet another turning point because you feel a personal responsibility for the comfort and feelings of your friends. And that was difficult because I thought, 'Am I going to lose them too?' At the moment we are all shifting and changing our positions. It's a bit like going into a new group of people and suddenly having to establish all the ground rules all over again. And that's quite difficult because early on I probably had the zeal of the convert and maybe overdid it a bit, but it's all about testing the water. You can't put on a new identity like a suit and just stroll down the street because the street has actually changed as well. Everything changes. If you change your view of yourself, you change your view of the world. It's quite scary, it's almost like being in a new place.

Having finished the course, that whole sense of guilt, blame and personal responsibility has been shifted although it hasn't completely disappeared. Being treated as an equal person, in an atmosphere of trust and respect, I've been able to see reasons why, in the past, I denied being disabled. I think age is important. I never thought at twenty-three that I had limitations. No way could I celebrate being disabled. I was twenty-seven before coming to terms with what being gay meant. It's all about trying to live your life as if you were normal, how you want other people to see you. But living in denial (in gay terms 'being in the closet') you're constantly performing and you can't be yourself. Now at forty-five things are different. It's easier to be myself, to say that I've got limitations and that I've got very valid reasons for them. And people don't think badly of me. I feel more friendly towards myself now. It has given me back a sense of control about my own life.

It's also changed the way I see disabled people. If you see yourself as a non-disabled person even though you are disabled yourself you see them as different to yourself. I didn't want to mix with disabled people. I wouldn't join a blind club or anything like that. I was afraid to identify with disabled people. They seemed to threaten me somehow. That resulted in isolation. All my friends were non-disabled people and I thought that that was OK. But, through the course and the people I've met, I'm now aware that disabled people share the experience of oppression along with others like black people, gay people, poor people, any people. Our lives are shaped by the way society sees us. So, I've not only changed my opinion, but I've made new friends.

But it's been more than just learning about disability. The course has opened up a complete new perspective for the future and a lot more choices. Before the course everything was narrowing, now everything is expanding. The whole business has made me very aware of what's going on all around. It's really about changing the fundamental nature of society. I feel that the Disability Movement has really acquired some clout in the last few years and I'm so pleased to be in on it. If you are part of the process that's all that matters. It's about personal change and being an agent of change. It's so fresh I can't really put it into words. I need a lot of time to really assimilate what's happened. At the moment it's great. I've got lots of opportunities, lots of work. There are people phoning me up saying, 'Would you like to come and do some training?' I can see now that how I was before was a result of society rather than my own limitations and that I can get out and do something about changing things.

If someone had said a year ago that being positive about being a disabled person will really help, will change your life, I couldn't have processed that at all. It's probably the best thing I'll ever learn in my life.

Note

I would like to thank the many people who, one way or another, have enabled me to write this chapter.

CHAPTER 20

REMIND ME WHO I AM, AGAIN

Linda Grant

Extract 1

The start of the end of my mother's life begins with a phone call early one morning from the home help, who we are now paying to come in every day. She says that my mother is not well, that the doctor thinks she might have had another minor heart attack and they are waiting for the ambulance to take her to hospital. She tells me not to worry, but there always has to be one of us who will drop everything and this time it is Michele who takes the day off work and drives from Oxford to Bournemouth to see her.

In the hospital Mum says to Michele, 'Come upstairs, I'll make you a cup of tea, I've got a kitchen upstairs.'

Where does she think she is? She thinks she might be in a hotel. Or she imagines she is still at home, though the evidence of her own eyes should have told her otherwise. This is a new confusion. Removed from the familiar surroundings of her own flat and the shop at the petrol station in the forecourt of her building, where, I suspect, most of her groceries are bought now, her brain no longer seems able to take in new information, assess it and make a judgement about what it contains. She looks at the hospital beds, the nurses in their uniforms, the doctors in their white coats, the sick people in their night clothes, and all these visual clues tell her nothing. Or perhaps they do, for a moment, and she understands, but then she turns her head away – looking down at the copy of *Hello* magazine Michele has bought her – and forgets what she knows.

The staff sister, however, understands exactly what *she* sees. After only a few minutes' evaluation she has decided that it is absolutely out of the

Source: *Remind Me Who I Am, Again*, Granta, London, 1998, pp. 185–93, 233–8.

question for our mother to go home. Under the hospital's own guidelines they are not prepared to discharge her back to her solitary flat and a paid visitor for only an hour a day. On the other hand, they need the bed; the heart attack is what? Perhaps only a particularly heavy bout of angina. Or another of those tiny strokes that continue to afflict her. Or has the whole incident been a superbly acted performance, a cry for help from a woman abandoned and deserted? For it is true: despite the best intentions of her daughters, we neglected her during that last year. We did not travel to Bournemouth every weekend and sit in her flat listening to the diminishing round of her conversation. We stayed at home not because we didn't care about her, but because it was unpleasant to be there. I could have gone more often but I didn't. That last visit to London, at Yom Kippur, I noticed that I spent much of the time sipping orange juice, heavily diluted with vodka. On my return train journey after taking her back, I bought two miniature vodka bottles, the equivalent of two doubles, and had consumed both not long after the train passed through Southampton. It was the stress, the irritation, the constant biting of my tongue that did me in and made me dread the thought of being with her. An hour was bad enough, but a day was a forever and a whole weekend required another day to recover from it. And anyway, a day wasn't enough for her. [. . .]

I was always hearing of people who gave up their careers to look after their elderly relatives, particularly childless daughters who some families breed and rear precisely so that one day they will be available to perform the task of caring for their parents in their old age. But if I had given up my work, it wasn't clear to me how, without an income, I would have been able to support us both. I suppose I could have sold my flat or hers and lived off the proceeds, but within six months I would have been an alcoholic and bankrupt three or four years later for neither of our properties was worth that much. Of all the scenarios for our mother's future, this was one that Michele and I *never* considered. And however badly others may think we behaved – those people who love their relatives and would not dream of putting them in a home – looking after her ourselves fell into the same category of the unimaginable as sharing all our secrets with her, having her as our best friend. The intimacy simply wasn't there to begin with.

[. . .]

The assessment

Michele rings Pat Tennuci (the social worker) and manages to persuade her to come back for a third assessment. How will our mother present herself to Pat, we wonder. Will she tell her that she has everything under control: her food, her medication, her memory of how to navigate the route from front door to shops? And so is Michele to remind her that once back home – though she isn't going, anyway – she would be picking up the phone to whichever daughter's number was first to hand, crying, saying, 'I can't cope any more'?

That night in the hospital Michele sits by our mother's bed and gives her what she calls 'a really hard talking to', perhaps the hardest she has ever had in her life. She tells her, 'Unless you say you can't cope you will *have* to cope, you will have to go back home on your own.' Then our mother starts crying and says what we have suspected for so long is the truth; she tells it like it is, at last: 'I don't want to go back to that flat,' she weeps. 'I never want to go back to that flat again as long as I live.'

Her own home had become a prison, a torture chamber.

Michele says to her, 'You have got to tell the truth about how you feel to the social worker.'

[. . .]

When Pat arrives for the meeting Mum bursts into tears and says, 'Don't make me go back to that flat, don't make me go back to that flat.'

Has she remembered her instructions? What, out of the previous evening's conversation, had lodged itself in her head? Has Michele managed to convey to her the enduring significance of her own misery so that she can recall it? Or has she known all along that the moment would one day come in which she would have to stop playing games, and it had arrived?

[. . .]

Now it is my turn to relieve Michele and go to Bournemouth, clutching a copy of *Hello* magazine which I am not then aware that Michele has already bought her and which is nowhere in evidence. It doesn't matter. She seizes mine eagerly, thirsty for celebrity gossip which goes in one ear and out the other.

[. . .]

I go to Social Services for a meeting with Pat, our first face-to-face, and understand at once that she is an intelligent woman whose hands are tied by the system, particularly that aspect of it which insists that the demented elderly are best left where they are, to be cared for by the community. We talk for ages. She's delighted at this resolution. Then I go back to the flat to find some clean nightdresses. The ones that are there are completely awful, torn nylon diaphanous garments from the early 1960s. Michele had noticed in the hospital how her dressing-gown was filthy, covered in stains. I can't believe how old the food in the fridge is.

When she had the first heart attack I had rented a portable television for her bedroom and now I go down to the showroom to sign the forms for cancellation. There's a rain-storm and I run, soaking wet, into Marks and Spencer's. I purchase the finest nightgowns money could buy as well as a quilted cream lace bag of toiletries. I want her to walk through the doors of wherever she is to go with her head held high, dressed as well as she has ever looked in her life, right down to the incidentals of the bathroom sink. When she enters Bayview Retirement Home or its clone, the other residents will see the mother *we* had known: the one for whom how you looked was who you are.

I go off to Spain and – not without guilt on my part and resentment on hers – leave Michele to it. Leave her to phone calls from our mother in hospital claiming that she has been kidnapped by the nurses and that Michele must come and get her at once.

Pat Tenucci's new assessment is that our mother has gone from not needing residential care at all to being an emergency case.

[. . .]

Extract 2

Michele's visits are less frequent than mine for she lives further away. She isn't sure if her mother knows exactly who she is any more, an idea I resist. Of course she knows Michele. Or is she just someone she recognises? Whenever Mum introduces me to anyone now, it is as a niece or a sister, never as a daughter. The niece is Marina, the girl she had grown up with. Reverting to her childhood, she is sloughing off later recollections. As her sisters Miriam and Gertie and Lillian had looked after her when she was the youngest child, so I'm now someone who looks after her. I'm a sister, she reasons, I must be.

What does she retain? She knows that Michele is getting married. She remembers this from visit to visit, but only when I remind her.

At the wedding itself, in her £209 outfit, she tells anyone who will listen, 'It's my niece that's getting married, you know.' Someone remarks that in this she reveals how entirely she has now repudiated the idea of herself as a mother. Except for the odd business of her saccharine sweetness when she sees a child.

She runs up and bends over: 'Hello, hello,' she tinkles in an ickle-baby voice.

I don't think it's that she feels a new sense of maternity that she didn't possess before. I think she relates to children as if she were part of their own tribe, people who have other people looking after them, called parents.

[. . .]

While the wedding is a success the aftermath is a disaster. A week later she has forgotten it.

'Don't you remember? The wedding. You were there, and Marina came and Jonathan and Lynne and Sefton.'

'Who are Jonathan, Lynne and Sefton.'

'Oh, never mind.'

'I'm very unhappy here. I want to go back to Bournemouth. I hate the Londoners, loathe them, they're horrible. I don't know anyone here. I've got nothing, I'm a nobody.'

A nobody. It's true. With her own past ripped away from her, and not just in her own mind, who is she? Who are any of us without a history? Buddhists long to move into a state beyond time, they want to rest in the moment. My mother has achieved this without any of the meditation and what state of transcendental bliss has it brought her?

At the wedding she was a somebody again, people knew who she was. She's forgotten the event itself, but the memory lingers of a single day in which she felt herself to be whole, an actor in a wider world. Then they all went away and she was brought back here, to her anonymity, to being Rose, from Liverpool, whom no one knows or remembers as a child or teenager or young mother. She's only Rose, who repeats herself, who has a daughter who comes in and takes her away for a few hours. That's another kind of prison we've put her in, not just the one with locked doors.

The Power of Attorney

But she is so angry, so aggressive – she took me by the shoulders and pushed me out of her room, once, when I told her I didn't have time to take her out. I want something to be done. What Michele and I are after is a chemical solution. How about Prozac, the happy drug?

At this time, also, we need power of attorney. Consulting a solicitor, we find that this can only be obtained if she is judged by a doctor to be sufficiently *compos mentis* to be able voluntarily to grant it. If not, the case will have to be referred to the Court of Protection.

I make an appointment with the home's GP.

Just before the meeting I say: 'Now Mum, we want to get power of attorney over your affairs so you won't have to worry about your finances any more.'

'Yes,' she says.

'For example, one of the things Michele is dealing with at the moment is Dorset Social Services who want us to sell your flat so we can pay back the money we owe them. But we don't want to sell just now because house prices are going up and anyway, there's a move by the residents to buy out the freehold on the whole building and that would add some value to your flat.'

'Oh, I'm past dealing with all that,' she says. 'You handle it.'

'That's just it, so we can, we have to have power of attorney and we're about to go down and have a meeting with the doctor to discuss it.'

In the office, the GP, an energetic, intelligent young woman, takes my mother through a set of standard questions they always give sufferers of dementia.

'Do you know what the date is?'

'No.'

'Do you know what day of the week it is?'
'No.'
'Do you know the name of the Leader of the Opposition?'
'No.'
'Do you know the name of the Prime Minister?'
'No.'
'Do you know the name of this place where you live?'
'No.'
'Do you know where it is?'
'No.'

Oh shit, I think, this is surely going to have to go to the Court of Protection.

'Do you know how to make a cup of tea?'
'Do you mean with tea bags or a strainer?'
'Your daughters want to have power of attorney over your affairs. That means you wouldn't have control any more. What do you think of that?'

'Well, I think it's a good idea,' my mother says, 'because someone wants to sell my flat and we don't want to because the house prices are going up and we'll get more for it. And we want to buy out the freehold, so that will make it worth more as well. I can't handle all that. I totally trust my daughters, they'll look after me.'

'I think your mother is *compos mentis* in her own way,' the GP says to me. 'Don't you?'

After the meeting we have a talk about her aggression. 'That's the emotional incontinence,' she says. 'It's a standard aspect of Multi-Infarct Dementia.'

'Isn't there any medication she could take?'
'I could consider one of the sisters of Prozac.'
'*One of the what?*'
'The sisters of Prozac. Not Prozac itself, but a drug in that family.'

And so she is prescribed something and it seems to work. The rages stop for a time. The Prozac Sisters and the Grant Sisters are the best of friends.

Why was it that my mother did not know where she was or what day it was or who the Prime Minister was, when she was able to recall the conversation I had had with her earlier, which contained what to many would be complex issues concerning property?

I concluded that she simply did not need the information about the date and place – why should she? She had no appointments. She never had to find her way back there. As for the name of the Prime Minister, what bearing did the government's disputes over entry into the European Exchange Rate Mechanism have on her chair and her place at the lunch table and her excursions to Marks and Spencer's? None.

With only so much room in her memory, she jettisoned anything she didn't need in order to retain what she considered to be important. Mention doctors or lawyers and her old immigrant's brain went on full alert. The authorities. You had to deal with them. You had to give them the right answer or who knows what ugly decisions they might make, not in your favour?

PART III

RIGHTS AND RISK

INTRODUCTION

Policies associated with care and welfare are typically referenced to the rights of the individual and the risks of intervention and non-intervention. For policy makers and practitioners there are many complex issues to be addressed, particularly as a result of the Human Rights Act 1998. Who has a right to what services? Who should pay for what? How should access be controlled and rights respected? Who is accountable for deciding who gets what? What should be the penalties following improper treatment or abuse? How can autonomy and dignity be promoted and maintained?

There is a burgeoning literature on the more formal aspects of these policy matters: legislation, standards, commitments, cost-effectiveness, quality, and so on. The chapters that follow adopt a less formal approach: informed discussions are interwoven with accounts of research.

Chapter 21 sets the stage with a review of how risk and dangerousness are managed in policy terms. Andy Alaszewski brings out the difficulties that care managers face in seeking to minimise risks. Michael Preston-Shoot in Chapter 22 draws on two case studies in order to examine how self-determination accords with social work values. A more detailed case study is based on the first-hand account provided by Jean in Chapter 23. Here she describes her long journey from institutional care to independent living 'in the world'. Contrasting with this, in Chapter 24, Jaber Gubrium, a US gerontologist, provides a powerful discussion and account of the prospective journey into residential care.

The next three chapters maintain the focus on residential care. In Chapter 25, the concepts of privacy, risk and independence are viewed from the perspective of the providers. Based on research in Scotland into the management of care homes, Rosemary Bland relates these three concepts to the 'hotel model' of residential care. During the 1990s, the late Tom Kitwood revolutionised the care for people with dementia by promoting the concept of personhood. Chapter 26 includes his narrative of a poignant case history, and the seventeen elements of the 'malignant social psychology' which underpins the 'depersonalising tendencies' of current practice. Then, in Chapter 27 John Burton provides a vivid account of how one individual, from a comparatively weak position, endeavoured to expose abuse and to reduce threats to vulnerable residents of care homes. Privacy is elaborated in Chapter 28 where Caroline Holland and Sheila Peace summarise their research into changes in how small care homes are inspected and regulated.

This overview of the rights and risk entailed in providing care and support concludes with two distinctive chapters. In Chapter 29, Luke Clements details the implications of the Human Rights Act 1998 for community care, and then, in Chapter 30, Simone Aspis, as someone with learning difficulties who has become a significant political figure, writes about self-advocacy and the changing relationship between users and providers.

CHAPTER 21

RISK AND DANGEROUSNESS

Andy Alaszewski

Risk and dangerousness are concerned with the harm that one individual or group of individuals can cause to others. While any individual can cause harm and therefore may be a danger to any other individual, the description of an individual or group as dangerous implies that the level of risk is seen as unacceptably high and that there should be collective action to assess and manage this risk. Thus drunken drivers are defined as dangerous and action is taken to identify them, for example by breath testing drivers, and to prevent them causing harm when they have been identified, including immediate action to prevent them driving while drunk and longer term action to remove their driving licences.

This discussion of dangerousness starts with the 'common sense' approach in which the nature of risk and danger are treated as self-evident and the role of professionals is to find out which risks are acceptable and then to manage unacceptable risks. I explore the limitations of this approach especially through evidence that risk and danger are socially constructed categories.

Risk has been around for a long time for, as Lupton (1999) points out, its use in the English language can be traced back to the seventeenth century. However, it seems to have only become a *key* concept in contemporary society.

Protecting the public

Concerns with dangerousness are particularly evident in criminal justice services. For example, Kemshall (2000) notes that preoccupations about dangerousness and public protection resulted in a major reconceptualisation of the role of probation officers in the 1990s, with a shift from case-oriented social work to the management of risk and dangerousness. A centralised controlling service was set up to test the use of explicit risk management strategies.

Similar concerns with dangerousness and risk can be seen in health and welfare services, especially those dealing with people with severe and enduring mental health needs. A number of high profile incidents in which psychiatric patients have killed others have contributed to a 'moral panic'. This has led to an emphasis on the dangerousness of ex-psychiatric patients and on risk assessment as a mechanism to identify and control 'dangerous' individuals. The killing in 1992 by Christopher Clunis of Jonathan Zito at a London underground station was particularly important in shaping media and official reactions. The inquiry highlighted repeated failures to assess the dangerousness of Clunis and emphasised the centrality of risk assessment to psychiatric services (Ritchie *et al.* 1994).

Underpinning the government's concern with the identification of dangerousness is the 'common sense' view that risk and dangerousness are self-evident and easy to identify (Kemshall, 2000: 148). It is seen as simple and straightforward to develop check lists to identify dangerousness and risk. Within this approach the emphasis is on ensuring that risk and danger are managed and kept within acceptable limits. Thus policy makers and practitioners need to be aware of public perceptions of risks and their acceptability.

The initial interest in and concern about public acceptability of risk started with environmental risk and dangers, especially the dangers to both the environment and to humans posed by new technologies. In the 1950s nuclear power for example was presented as an inexhaustible source of safe and cheap energy. This optimism evaporated with a number of major accidents such as the explosion of the Flixborough chemical works in 1974 and the large scale contamination following the Chernobyl accident. These major events stimulated the development of environmental groups which challenged the current orthodoxy about the safety and social benefits of technologies.

A major difference between industrial and human services lies in the source and nature of the dangers or hazards. In the industrial sector the processes used are seen as the major source of danger. Human error does play a major part. For example, the nuclear plant at Chernobyl would not have exploded if technicians had not undertaken unsafe experiments. However the response to such accidents is to analyse the nature of the human errors and to 'design them out of the system' through improved safety technology. Thus the response to the Piper Alpha explosion on the North Sea has been to change the design of oil drilling platforms. In human services in contrast, it is virtually impossible to separate the human component from the technical process, as the core activity involves person-to-person working. The main hazards are seen to be people who are less predictable and more difficult to control than technologies.

Recognising people as potential sources of hazard creates a number of tensions in human services that are difficult to resolve. The first tension relates to values and can most clearly be seen in health and safety issues. Under Health and Safety legislation employers have a legal duty to protect their employees from hazards. This creates tensions when service users are the source of danger.

The tension between protecting employees and others from danger and empowering clients results in inconsistencies and fluctuations in agency and professional responses to dangerous behaviour.

In our study of welfare agencies we could find little evidence that practitioners either recognised the risk policies of their agency or that they used them as the basis of their decision making (Alaszewski, Harrison and Manthorpe 1998: 72–86). There were therefore inconsistencies both between agencies but also within agencies in responses to risk and danger. These inconsistencies can create inequities in the treatment of individuals. They can result in harm not only for others but also for users themselves. This can be seen in the inconsistent response to men with learning disabilities whose behaviour is dangerous because they sexually abuse.

Responses to abuse relate more to the context of the act than its harmfulness and, paradoxically, agencies often fail to protect other vulnerable individuals:

> *responses are not correlated to the nature of the act but to the social context of the act, especially the status of the victim. Services tended to be more tolerant of sexually abusive behaviour if the victim was another person with learning disabilities or a female member of staff ... services have been found deficient, commonly failing to prevent men with known histories of abusing from committing further assaults.*
>
> *(Thompson 2000: 38)*

Thompson argues that this inconsistency can be harmful to the men themselves. If there is a weak and tolerant response to their abusive behaviours they are likely to persist and, if they reach the limits of tolerability, they may find themselves more harshly treated than other men who have behaved in the same ways (Thompson 2000: 39). He argues that it is both legitimate and necessary for agencies to intervene to manage dangerousness, but:

> *The challenge is how best to do this work of risk assessment and management in any specific situation and how to ensure a consistency of approach regardless of which service a person with learning disabilities is accessing.*
>
> *(Thompson 2000: 44–45)*

As Thompson points out, denying that users of human services may behave in harmful or dangerous ways can result in inconsistent and inequitable responses which not only can threaten the public and staff, but can also be harmful for users themselves. The issue is how dangerous behaviour can be effectively prevented or managed and it is to these questions I turn next.

First I consider the limitation of the industrial approach to risk and dangerousness, and responses to these limitations. Then I will consider the official response which we label *bureaucratic*, a *critical* approach emphasising a change in the ways in which agencies and professionals work and, thirdly, the *radical* response.

Responses to dangerousness

The limitations of industrial models are exposed when they are used within human services. Implicit in these models are a number of 'common sense' assumptions, for example that hazards can be objectively identified, that an objective level of tolerability can be established, and that there is shared and common interests in minimising harm. As I have already shown, within human services these common sense assumptions are difficult to sustain. Technical definitions of tolerability in particular are based on expert assessments of the risks to which a defined population is exposed over a period of time. These estimates are based on evidence such as actuarial information drawn from recorded events. Non-experts are more concerned about the personal implications and estimates of risk. They use a variety of sources of information which they evaluate in terms of relevance and trustworthiness. Their willingness to tolerate risk depends not only on their assessment of the magnitude of the risk but also on its relationship to other risks.

The social factors involved in non-expert assessment of risk can be seen in perceptions of mental health and in food panics such as those associated with BSE.

Reilly notes how the announcement by the government of the link between eating beef and *nv*CJD caused a major shift in public perceptions as respondents treated the government as an authoritative source of information (Reilly 1999: 137). Not only do expert and lay assessments of dangerousness and risk differ, but the ways in which information is used also differ. Experts are usually specialists and concerned with specific risks. Lay people do not respond to one risk in isolation; they set an individual risk within the context of other risks and their overall lives. Thus Reilly notes that while respondents in her study seemed to experience the same shift in perceptions, the response in behaviour was not uniform: some individuals stated that they had stopped eating beef, while others still ate it even though they accepted this was dangerous behaviour. The differences seemed to be explained by different social contexts. Individuals who were responsible only for their own lives tended to persist with their behaviour while individuals who were responsible for others, especially parents of young children, tended to behave 'responsibly' and stopped eating beef (Reilly 1999: 140–142).

The difference between expert and lay perceptions of, and responses to, risk is a serious problem if 'tolerability' of risk and dangerousness is defined solely in expert terms. What are the official responses to this risk 'gap'?

The bureaucratic solution

Within current government reports on health and welfare, there is a concern to create and maintain public confidence in services by ensuring that the public are adequately protected from danger. For example, while the White Paper on social services acknowledges that 'In many areas, social services are doing a good job', it continues: 'but there are too many cases where they are not' (Department of Health 1998). The government's response to this perceived problem has been essentially organisational: more control over practice linked to better communication.

Its main focus of attention and action has been on professional decision-making. In the NHS, for example, there has been increasing concern about the dangerousness of medical decision-making prompted by evidence of serious harm to patients. The government's response to a series of disasters has been to try to establish control over decision-making. In its drive to modernise the delivery of health and welfare, government has emphasised the importance of the collection and use of scientific knowledge or 'evidence'. In the White Paper on the modernisation of the NHS there are three interlinked elements designed to ensure the development of evidence-based practice (Department of Health 1997: 57–59). The government wishes to use this new system to counteract danger and to improve outcomes by reducing levels of harm.

There is a more fundamental problem. Implicit in the outcomes approach is the 'common sense' view that safety is the prime objective of service provision. Harm, especially death, is self-evidently bad and should be avoided at all costs. The best decision is the safest. Professionals and government ministers share this view but it is not clear that the public and users of services view risk in the same way.

A simple example will illustrate the difference. As Cox *et al.* (1992) point out, measured in fatalities per kilometre covered, the safest way to travel is by public transport, especially scheduled air service, and the most hazardous is by private transport (including using a car, walking and cycling). However it is clear that 'user' perceptions of the dangerousness of, and preferences for, different types of travel are very different. Not only does the public prefer private means, but there are anxieties about the safety of public transport. There is a well-established 'fear of flying'. People who walk or cycle use a simple technology that they both understand and control. They feel safe and have a sense of security. Moreover, many health promoters advise them to take such exercise. So policy based solely on harm or accident minimisation might reduce fatalities but would be neither practical nor acceptable to the public.

This difference between expert and public assessments of risk tends to be addressed as a problem of communication. For example, the government's former Chief Medical Officer, Sir Kenneth Calman and his colleagues have expressed concern about excessive public reaction to 'risk' such as 'food panics'. They argue that the most effective way of preventing such panics is to involve the public in decision-making through improved risk communication. While they acknowledge both that risks involve values as well as technical issues and the importance of the decision-making process, their main emphasis is on the technical dimension, a greater openness so that the public has improved access to information while experts have a greater opportunity to identify and allay public anxieties (Bennett and Calman 1999).

While there is increased demand and pressure from governments for more effective assessment of and communication about risk and dangerousness, sociologists have raised doubts about the whole enterprise and it is to their concerns I turn next.

The radical response

The 'common sense' approach to risk and dangerousness is based on the assumption that these phenomena can be objectively measured by experts. Social scientists argue that this 'objectivity' is an illusion. Lupton (1999) has reviewed risk from a sociological perspective. She rejects 'objective' representation of risk which underpins much current psychological research on risk, seeing risk in terms of power and domination. Drawing on the work of the French sociologist, Foucault, she sees risk in terms of 'discourses', as a technique for establishing and creating social control developed during the eighteenth century. During this period governments increasingly saw their populations as resources that could be exploited for economic and military superiority. The emerging professions developed forms of knowledge that facilitated this exploitation. Thus 'threatening' elements in the population created a danger that needed to be identified. Once identified, these elements could be isolated and 'reprogrammed' in new institutions such as prisons and mental hospitals. The remainder of the population internalised control through 'responsible' behaviour based on professional advice about safe and hygienic practices.

This Foucauldian approach has been influential in the health and welfare services and especially in the ways in which professionals create and manage risk. Analysts using this approach seek to identify discourses through which experts create knowledge and power. These usually involve some form of binary opposition based on normal/abnormal, safe/danger-ous and good/bad. They may be applied in various areas of human experience, for example, heterosexual/homosexual, sane/mad. There is also a psychological dimension to these discourses as the 'self' seeks to align to 'normal' and separate from 'other', but is both attracted to and threatened by the latent 'other' which has to be psychologically policed and repressed.

The 'factories' of the welfare system, the asylums which disciplined inmates in the interest of public safety, have been increasingly replaced by more individualised and 'risky' forms of care. However, Foucauldians would see this liberation as a new and sophisticated form of repression, a sort of 'false consciousness'. In this context, liberation can take the form of deliberately disregarding professional advice and living dangerously. Radical individuals in the disability rights or the gay movement challenge expert definitions of normality and abnormality. They welcome and are happy to live in a complex, uncertain world in which risk taking and 'living on the edge' is fun, for example by practising what professionals might label unsafe sex (Lupton 1999).

The critical approach

Douglas argues that, for individuals and groups, risk and dangers are important realities, but that different groups and individuals define this reality in different ways. For example, she reports on lay responses to health risks in a study of perceptions and responses to HIV in Brittany. She argues that professional models and information had little impact on some members of the community:

> The most baffling thing about the pattern is that a large number of the community at risk are impervious to information; either they know unshakeably that they themselves are immune, or recognizing that death is normal they draw the conclusion that to live trying to avoid it is abhorrent.
>
> (Douglas 1992: 111)

Douglas argues that perception of, and responses to, risk are related to an individual's position in a cultural system. If different groups and indi-viduals define risk and danger in different ways, how can it be possible to develop socially agreed and accepted definitions of 'acceptable' or 'reason-able' risk and methods of managing risk? Kemshall argues that the only way of doing this is to recognise different definitions and to see risk management as a process of negotiation between different groups and individuals with their different assessment of risk and its acceptability (Kemshall 2000: 152).

It should be clear from this discussion that risk and dangerousness have become central issues in human services and that agencies and their employees are expected to assess and manage risk and danger effectively. However the current approach to risk and danger is muddled, some services have imported industrial models without realising they have imported the assumptions that go along with them. Others seek to develop distinctive human service approaches to risk while some professionals and commentators see these debates as discourses creating repressive and invidious forms of surveillance.

There is great merit in Kemshall's approach. She both recognises differences in assessment of risk and argues that effective risk management requires mutual respect and negotiation. While public and service users have become more cynical about expert assessment of risk and are less willing to take them 'for granted', they are still willing to accept and trust these assessments if their own perceptions are acknowledged, and if they are involved in the process of decision-making and risk management.

REFERENCES

Alaszewski, A., Harrison, L. and Manthorpe, J. (eds) (1998) *Risk, Health and Welfare: Policies, Strategies and Practice*, Buckingham, Open University Press.

Bennett, P. and Calman, K. (1999) 'Pulling the threads together', in P. Bennett and K. Calman (eds) *Risk Communication and Public Health*, Oxford, Oxford University Press.

Cox, D., Crossland, B., Darby, S.C., Forman, D., Fox, A.J., Gore, S.M., Hambly, E.C., Kletz, T.A. and Neill, N.V. (1992) 'Estimations of risk from observations on humans', in The Royal Society (ed.) *Risk, Analysis, Perception and Management: Report of a Royal Society Study Group*, London, The Royal Society.

Department of Health (1997) *The New NHS*, Cm 3807, London, The Stationery Office.

Department of Health (1998) *Modernising Social Services*, London, The Stationery Office.

Douglas, M. (1992) *Risk and Blame: Essays in Cultural Theory*, London, Routledge.

Kemshall, H. (2000) 'Conflicting knowledges on risk: the case of risk knowledge in the probation service', *Health, Risk and Society*, 2, 143–158.

Lupton, D. (1999) *Risk*, London, Routledge.

Reilly, J. (1999) 'Just another food scare?', Public understanding and the BSE crisis', in G. Philo (ed.) *Message Received: Glasgow Media Group Research 1993–1998*, Harlow, Longman, pp. 128–145.

Ritchie, J.H., Dick, D. and Lingham, R. (1994) *The Report of the Inquiry into the Care and Treatment of Christopher Clunis*, London, HMSO.

Thompson, D.J. (2000) 'Vulnerability, dangerousness and risk: the case of men with learning disabilities who sexually abuse', *Health, Risk and Society*, 2, 33–46.

CHAPTER 22

EVALUATING SELF-DETERMINATION

Michael Preston-Shoot

Self-determination is invariably regarded as a core social work value. Not surprisingly, therefore, it features strongly in the literature on elder abuse. Indeed, practitioners are castigated for any tendency to want to rescue victims from abusive situations rather than to assist them to disclose their concerns in their own way and to make their own choices (Pritchard 2000).

Penhale (1993) asserts that it can be difficult for professionals, often holding strong protective instincts, to accept that older people have the right to refuse assessment and intervention. She does, however, allow an exception, when an individual is either at very grave risk or severely mentally impaired. Hargreaves and Hughes (1996) note that older people are adults and that their rights to self-determination, including the right to refuse intervention, therefore demands a different framework from that applied to children. They comment that some professionals appear to view self-determination as more of an inconvenience than a right. However, can the case for protection be so summarily dismissed?

A clear tension exists between protection and self-determination, paternalism and autonomy (SSI 1993). Equally, a danger exists that values-talk can become disguised as factual discourse and used to justify action when it should only inform (Cheetham 1989). The purpose of this chapter is to review whether self-determination has been overly inflated or privileged in

Source: Adapted from 'Evaluating self-determination: an adult protection case study', *Journal of Adult Protection*, 3.1 February 2001, pp. 4–15.

theory and practice concerning elder abuse cases. How might the balance between protection and self-determination, between individual freedom and professional intervention be calibrated?

In recent research (Preston-Shoot and Wigley 2000), several cases such as Case Study 1 raised the issue of who should be responsible for making decisions about police involvement. Usually the victim's views prevailed, even where clear evidence of abuse and crime was apparent. In some cases social workers did not investigate because the 'client' did not want any action taken. Many staff privileged self-determination over protection, in some instances even where the older person had been assessed as being confused and unable to make decisions. There were, however, examples of indirect directive behaviour, characterised by the statement: 'I am not allowed to leave you in this situation because it is not safe for you.' In the main social workers attached considerable weight to the expressed views of the older person, even when this left them in a dangerous situation.

Case Study 1

The referral came from the police and the woman victim, aged 68. She lives with her family. She alleges physical abuse and food deprivation. An earlier community care assessment found the 'client' to be doubly incontinent, with poor mobility and very limited ability to complete personal care tasks. The family dynamics are noted as difficult, with reference to alcohol abuse by the son and his partner, aggression when drunk, poor relationships and a risk that care will breakdown.

Two social workers visit and find her distressed but wanting no action taken. Daily domiciliary care is arranged, a GP assessment requested and a housing transfer request initiated. The victim refuses temporary residential care and police involvement. The social workers speak to the victim's son and partner, who state that the victim is unreasonable and demanding. They admit throwing a commode at her. Regular contact is maintained for four months, with further complaints by the victim of arguments, verbal abuse and of her son's aggression. Social workers ask regularly if she is safe but her message is the same: she refuses to move out, being concerned about whether she would manage alone; she does not want the police involved; she refuses day care but accepts home help; she will not evict her family.

Then the home helps withdraw because of the family dynamics. There is concern about the welfare of a two-year-old grandchild. A few days later, following further family arguments and a 'fall', the victim agrees to move into temporary residential care but later declines. Two months later she is beaten up and almost strangled. The domiciliary care staff, who had agreed to return, are also assaulted. Police officers visit but she will not press charges. There are marks on her neck, caused by the son's partner pulling telephone wires around it. However, she refuses to leave home or to evict her family. A multi-agency case conference is held at which daily monitoring is agreed, because of the risk of harm. The pattern continues.

This case raises many issues. However, for the purposes of this discussion, those relating to self-determination will be highlighted. First, there is clear evidence of a crime on first contact but the police are not automatically involved. This was not consistent with the inter-agency procedures operating in the area and is outside current policy guidance (DoH 2000). Rather, the victim's self-determination is given precedence. However, this takes a short-term rather than a longer-term view and adopts a negative rather than a positive freedom perspective.

The 'client' oscillates in her views about the acceptability of some of the proposed options but no one outside the immediate multi-professional system questions how the case is being managed. The interventions are, therefore, characterised by 'more of the same' and no change is being effected. The abuse continues and, indeed, escalates. No one appears to question why the victim might be reluctant to move or to request police intervention. At several points, if not throughout, there is evidence of immediate danger but it is difficult to see how the intervention plan could keep the victim safe.

The status of values

Clark (1998) argues that practitioners are not taking difficult and problematic judgements in dependably fair and consistent ways but are relying on intuition and slogans. Davis and Ellis (1995) suggest that, to survive difficult dilemmas, practitioners exercise their discretion in irrational, covert and punitive ways, sometimes basing decisions on stereotyped responses or moral judgements. Indeed, there may be little time within social services departments currently to debate value issues (Marsh and Triseliotis 1996) and doubts about whether a values-based approach to practice remains possible (Preston-Shoot et al. 2001). Nonetheless, values may provide one framework for situations where choice of action requires a decision between competing principles.

Social work values and accompanying codes of ethics have been criticised for:

- being an idealistic set of abstractions, providing inadequate guidance on the dilemmas that practitioners encounter (Clark 1998; Payne 1999). Since the same facts can apparently support incompatible value judgements, values may not be able to resolve conflict between different valued courses of action, such as protection versus self-determination.
- being weak or irrelevant when confronted with agency and Govern-

ment imperatives (Cornwell 1992/93; Preston-Shoot 1996; Clark 1999) and insufficiently strong to guarantee ethical individual and/or agency practice.

■ lacking coherence and clear meaning (Timms 1986, 1989; Clark 1999).

Practitioners have been criticised for using values statements uncritically (Timms 1986). Values are not fixed directions (Timms 1983). They are less universal or absolute truths than informative signposts, determined by what society will sanction, define and limit (Horne 1987; Biehal and Sainsbury 1991; Banks 1995). Similarly, Clark (1999) views codes of ethics as points of reference, warning of danger, rather than as destinations. He describes the debate between Kantian and utilitarian ethics as 'a draw', while Horne (1987) notes that values, such as self-determination, raise questions unresolved among philosophers. This suggests that different value positions can at best simply enlighten issues and controversies, and identify the different arguments that could be deployed by practitioners when evaluating which course of action to take where a range of actions is possible.

Thus, a 'right' course of action can only be determined by reference to the situation confronted. Values cannot dictate what practitioners ought to do in each and every situation since their approach will be influenced by how they conceptualise the ethical choices facing them.

[...]

Self-determination

Self-determination is a long-established social work value, to which practitioners retain strong attachment (Clark 1998).... 'Clients' have the right to make decisions about what help to accept and about their future, even if their choices involve risk. Potential self-harm is not, in principle, grounds for constraining choice.... Wilmot (1997) comments that autonomy is widely valued as a right that takes priority over most other considerations. Thus, while autonomy may be qualified to some degree, any departure from it requires very good reasons....

Social work codes of ethics acknowledge that self-determination may be qualified. For example, NASW (1996) qualifies the value when, in their professional judgement, practitioners believe the actions of 'clients' or their proposed behaviour pose serious, foreseeable and imminent danger to themselves or others. [...]

Self-determination is problematic as a sole guiding principle (Wilmot 1997; Clark 1998) because:

■ it does not take into account the restraints on choice necessary to protect other individuals' equivalent rights; one person's autonomy might compromise another person's self-determination. One individual's actions will invariably affect others. In a family, therefore, is a focus on self-determination for one individual meaningful?

■ it presupposes the existence of opportunity and freedom to choose between options. An individual's perception of their autonomy, their view of their right to exercise choice, may be limited. Should a practitioner accept this as defining this person's situation? An individual's choice or freedom to decide may be constrained by their own belief system (for instance, about options available) and by the actions of and pressure exerted by others. How should practitioners respond when an individual's decision appears constricted in the face of intimidation or exploitation? Experience as a victim or as helpless may make a right to self-determination seem non-existent (Perlman 1975).

■ it does not deal satisfactorily with people who seem likely to make self-damaging choices. An individual may be competent but ill-informed. If they implement misconceived decisions, promotion of self-determination may result in unhappiness. Equally, determining mental competence is itself problematic . . .

■ it is possible to distinguish between a person's short-term and long-term interests. Where these differ, Horne (1987) advises that practitioners should prioritise the individual's longer-term interests, even if this means violating self-determination in the short term.

[. . .]

It is also possible to distinguish between negative freedom (self-determination as a right, meaning that individuals should be free to do whatever they choose, unless another individual's interests are threatened) and positive freedom (intervention to enable individuals to become more self-determining) (Horne 1987; Banks 1995). It is a perspective of self-determination as negative freedom that lies behind the view that concern for an individual's welfare should only be activated where their capacity to act responsibly is severely diminished. A perspective of self-determination as positive freedom may have the goal of liberating people from oppression and ignorance but risks coercion and manipulation towards behaviours that other people define as rational and constructive (McDermott 1975).

Moreover, self-determination is not the only ethical principle for practice (Banks 1995), such that it is simplistic to assume that autonomy is automatically good and paternalism bad (Sainsbury 1989; Braye and Preston-Shoot 1995). . . . Self-determination may also be constrained by factors such as the level of agency resources and by how 'clients' perceive a practitioner's authority (Braye and Preston-Shoot 1995). This suggests that social workers cannot avoid affecting a client's behaviour, all of which suggests that it is difficult to negotiate the path between uncritical acceptance of an individual's decision and of one's own interpretation of the needs in a situation.

Elder abuse

The literature here appears somewhat less circumspect about self-determination as a concept. Pritchard (1999) is forthright: practitioners must accept that self-determination is a basic principle of good practice and must avoid the concept of rescuing people. Everyone has the right to take risks and to choose. Bennett and Kingston (1993) view coercion as ageist and argue that older people value autonomy above personal safety. They do not, however, offer evidence for this view. Slater (1999) cautions that a specific elder abuse policy, as opposed to a generic adult abuse policy, can create a culture of paternalistic over-protection, a concern with harm rather than respect for individual freedom. In similar vein, Anderson (1999) argues that intervention and monitoring must be acceptable to the victim, even where they choose to remain in or return to an abusive situation, while Fearns (1999) suggests that the wishes of the victim are paramount.

Not everyone is unequivocal but here commentators vary in the degree to which they will depart from an apparently absolute principle. For example, Lawson (1999) states that it may be necessary to override the wishes of a vulnerable adult if they are being intimidated, if their safety is jeopardised, if other people are at risk, or if they are incapable of consenting. Penhale (1993) refers to individuals at very grave risk or severely mentally impaired, and to a reluctance to report borne of dependency on the abuser, fear of making the situation worse, assuming blame and concerns about jeopardising the family's standing in the community. Quigley (2000) argues that, where a mentally capable person makes a free and informed choice to decline some or all of the interventions offered, their wishes should be respected. However, professionals may impose their judgement of a person's best interests where the public interest necessitates intervention. This arises where the abuser poses a risk to other vulnerable people, or the injuries are so severe that the police must act, or the victim's decision is based on an unacceptable degree of intimidation or exploitation that affects their personal safety. Similarly, Hugman (1995), Lawson (1999) and Wilson (1994) advise that otherwise competent people may be intimidated and prevented from acting, thereby jeopardising their own safety or exposing other people to risk. Thus, a decision that might appear free and informed can be heavily constrained by power and dependency, both emotional and economic.

The aforementioned research (Preston-Shoot and Wigley 2000) undertook a comparative analysis of procedures devised by different local authorities in partnership with other agencies. A survey of five inter-agency procedures relating to adult abuse illustrates the difficulty with the concept of self-determination and, arguably, the inadequacy of guidance for practice. . . .

Procedure One states that, where individuals choose to accept risk, their wishes should be respected within the context of their capacity to anticipate and understand the risk. The document gives some attention to assessment of mental incapacity but not other factors that may impact on decision-making. It does not provide a framework to assist practitioners to determine exceptions to 'the rule'. Practitioners are advised that common law allows for intervention, without consent, to save life or avoid serious harm, if the action is reasonable and can be professionally justified as immediately necessary. This is also mentioned in the next two sets of procedures.

Procedure Two includes a specific section on values, clearly emphasising empowerment and participation of the victim. Practitioners are advised that the right of vulnerable adults to make decisions about their own safety should be respected, but the guidance recognises that difficulties arise when it is unclear if the victim is capable of making decisions or if their decision is being made under duress. Practitioners are advised that, when a victim with capacity refuses intervention, this should be respected unless a failure to act will leave other vulnerable people at risk. This appears to negate the common law principle noted above and to privilege self-determination among ethical principles. It also adopts a negative freedom perspective on self-determination. Where intervention proceeds, in the guise of best interests, the victim's past and present feelings and wishes should be ascertained if possible (the third procedure also mentions this), and intervention should be limited to maintaining the person's safety.

Procedure Three, again in a specific section on values, opines that people should have the greatest possible control over their lives and should be able to make informed choices about their lifestyles, including taking risks. People who are afraid or are being intimidated should be offered realistic alternatives. An individual's wishes should only be overridden when it is necessary to protect other vulnerable adults from abuse, again limiting the use of common law. Assessment of capacity focuses exclusively on mental competence, excluding broader interpersonal dynamics, by considering a person's ability to understand and retain information relating to the required decision, and to weigh it in the balance. The procedure does state that the decision should be free but does not elaborate on what action to take if there is doubt on this point.

Procedure Four states that, when individuals can make an informed decision concerning their circumstances where risk has been identified, and when they reject intervention, their wishes must be respected except where a statutory responsibility to intervene exists. These are narrower grounds than in the previous two procedures. In such instances intervention should be at the minimum level required to provide necessary support and should be aimed at allowing individuals to achieve the highest level of independence, consistent with mitigating the perceived risks. The procedure then invites confusion by appearing to depart from its opening stance in relation to adults who are judged not competent and where immediate intervention is thought essential to reduce risk. Practitioners are advised to take action to remove or reduce the risks and to safeguard the individual, involving statutory powers if possible.

Procedure Five, as in the third procedure, adopts mental competence as the determinant of capacity but also recognises the presence in some cases of undue pressure to take a particular course of action. The principle of self-determination is seen as central but allows for exceptions where the decision follows an unacceptable degree of intimidation or exploitation, or where others may be at risk, or where an individual's own safety may be jeopardised unless the abuse is stopped.

Newly issued policy guidance (DoH 2000) is inconsistent in its approach to self-determination. At one point it unequivocally supports the principle, requiring agency policy to support an individual's right to independence based on choice and self-determination, recognising that this involves risks which should be discussed with the victim. Elsewhere it is more equivocal, suggesting that intervention may be justified following an assessment of seriousness, which includes the victim's vulnerability, the nature and extent of the abuse, the length of time it has been occurring, the impact on the victim, and the risk of repetition and escalation. The guidance stresses the importance of assessing context because exploitation, deception, misuse of authority, intimidation or coercion may render an individual incapable of making decisions. In such situations, the policy guidance recommends removing the victim from the sphere of influence so that they may reach a free (or freer) choice about how to proceed. Elsewhere, it appears to endorse intervention, noting that referral to the police should be made as a matter of urgency when complaints indicate that a criminal offence may have been committed. Practitioners may, however, circumvent such guidance if they perceive elder abuse through a welfare rather than criminal justice lens.

[. . .]

Finally, there are three particular problems with the concept of self-determination in relation to elder abuse as articulated in the literature. First, the focus is on the victim and the aim of intervention is often to move the victim away from the abuser (Wilson 1994). As has recently occurred in child care (Family Law Act 1996), perhaps the focus should shift to removal of the abuser.

Second, the focus on decision-making, and balancing the right to autonomy with the right to protection, has emphasised mental capacity but this leaves other older people at risk because they are judged mentally capable but may be intimidated or otherwise prevented from acting (Hugman 1995). As policy guidance now recognises (DoH 2000), the assessment of competence should include emotional alongside mental capacity.

Third, prioritising self-determination may lead to under-reporting (Penhale 1993).

The net result is that the application of self-determination in practice remains inconsistent (Whittington 1971). Case Study 2 illustrates how practice can veer between empowerment and protection, and alternately emphasise an individual's competence and incapacity.

Case Study 2

The referral came from a daughter concerned about her father, aged 70. He is looked after by his son who has a history of alcohol abuse and mental disorder. The victim sleeps on a soiled mattress, has lost weight and is malnourished. The daughter believes that the son physically abuses him. The house is filthy and devoid of food. The victim appears disoriented and confused.

The social worker and daughter want to contact the general practitioner and the police but the victim refuses, becoming anxious and upset. He does, however, agree to move temporarily into residential care, admission being achieved the same day. Following concern expressed by residential care staff, which threatens to disrupt the emergency placement, the victim is asked to sign a note agreeing that the son should not be informed of his whereabouts. This he does.

The general practitioner is asked to arrange a psychiatric assessment, again following concern from residential care staff about the victim's behaviour and capacity, which diagnoses moderate dementia. A review recommends permanent residential care, noting the subject's improved mobility and weight gain. The subject agrees.

Here the social worker's initial strategy was guided by not wanting to upset the 'client', hence the non-involvement of the police. However, the practitioner would have used statutory powers of removal (National Assistance Act 1948, section 47, rather than the provisions of the Mental Health Act 1983) if admission into residential care could not have been achieved 'voluntarily'. At times the subject is viewed as mentally competent to make decisions, even though there is concern about his confusion – for instance, about contact with the general practitioner and disclosure of his whereabouts to his son. At other times, his choices appear to be over-ruled. Once again, the strategy involved removing the subject rather than the abuser, despite knowing the dangers of moving vulnerable older people and having the option of using the law to remove the perpetrator of neglect and physical abuse.

Conclusion

Pritchard (1995) accepts that there are no right or wrong answers when faced with the kind of dilemmas encapsulated in Case Study 2. However, she argues that, when victims are mentally competent, social workers can only offer support and explain available options. They cannot impose solutions. One problem with this approach is the narrow view taken of self-determination. Another is the assumption that victims can exercise control over decision-making. Duress from others, or passive acceptance and personal blame, borne of internalised negative valuations people have experienced, lead to a subordinate position. A third is the absence of balance. Bennett and Kingston (1993) refer to compassion and control; the SSI (1993) to preventive *and* protective aspects of intervention. The former alone may risk further violence; the latter unnecessary rapidity in long-standing situations. Hence, the importance of assessment skills to identify levels of risk. Even so, for competent elders in immediate danger but refusing intervention, they, in common with others (for example, Lawson 1999), suggest maintaining contact, involving the victim in decision-making, activating support networks, advocacy and peer interaction and exploring fears and expectations. More, however, may be necessary, as the various legal provisions legitimate.

[...]

As Pritchard (2000) found, victims frequently remain in abusive situations because they do not know how or where to access practical advice and the information they need about accommodation and benefits. They identify their needs as supportive discussion, practical advice, and appropriate housing. I am not calling for authoritarian practice, or for defensive practice borne of an urge among practitioners to protect themselves or their agency.

[...]

Implicit, therefore, in this chapter is the importance of a values literacy. This connects values with social work law (Preston-Shoot *et al.* 2001), articulates the extent of and limits to a value principle, and outlines a way forward when interests collide. It suggests that practitioners should acknowledge their own orientation in relation to values, whether Kantian, utilitarian, or other (see Wilmot 1997, for a discussion about how these value positions differ), for this will influence their configuration of needs, rights and competing interests. It will shape their choice of options and outcomes. The new requirements of accountability require that the thinking underpinning decision-making must be transparent and credible. This requires practitioners to deconstruct concepts like self-determination in order to articulate considered arguments for the efficacy of particular actions (Payne 1999; Aymer and Okitikpi 2000). For instance, in relation to self-determination, it requires a sophisticated understanding of the difference between a positive obligation to provide good and a negative obligation to cause no harm. In relation to elder abuse work generally, it indicates the importance of reconsidering the balance between welfare and criminal justice discourses. If this is accompanied with a decision-making literacy, which offers different models for approaching situations where different interests collide or where dilemmas result in having to choose between 'disagreeable' options, then this will not erase tensions between self-determination and protection, but it may give a clearer direction to practice.

REFERENCES

Anderson, A. (1999) Elder abuse: the clinical reality. In: J. Pritchard (ed.) *Elder Abuse Work. Best Practice in Britain and Canada*. London: Jessica Kingsley Publishers.

Aymer, C. and Okitikpi, T. (2000) Epistemology, ontology and methodology: what's that got to do with social work? *Social Work Education* 19 (1), 67–75.

Banks, S. (1995) *Ethics and Values in Social Work*. London: Macmillan.

Bennett, G, and Kingston, P. (1993) *Elder Abuse: Concepts, Theories and Interventions*. London: Chapman and Hall.

Biehal, N. and Sainsbury, E. (1991) From values to rights in social work. *British Journal of Social Work* 21 (3), 245–257.

Braye, S. and Preston-Shoot, M. (1995) *Empowering Practice in Social Care*. Buckingham: Open University Press.

Cheetham, J. (1989) Values in action. In: S. Shardlow (ed.) *The Values of Change in Social Work*. London: Tavistock/Routledge.

Clark, C. (1998) Self-determination and paternalism in community care: practice and prospects. *British Journal of Social Work* 28 (3), 387–402.

Clark, C. (1999) Observing from the lighthouse: from theory to institutions in social work ethics. *European Journal of Social Work* 2 (3), 259–270.

Cornwell, N. (1992/93) Assessment and accountability in community care. *Critical Social Policy* 36, 40–52.

Davis, A. and Ellis, K. (1995) Enforced altruism in community care. In: R. Hugman and D. Smith (eds) *Ethical Issues in Social Work*. London: Routledge.

Department of Health (2000) *No Secrets: Guidance on Developing and Implementing Multi-Agency Policies and Procedures to Protect Vulnerable Adults from Abuse*. London: The Stationery Office.

Fearns, B. (1999) 'It is better to talk of bulls than be in the bull ring': elder abuse – a police perspective. In: J. Pritchard (ed.) *Elder Abuse Work. Best Practice in Britain and Canada*. London: Jessica Kingsley Publishers.

Hargreaves, S. and Hughes, B. (1996) The abuse of older people: an evaluation of the care management model and the impact of anti-discriminatory practice. *Practice* 8 (3), 19–30.

Horne, M. (1987) *Values in Social Work*. Aldershot: Wildwood House.

Hugman, R. (1995) The implications of the term 'elder abuse' for problem definition and response in health and social welfare. *Journal of Social Policy* 24 (4), 493–507.

Lawson, J. (1999) Developing a policy on abuse in residential and nursing homes. In: J. Pritchard (ed.) *Elder Abuse Work. Best Practice in Britain and Canada.* London: Jessica Kingsley Publishers.

Marsh, P. and Triseliotis, J. (1996) *Ready to Practise? Social Workers and Probation Officers: Their Training and First Year in Work.* Aldershot: Avebury.

McDermott, F. (ed.) (1975) *Self-Determination in Social Work. A Collection of Essays on Self-Determination and Related Concepts by Philosophers and Social Work Theorists.* London: Routledge and Kegan Paul.

National Association of Social Workers (1996) *Code of Ethics.* Washington, DC: NASW.

Payne, M. (1999) The moral bases of social work. *European Journal of Social Work* 2 (3), 247–258.

Penhale, B. (1993) The abuse of elderly people: considerations for practice. *British Journal of Social Work* 23 (2), 95–112.

Perlman, H. (1975) Self-determination: reality or illusion? In: F. McDermott (ed.) *Self-Determination in Social Work. A Collection of Essays on Self-Determination and Related Concepts by Philosophers and Social Work Theorists.* London: Routledge and Kegan Paul.

Preston-Shoot, M. (1996) A question of emphasis? On legalism and social work education. In: S. Jackson and M. Preston-Shoot (eds) *Educating Social Workers in a Changing Policy Context.* London: Whiting and Birch.

Preston-Shoot, M., Roberts, G. and Vernon, S. (2001) Values in social work law: strained relations or sustaining relationships? *Journal of Social Welfare and Family Law* 23 (1).

Preston-Shoot, M. and Wigley, V. (2000) *Evaluation of 'Abuse of Older People in Domestic Settings' Inter-Agency Procedures. Report to the Inter-Agency Group for Adult Protection.* Liverpool: John Moores University, School of Law and Applied Social Studies.

Pritchard, J. (1995) *The Abuse of Older People* (2nd edition). London: Jessica Kingsley Publishers.

Pritchard, J. (1999) Lessons learnt in working with elder abuse in the last decade. In: J. Pritchard (ed.) *Elder Abuse Work. Best Practice in Britain and Canada.* London: Jessica Kingsley Publishers.

Pritchard, J. (2000) *The Needs of Older Women: Services for Victims of Elder Abuse and Other Abuse.* Bristol: The Policy Press.

Quigley, L. (2000) Screen test. *Community Care* 16–22 March, 26–27.

Sainsbury, E. (1989) Participation and paternalism. In: S. Shardlow (ed.) *The Values of Change in Social Work.* London: Tavistock/Routledge.

Slater, P. and Eastman, M. (1999) *Elder Abuse: Critical Issues in Policy and Practice,* London: Age Concern England.

SSI (1993) *No Longer Afraid. The Safeguard of Older People in Domestic Settings: Practice Guidelines.* London: HMSO.

Timms, N. (1983) *Social Work Values: An Enquiry.* London: RKP.

Timms, N. (1986) Value-talk in social work: present character and future improvement. *Issues in Social Work Education* 6 (1), 3–14.

Timms, N. (1989) Social work values: context and contribution. In: S. Shardlow (ed.) *The Values of Change in Social Work.* London: Tavistock/Routledge.

Whittington, C. (1971) Self-determination re-examined. *British Journal of Social Work* 1 (3), 293–303.

Whittington, C. (1977) Social workers' orientations: an action perspective. *British Journal of Social Work* 7 (1), 73–95.

Wilmot, S. (1997) *The Ethics of Community Care*. London: Cassell.

Wilson, G. (1994) Abuse of elderly men and women among clients of a community psychogeriatric service. *British Journal of Social Work* 24, 681–700.

CHAPTER 23

OUT IN THE WORLD

Jean

I want to say a bit about where I used to live and my home from when I was a little girl. I was born in 1942 and I used to live in the country with my mother and father and brother in Banham, Norfolk. We had a thatched house and I can remember we had candlelight, and the tin bath in front of the coal fire. I used to do messages for my Mum to the newspaper shop, and I played with my brother Charlie in the garden – he used to chase me. I went to the village school which I liked and I made good friends there who used to come home to play.

When I was about twelve I went to boarding school which was a special sort of boarding school. I went there for reading and writing and everything. It was alright there. They were very kind to us in the Hall where we lived, but at the school down the lane it was very strict. I got whipped with the cane, the cane, the cane! for being a nuisance. They used to in them days, you know ... and after that I was alright. We used to get squared up and get told off ... and sometimes I were a little devil! Then I used to go home for leaves and things like that, backwards and forwards. But I used to stay there sometimes. I didn't used to go home, I used to stop there when the school term had finished. That was a nice school though. The caning didn't worry me too much, but I just used to go through it. I used to get wrong for not doing writing properly. You see, I couldn't grasp it ... but they said I'd get better and better, which I have.

I had to go away to boarding school because my father was violent, he was drunk, really drunk. He used to go out drinking really a lot ... you see, he couldn't stop. He hit me once or twice, several times when I was small, with a belt, with a strap, really violent. He used to shut me in a cupboard, and he put my head down our well once ... you know, one of these old-fashioned wells. Course, I had to go away ... that's how I got in them places ... I should never have been there, I should never have been there from the start. I felt safer in boarding school . . . I went there for protection. They told me they were going to put him away, but they couldn't keep him in prison.

From boarding school I had to go into a hospital when I was thirteen. I can remember my Mum taking me. I know why I went in there, that's because of my father . . . that's why I had to leave home. My Mum thought I'd be better off in there for a little while. She used to write me letters, and she used to come and visit me a lot . . . every weekend. And she had two enormous black eyes what my father gave her. We were very close, I was, to my mother . . . I was very close to her. But then I never made it out again, because she died. She had sugar diabetes . . . yes, that and other things, like being bruised. I think I was about nineteen when she died.

I went to school in the hospital and then I used to work there. There's one nurse who still pops round to see me. She knew me since I was a little girl. She used to beg me to get into the bath, because I never used to get in the bath till she was on duty . . . there had to be that certain nurse on. Oh, she said I was a little terror! I used to help her. I was her right-hand woman on the wards. F6 and F3 – they were my wards. I used to look after the children, used to bathe them and make the beds and used to go back at night and feed them. I loved that work because it was children . . . they needed looking after and I felt sorry for them. I was able to communicate with some of them, but it was a bit hard . . . they couldn't speak a lot. And then I used to work in the laundry, folding up and ironing the sheets. I liked the laundry work and meeting the laundry-men who used to chat me up!

I met my husband John in hospital when he was fifteen, and we used to meet in secret the other side of the laundry when no-one was looking! They weren't very keen on us mixing. We weren't together, that weren't allowed. But we still kept it up. We used to sneak out! I remember when we used to go to church we used to sit with me on one side and John would be on the other. So we used to wave 'Toodle-oo'! There weren't nothing in hospital so why not make a life while I was in there?

Mind you, while I was in there I lost my temper a lot . . . that was just being in there and that was one thing I couldn't help. It was agitation, frustration, anger really, from being there. But as soon as I came out, I controlled it. I was put on F8 and I hated it in there. You could go out, but you had to be back at a certain time or the doors were locked. I didn't like that. I didn't understand it, because I wasn't a bad case. Then I did get my own key for F8 because I was trustworthy. I met my great friend while I was in there. She was a student nurse and we were the same age! We go back a long way – she helped me a lot – and she still comes to see me now.

In 1966 when I was about twenty-four I moved from the hospital into a hostel. There was a doctor in the hospital, Dr S. and she gave me a lot of help. She said, 'You understand now, Jean, that you can't be here much longer ... it's about time you had your discharge'. And when she told me that, oh my goodness, I didn't know where to put my face! I couldn't believe it ... And I still can't! Oh I was happy, I was pleased! I said 'Hip hip hooray!' And my brother Charlie helped to get me out too, as he had spoken to Dr S. She checked on my I.Q. I had to go through all that before I came out. They do it to everybody, just to see how intelligent you really are. I had to do all these old bricks on this table. I think that's childish really. Those bricks! You had to pile them all up. I said to Dr S., 'Do you think I'm a child?' She said, 'Your I.Q.'s alright, you shouldn't be here. I'll give you your freedom, you can be free.'

It was much better in the hostel because that's more homely, you can get out when you want, come home when you want. It was like your own home. I couldn't believe it. The doors were open. They weren't closed and they weren't locked. That was one blessing. I felt relieved. It just felt like freedom. It wasn't so strict. But when you leave them places, you come out in the world, and that's hard to grasp. In the hostel I still kept up with John. He used to phone me and I used to meet him up the city ... on the quiet.

I went out to work from the hostel. I did two house jobs and also worked part-time at Macintoshes [Chocolate Factory]. I liked my house jobs because you could sit and have a coffee – they'd give you a break and you used to sit there and talk. I liked that. They were very friendly. I used to do cleaning up, dusting and things like that and sometimes they'd pop out and leave me in the house on my own. But crossing roads! That was the worst of it! I used to dread crossing that road. When it came to crossing roads, I had to get myself out of it, because that was making me nervous ... even more ... to think I'd got to be out in the world on my own. Yes that was the worst thing in my life then. Because I'd had no traffic where I was, did I? How on earth did I get across that road? But I helped myself. I had to do it myself.

At the hostel I still felt I was closed in, and wanting to get out, right out. I had more or less freedom there, but not the freedom I'm getting now. Then my father died. I wouldn't be out if he was still alive because he'd chase me up. If he didn't pass on, I'd want to stay in the hostel. Soon as I knew he'd gone, I wanted to come out. So I made another step forwards instead of backwards, and after the hostel, I went into a Group Home in about 1975. I was allowed to leave the hostel because I got on, didn't I? And then John also came to the Group Home and we stayed for a while until we got this flat. I worked myself up to get this ... I helped myself. I'd rather have my own place. I couldn't believe my eyes when I saw this flat ... I mean I'd been in those places all that while. And we got married! You wouldn't believe this, but we took ourselves down to City Hall without anyone knowing. But mind you we had to tell people in the end and the social worker helped us. The date was 24 January 1980! I used to wonder how we did it!

At first when we moved into the flat we had a Warden. I was told that we were going to be living on our own, but apparently there were two wardens up here ... I never dreamt that ... I thought we were going to be completely on our own. I put up the flags when they went! We're quite capable of looking after ourselves. What I do in my place is my business and nothing to do with anyone else. I don't need social workers now! We've grasped it!

In 1996 I started talking to Sheena about my life. I'm interested in research now, and I had the idea of starting a 'Memories Group' to talk about our memories of hospital and the hostel. I wanted these meetings to carry on to talk about different things and they did.

My life has had lots of changes. It's interesting to talk about it. It's made us think we're not, what can I say, not shut in any more. I feel as though I'm opened ... I feel as though I'm out, I'm not in. I feel happy the way I am. I didn't realise then what I do now and the situation what I've been through in the past. It was important to tell my story so people can understand. It has let people know what I have been through in my life ... and just to let them know I've been pushed from pillar to post! I want people to know the life I've had – but they don't believe me, you know. I've had a life! People think that when you've been in them sort of places you need someone to look after you ... they think we're stupid but we're not! Just because I can't read or write very well that don't stop me from doing things, do it? But we can manage on our own and come out in the community.

CHAPTER 24

THE PROSPECT OF RESIDENTIAL CARE

Jaber Gubrium

The phrases 'shake the past' or 'forget the past' are regularly used as a guide for positive personal adjustment. This is based on the idea that time and experience can be divided into distinct portions, which can be selectively emphasised, suppressed, or eliminated. Given effective management of life history, one can successfully dwell in a particular portion of a lifetime. Commonplace remarks such as 'You're living totally in the past' and 'You're always thinking about the future' suggest as much.

Intervention conveys preference for living in the present. Tradition is viewed as a likely cause of many troubles in daily life, preventing those affected from casting off troubles linked with past ties and forming relations appropriate to present conditions. By and large, living in the past is a negative adjustment. A caregiver's living in the past suggests a lack of realism about present responsibilities. The care receiver who expects treatment in accordance with past obligations or sentiments places an unrealistic burden on the caregiver. Positive adjustment means being 'realistic', which, in turn, means being oriented to present realities. The idea that one might be positively adjusted by placing past obligations to the care receiver at the centre of one's current relationship with him or her is unrealistic.

The problem with the future is not that one is likely to 'live there', which would be the future equivalent of living in the past, but that one might persist in dwelling on positive times to come. Chance is best figured in terms of present conditions rather than in terms of uncertain future prospects. In other words, the future is best treated as an extension of the

Source: *The Mosaic of Care: Frail Elderly and their Families in the Real World*, Springer, New York, 1990, pp. 72–4, 88–92.

present. Given the frailty of care receivers, the ageing process, and the increasing burden of care, the future bodes negatively unless it is faced realistically. Present conditions are likely to get worse. For a positive adjustment it is altogether reasonable to raise the question of the care receiver's institutionalisation.

A present-centred preference applies to all, not just the caregiver. Ideally, frail elderly are expected in time to make the transition from avoiding the prospect of nursing home placement to the realisation that increasing impairment is beyond the capability of the most devoted caregiver. The much used phrase, 'the second victim', aptly conveys a negative outcome. Frail elderly who are not lucid enough to take stock of caregiving in support of ostensibly realistic decisions can be spoken for. Statements like 'Martha [a demented care receiver] would realise the burden of care if she could and would want you [the caregiver] to think about a nursing home' are commonplace. Even the caregiver can be spoken for. A former caregiver who has placed her husband in a nursing home and is now a facilitator puts it this way in explaining to Katherine, a caregiving wife, what the wife 'really' feels, despite heroic efforts and claims to the contrary:

Katherine, we all know what you're saying. Each of us has been there, believe me. Oh, how we've been there! But have you asked yourself what you're saying? Have you really, really listened to yourself lately? My dear, you sound a lot like I did last year when Bill [her now institutionalized husband] was at home vegetating. He didn't even know my name. I kept saying to myself, 'I'm his wife. I love him. I know he'd do the same for me if I was in his shoes.' Katherine, face it. You're not that different. Face up to what you're really feeling right now. Forget the past for a minute. I know now that what I was really saying to myself underneath it all was, 'Bill, I'm sorry, really sorry, but it's just too much for me now and I need to do something before I fall apart.' I just know that's what you're feeling Katherine, but I know, too, how you don't want to admit it.

Of course not all caregivers accept such interpretations of their presumed 'real' thoughts and feelings about the past, present, and future. In practice, the question of institutionalisation presents caregivers and family members with diverse ways of addressing the future as it weighs on the present.

While sympathy is extended to anyone burdened by caregiving, ideally, in due course the realistic caregiver comes around to display the proper attitude. When the proper attitude is not forthcoming, the caregiver or family member is said to be unrealistic and, in the final analysis, a 'martyr' or 'denying'. The martyr does not accord with the linear view of personal adjustment because he or she is said to 'need' to prove that a tradition of filial responsibility is dutifully in effect. The denier does not accord with the linear view because he or she does not realise what really is being felt 'underneath it all'. The martyr gives priority to tradition while the denier unwittingly ignores the significance of newly emerging ties with the care receiver.

From the nursing home and support groups to family homes, attendant professional workers by and large take formal account of responses to the question of institutionalisation in linear terms. Dora's four-stage interpretation of Harry's adjustment to the care of his wife Ruth is exemplary. References are made to both popular and professional literature conveying the same point of view. Professional competence is signalled by references to 'models', 'theories', and other formal designs claimed to represent the course of personal adjustment in the broader context of the institutionalisation decision.

Professional workers can be annoyed by the conceptual obligations of their competence (Gubrium, Buckholdt and Lynott 1989). For example, a nurse who, despite a professional commitment to represent adjustment in linear terms, pleads with her colleagues to attend to experiential timings, informing them she is aware that there is more to the care experience than a course of adjustment. But, like the past that is said to tell only of things long gone, thereby constituting the realistic present, the linear view is not simply set aside for what is sensed to be more diversely organised. Dissention risks casting doubt on professional competence itself.

The language of stages, adjustment, past abnegation, current reality, and future forecasting based on the present is virtually in the air everyone breathes about the why's and wherefore's of responding to caregiving. In this regard, what the service provider conveys in the capacity of a professional merely reflects what is generally understood (Gubrium 1986a, 1989). [...]

Mary's story

Mary is the sixty-two-year-old caregiver of her mother, Nina, who is eighty-four and suffers from Alzheimer's disease. They live across the street from each other in separate houses. After Nina's husband dies, younger members of the extended family move in with Nina at various times. It offers a modicum of independence from parents for the young people and provides live-in supervision for Nina. Mary is the primary caregiver.

Mary always has lived near her mother, either in the same neighbourhood, in each other's homes, or, currently, on the same street. They have been best friends. As Mary remarks, 'When Mother was up and about, people used to think we were older and younger sisters; we were always together.' Nina's forgetfulness, confusion, and occasional incontinence cause Mary as much emotional distress as it is physically burdensome. Mary misses the 'old Nina', the company they kept, and the bosom companionship they provided each other.

Mary's husband, Don, always has been cool to Nina. As Nina's dementia, physical health, and her presence in and about his home increasingly takes Mary away from him and the family, Don's resentment flares. But Mary understands:

> Poor Don. I know what he's going through. Who wouldn't? I'm torn between having to tend to Mother and keeping him company. A man needs a wife around. It's his companion. Still, she's my mother and I really, really feel that, as long as she's with us [Mary knocks on wood], I'll try to make her life as comfortable as possible. [Details her daily cares for Nina.]
>
> Mother and I were always very, very close. I think you'd say we were best friends. Don was pretty good about it, but I think underneath he really resented it, especially when I took time away from him and the boys [their three children]. In a way, I was lucky to have boys, because the men in the family did a lot of men things together anyway. I always wished I had had a daughter though, like Mother.

Judged by the literature on social support, home care, and institutionalisation, Nina's situation gets high marks for keeping her in the community and out of a nursing home (Johnson and Grant 1985, chap. 4). A major factor in institutionalisation is the lack of a support system. In Nina's case, various adult grandchildren reside with her offering supervision and a daughter is conveniently available for personal cares and home management. But Nina's home care is not only affected by a support system. A wider social network of ties indirectly impinges on the support system.

While a social network is a configuration of ties, it is not necessarily supportive. As Morgan (1989) points out in a study of adjustment to widowhood, social networks do not always 'really make it easier'. The implication is that the broader network of social ties should be paid closer attention in examining the effect of social support on the chance of institutionalisation. On balance, part of a network of social ties actually may 'push' a care receiver out of the home while another part may only weakly 'pull' the receiver back in (Gubrium and Lynott 1987).

In Mary's story, Don is exasperated with what he sees as his wife's and children's unrealistic devotion. It requires unacceptable time commitments. To complicate matters, Mary's active participation in a local support group for caregivers of Alzheimer's disease victims conveys mixed messages about whether the time for nursing home placement is rapidly approaching in Nina's case. Certain support group friends suggest that it is unrealistic for Mary to continue carrying the daily load of her mother's care, while others feel differently.

Nina's support system is virtually under siege as members of her broader social network variously perceive looming troubles, not mere inconveniences, in the home care situation. Mary has become the proverbial 'woman in the middle', caught between the claims and commitments of separate generations and the contrasting sentiments of respected friends and acquaintances (Brody 1981). In this context, the question of whether 'it's time' is not simple and straightforward. The many versions of her story confuse Mary: what she has always told herself, what her husband is now vociferously demanding, and what others variously convey.

Mary's story also shows that the question of institutionalisation is as much imaginatively addressed as it is figured in relation to versions of particular concrete conditions of care. Mary contemplates 'both sides' – what it would mean for both her and her mother if Nina were placed in a nursing home and what it would mean for them if Nina remained at home in Mary's care. In a related conversation in her home, Mary talks about the dilemma. She starts by poignantly reminding me of what she knows we both have heard, time and again, concerning how one placed in a nursing home 'must feel' leaving a home and lifelong ties behind, to spend his or her remaining days alone in an institution.

> You can imagine how it must feel to leave your family behind – all your friends, your kids, your home, all of it. Think about it. It's done. It's over. There you are, all alone, nothing of yours around to remind you that you're Jay or you're Mary. It must be awful. That's what I think of, day in and day out, when I think about what Don and the others say I should do. I know they mean well ... and poor Don ... what am I going to do with him? He's suffering too.

I remind Mary that we both also have heard caregivers say that there gets to be a point when 'it's time', when the Alzheimer's disease patient does not recognise the caregiver any more, or even those known a lifetime. When I mention that perhaps such persons would not suffer so, Mary sharpens the image presented earlier:

> Yes. I know. But did you ever stop to think, like I have, that maybe ... I know she [Nina] sounds very confused and she can't tell us much.... Maybe deep, deep down inside, maybe she knows what's going on, like she's trying to reach out but isn't able to say it so it comes out right? Who really knows? I thought about that real hard

when Cathy [a support group participant] ... that poor woman. I really feel sorry for her. Since she put Hal [Cathy's husband] at Mill-haven [a nursing home], she just cries and cries every time she thinks about how he feels in there. I think about it ... Mother in there and she's in a wheelchair, and like she calls out something nobody can understand and what she wants to say is like 'Mary, Mary, please help me. Mary, come and get me. Mary, hug me because I'm so alone.' [Long pause.] Everyone has a soul, you know. We can't just forget that. [Mary weeps.]

Mary of course knows that there is another version to the story. She hears it told in varied detail in her support group. It is a story of a caregiver who cannot admit, despite all evidence to the contrary, that a loved one has, for all practical purposes, died as a person. Mary has heard others describe how the Alzheimer's patient, in time, becomes an 'empty shell' and how life for those who insist on caring for such an individual is like a 'funeral that never ends'. Mary knows, too, that this story has holes. As she asks implicitly in the preceding extract, is that so-called empty shell really empty? How can one know for sure? Maybe Alzheimer's is an incapacity to communicate, not the death of a soul. What is known of such matters in the final analysis (Gubrium 1986b, 1988)?

Mary says that there are times she believes what the evidence suggests, which is that Nina is no longer that mother Mary once knew. On these occasions, Mary wants to believe that Don, her husband, is right. She wishes desperately to be rid of her alleged denial. As she has so often been told, she wants to put the past behind, look to the future, and begin to think about her own health and well-being. She hopes to be on her way to making the 'right decision'. Yet a particularly telling comment of hers suggests that the process of adjustment is more an idea she has to convince herself of than it represents what caregivers actually go through: 'Maybe if I keep telling myself that that's the way it is [the various stages one goes through], I'll eventually believe it and things'll work out like they say they should.' Again we find that linear time and personal adjustment are as much themes applied to experience as they are facts of caregiving.

REFERENCES

Brody, Elaine. 1981. 'Women in the middle and family help to older people', *The Gerontologist* 21:271–282.

Gubrium, Jaber F. 1986a. *Oldtimers and Alzheimer's: The Descriptive Organization of Senility.* Greenwich, CT: JAI Press.

Gubrium, Jaber F. 1986b. 'The social preservation of mind: The Alzheimer's disease experience', *Symbolic Interaction* 6:37–51.

Gubrium, Jaber F. 1988. 'Incommunicables and poetic documentation in the Alzheimer's disease experience', *Semiotica* 72:235–253.

Gubrium, Jaber F. 1989. 'Local cultures and service policy'. In Jaber F. Gubrium and David Silverman (eds), *The Politics of Field Research: Sociology Beyond Enlightenment*. London: Sage.

Gubrium, Jaber F., David R. Buckholdt and Robert J. Lynott. 1989. 'The descriptive tyranny of forms'. In James A. Holstein and Gale Miller (eds), *Perspectives on Social Problems*, vol. 1, Greenwich, CT: JAI Press.

Gubrium, Jaber F. and Robert J. Lynott. 1987. 'Measurement and the interpretation of burden in the Alzheimer's disease experience', *Journal of Aging Studies* 1:265–285.

Johnson, Colleen L. and Leslie A. Grant. 1985. *The Nursing Home in American Society*. Baltimore: Johns Hopkins University Press.

Morgan, David L. 1989. 'Adjusting to widowhood: Do social networks really make it easier?' *The Gerontologist* 29:101–107.

CHAPTER 25

INDEPENDENCE, PRIVACY AND RISK

Rosemary Bland

Residential care for older people in the UK originated in the nineteenth-century Poor Law asylums, which provided a harsh regime of custodial care designed to deter and stigmatise people in need. Common elements of their institutional routines have been identified as batch treatment, regimentation, depersonalisation and segregation (Booth 1985). With the break-up of the Poor Law in 1948 (Means and Smith 1983), it was suggested that the 'master' and 'inmate' relationship which had previously existed between Public Assistance Institution managers and older people should change to resemble that between a hotel manager and his or her guest (Townsend 1962). A 'hotel relationship' would become feasible because people would no longer go into homes because of destitution but from choice, using their retirement pension to pay local authorities for their care (Means and Smith 1983). If an economic rent was charged, 'any old people who would wish to go might go there in exactly the same way as many well-to-do people have been accustomed to go into *residential hotels*' (my emphasis) (Bevan quoted in Sinclair 1988: 244).

However, given the limited finance available for new buildings the parliamentary and media enthusiasm for the 'hotel' relationship was unrealistic (Means and Smith 1983). Pensions were too small to enable most people to pay the full costs of care so public subsidy was required and 'need' remained the determinant of admission (Sinclair 1988). Need was defined by professional gatekeepers not, as Bevan had intended, by older people themselves. So the 'guest and hotel keeper' relationship never

Source: 'Independence, privacy and risk: two contrasting approaches to residential care for older people', *Ageing and Society* 19.5, pp. 542–60.

developed. Research published fourteen years later found that, despite post-war aspirations, many former Poor Law buildings, standards and staff attitudes to residents were unchanged (Townsend 1962). Attempts were made to improve the situation and promote the desired model of new residential homes to local authorities [. . .]

These documents gave confused and sometimes conflicting messages to local authorities about the care they were expected to provide. On the one hand guidance stressed that older people moving into care would lose no more rights or privileges than if they entered 'other establishments such as hotels' (DHSS 1977: para. 4); yet recommended that staff assume responsibility for residents' medicines and encourage them in 'meaningful activity' (etc.). Thus the approach to care and the reality of resident status were more like that of hospital patient than autonomous adult or hotel guest.

[. . .] The debate about the role of homes as hotels or places for 'needy' people was revived in the 1980s by the significant growth in private sector care, fuelled by alterations in state funding arrangements for residents. The quantity and type of residential provision expanded and, theoretically at least, increased choice for older people – as Bevan had originally intended (Sinclair 1988; Phillips 1992). The less prosperous majority of older people had a brief opportunity to opt for residential care using social security funding, since eligibility was based solely on income rather than any defined 'need for care'. [. . .]

The small social science literature on hotels (Wood 1994) does not indicate any of the ambiguity or uncertainty of purpose which surrounds residential care. Hotels are defined as public organisations which offer individualised service in return for payment (Mars and Nicod 1984). [. . .] The commodity that hotels of all kinds trade in is personal service. The stratification in the hotel industry only serves to create 'different expectations of the extent and quality of [that] personal service' (Wood 1994: 70). Whether hotels meet their customers' expectations or not is a crucial element of satisfaction. [. . .]

At the individual hotel level, hospitality is 'managed' in order to maintain the decorum and privacy which underlie acceptable social relations in public. Guests expect hotels to treat them as private individuals. The challenge for the hotel lies in meeting this expectation whilst continuing to operate a generalised business function to *sets* of individuals. [. . .]

The case study home

The married couple who owned the case study home had both previously worked as hoteliers. [. . .] The home's approach to its residents resembled the personal service orientation of hotels. There was a sense that residents expected to be and were treated by the owners as individuals. There was no obvious emphasis on 'the resident group' or any sign that the home functioned as a surrogate community as in some local authority homes (Davies and Knapp 1981). The residents appeared to have retained a considerable measure of independence, control and privacy in their lives. We sent residents a brief postal questionnaire about aspects of their care, and used subsequent individual interviews to find out how far our impressions of the home were a reality for them. We asked about aspects of life which previous research had identified as important to users (Sinclair 1988; NISW 1988) as well as addressing the core values promoted by the Social Services Inspectorate (DoH/SSI 1989). Residents were asked how far they could safeguard their privacy and control their immediate physical environment; whether enough activities were provided, whether they could gain access to community health services when they wanted and whether staff respected residents' privacy. All twelve residents who responded to the survey replied affirmatively to these questions. All but one were satisfied with the food and the activities offered, and ten of the twelve were satisfied with the level of heating.

The questionnaire invited residents to identify aspects of home life which they liked, disliked or would change. Again, they recorded high levels of satisfaction in their responses. Most did not mention any dislikes. One person was critical of staff and three people criticised the quality and quantity of the food at tea-time and the heating, which was sometimes inadequate. The highest number of positive comments was made about the owners, the care staff, the services and the atmosphere in the home. Other valued aspects were the freedom, privacy and cleanliness of the home, and the gardens. This home received the highest level of positive endorsement from residents in the six homes visited. All the residents in the case study home who returned the questionnaires gave positive responses to six of the nine questions asked about life there.

In the subsequent individual interviews, two interesting differences with public sector resident interviews emerged. First, the private home residents expressed particular appreciation of the owners' flexibility and attention to them as individuals, giving numerous examples. These included providing vegetarian meals made from home grown vegetables for one resident; and accepting another resident's pet dog as well as her grand piano, on which she was able to continue giving music lessons. Public sector residents were appreciative of staff in general rather than commenting about the quality of their relationship as individuals with the homes' managers. Secondly, the case study home residents responded confidently to questions about the way dissatisfactions or complaints were handled. The owners had asked them to raise any dissatisfactions with them direct rather than discussing them among themselves. This gave residents three important messages. First, that they recognised that there would be elements of home life which would displease individual residents from time to time; secondly, that residents had a right to voice these displeasures and thirdly, that the owners wanted residents to mention any dissatisfactions to them direct in order to address them straight away. Half the residents interviewed had raised matters at some time and declared themselves satisfied with the owners' prompt response. This contrasted with residents' awareness of whom they should address complaints to in the public sector homes, but their general lack of experience of actually doing so, despite some dissatisfactions with aspects of their care expressed during the research interviews.

Residents' relatives were also asked to complete a brief postal questionnaire on aspects of quality in the six homes. They showed similarly high levels of satisfaction with the case study home and the care given to their relatives. All relatives enjoyed privacy on their visits and knew where to address complaints if not satisfied in any way. Ninety per cent of those who responded did not want any changes to the way the home was run. This was the strongest expression of relatives' satisfaction across the six homes. Again the largest number of positive comments made were about staff (more than in the other five homes). These questionnaire responses from residents and relatives confirmed the high scores obtained by the home on the quality of care questionnaire administered in the survey phase of the research and our impressions during the field visits.

Contrasting approaches

I now want to examine how the private home's *service approach* to the care of its residents differed from *the social care approach* of local authority homes in certain key respects; notably in the home's attitude to residents' privacy, freedom of choice and independence and in the way it managed risk. [. . .]

The case study home provided residents with individual rooms which were lockable, all with en-suite facilities; the only home in the region offering such a high level of amenity when it had opened three years previously, and still comparatively rare. The postal questionnaire asked residents about using and securing their privacy within their rooms. All twelve residents who returned questionnaires responded positively to these questions. When a resident's GP visited them, they did so in the resident's own room and a member of staff was present only if the resident wished. The home was successful in according residents their privacy because it provided the physical accommodation for them to do so and because the owners applied the normal social conventions of privacy between strangers as hotels do, and transmitted these to the care staff. Residents respected the staff's right to their privacy by not going into the kitchen and were able to maintain control over their privacy and exercise choice in terms of personal care. When they moved into the home, the owners discussed with residents the kind of assistance they wanted, such as whether they wished to be helped with bathing and whether they wanted to have breakfast in bed. This discussion was the basis on which individualised care was provided.

The social care approach does not adhere to the normal social conventions about preserving privacy between strangers in public places because these conventions differ from those which exist in two settings which it tries unsuccessfully to combine in residential care. These are the hospital setting, where the patient may temporarily forgo their normal, conventional expectations of privacy in pursuit of treatment, and the domestic home which is quintessentially private, where the adults in the family are not strangers and where expectations of privacy between family members are less clear-cut. The attitudes of staff implementing the social care approach to residents' privacy are therefore governed by a social construction of the resident as 'patient' or 'family member', even 'child', any of which roles do not imply a guaranteed right of privacy. The prime function of the residential home is 'to care', that is to take responsibility for or take charge of people who are deemed unable to care for themselves, an ideology of caring which Morris (1993) suggests underpins practice in both health and social services. Normal social conventions surrounding privacy are therefore seen as inappropriate or impracticable at best or dangerous at worst, since residents need to be under staff surveillance if their welfare is to be safeguarded. This highlights the gap between the rhetoric of policy documents which place great emphasis on resident privacy and choice and the reality of care in practice.

Acknowledging residents' independence or autonomy involves staff in homes giving up some of their power and control, thereby incurring an element of calculated risk (Adams 1996). This is not something local authority homes find easy to do because they see their primary function as to carry out their statutory 'duty of care' which may be deemed incompatible with allowing residents to take risks and possibly come to some harm by doing so. In the case study home, the residents' right to retain their independence seemed to be taken for granted by the owners. This autonomy extended to residents engaging in some potentially risky activities if they chose. For instance, there were no rules about smoking and residents were free to smoke when and where they wished, including in their bedrooms. The owners appeared to respect what Wood chooses to call 'the bourgeois notion of the sovereignty of the self' (1994: 74). The owners knew which residents smoked. They included one very heavy smoker who had epilepsy, which constituted an even greater potential risk. The owners described how they had assessed the risk involved and taken a number of precautions to minimise it, with help from the local fire officer. Safety was promoted through fire doors and by installing smoke alarms in each room and by dividing the house into a number of zones and assembly points. Waste paper bins in the smokers' bedrooms were not lined, as an additional precaution. The owners were aware of the potential risks involved in giving residents that degree of autonomy but because they were in the home most of the time, they were able to manage, monitor and carry that risk themselves. Hotels cannot prevent guests smoking in the privacy of their bedrooms and must manage the risk of fire, relying on technical means to minimise it. The private home owners adopted a similar approach, whereas local authority homes minimise the risk by restricting smoking to one area of the home or by holding residents' smoking materials on their behalf. Smoking in bedrooms is usually forbidden. The social care approach tends to be more directive and paternalistic, focusing on the health and safety of the resident group as a whole rather than on maintaining the autonomy of the individual.

The private home used technical means to manage the potential risk surrounding another activity, namely that of bathing. The en-suite facilities in all bedrooms reinforced the possibility of the initiative and control over bathing or showering remaining with the resident. Residents decided when they wished to take a bath, and help from staff was available for those who wished it but was not routinely imposed. Residents who bathed or showered without assistance were therefore able to safeguard their dignity and their privacy when performing these intimate personal care activities. Hotels are preoccupied with maintaining a state of normality and with respecting guests' rights to their privacy. For the private home residents who chose to bathe without help, technical means were again used to manage the risks involved. Each bathroom was equipped with grab rails, seats and pull cords so that the resident could summon help if it was needed.

Although local authority homes usually have mobility aids and alarm mechanisms in bathrooms, these do not appear to minimise risk enough for staff to feel able to let residents be the judge of whether they can bathe safely without help. Moreover, staff have made a 'professional' assessment of the individual's need for assistance with which the resident may feel unable to disagree. A tendency towards risk avoidance rather than risk management, by assisting all residents to some degree, undermines their independence, privacy and dignity. [. . .]

The service approach in the case study private home offered residents choices about their everyday lives within a range set by the home but which largely matched their expectations. Thus, market segmentation and a diversity of approaches to care can enable a closer fit between the kind of care residents (and their relatives) are seeking and that which homes are able to provide. In the service approach the 'expert' about needs and wants is ostensibly the resident, so long as they and the owner/manager have shared expectations about what the home is offering. Homes which operate the social care approach may put less emphasis on the importance of residents' wants or expectations, since it is the staff's professional definitions of what constitutes residents' welfare which have the greatest influence on the overall approach to care.

The statutory model of care expects homes in all sectors to enable residents to enjoy privacy, dignity, independence, choice and fulfilment in residential care and for their rights as adult citizens to be safeguarded. The approach to caring is supposed to derive from these values. However, in the social care approach the values themselves may be open to varied inter-pretation by staff (Dixon 1991). The central concern of the service approach is to manage the hospitality it is providing successfully. This is achieved by ensuring that guests' privacy, independence, dignity and freedom of choice are maintained. These are normal, taken-for-granted elements of hospitality in hotels. The core values associated with the statu-tory model of care are more akin to the hospitality model of hotels than to those associated with hospital or domestic or familial models of care. Some local authorities have now moved from producing generalised state-ments about residents' rights in homes to individual service agreements or contracts with residents. These cover the basis on which they are resident and their care is provided, as required of independent sector homes by inspection units. However, residential care 'is still one of the most insecure forms of accommodation, with no legal framework for security of resi-dence or rights to a contract' (Wagner Development Group 1992: 77).

Conclusion

This paper has compared two approaches to the delivery of residential care for older people, principally in terms of their success in treating residents as autonomous adults and managing any associated risk. I have suggested that the service approach adopted in the private home derived from the owners' previous experience of providing a residential service and manag-ing hospitality in hotels. This approach appeared to be more successful in realising the core values of independence, choice, privacy, and dignity for residents than the social care approach adopted in local authority homes. It is suggested that four main factors account for this. First, the right of residents to retain their autonomy and independence was not contested by the owners or care staff. Risks were calculated and managed using tech-nical means, rather than by restricting residents' freedom of action through the imposition of rules and sanctions. Secondly, residents were able to maintain control over their lives because they and the staff had a shared understanding of, and mutual respect for, the normal social conventions of privacy which they applied to both residents' rooms and staff quarters. The provision of television and tea-making facilities in bedrooms encour-aged residents to use them during the day as bed-sitting rooms rather than solely for sleeping at night. Residents could therefore choose to spend time in the company of other residents or enjoy the privacy of their room. Thirdly, residents were primarily responded to by the home owners as socially competent adults who were paying for (or contributing to the cost of) a service, rather than as frail, vulnerable people who had been identi-fied as needing to be cared for and protected like children. The home responded to its residents who had dementia with the same respect for the adult 'self' shown to other residents, not as children. Fourthly, because the home owners had a background in hotels rather than the caring professions, they had no difficulty in seeing residents as the 'experts' about their needs and wishes. Residents retained greater control over their lives because the owners had no sense of their own professionalism or role as 'carers' being undermined or threatened. They worked to a model of hospitality which included assistance with personal care as part of the overall service rather than being seen as the central function of the enterprise.

Although the social care approach emphasises privacy as a core value in homes, this is in conflict with the overriding need for staff to minimise or avoid risks by keeping residents under surveillance. The approach denies privacy to residents who have to share bedrooms, cannot lock their rooms or who have to submit to assistance with bathing. Such arrangements resemble the model of care delivered by hospitals or a domestic model of parenting, rather than the normal cultural expectations surrounding the privacy and dignity which would apply in hotels and the home operating the service approach. There is uncertainty as to whether residential care homes are supposed to be run like hospitals, hotels or domestic residences. This leads to a lack of shared expectations and understandings between staff and residents about the objectives of the service and what are 'normal' conventions of social behaviour for each group.

There is some evidence from this case study to suggest that both the residential service model of hospitality used by hotels which respects the right of guests to their privacy and autonomy, and the use of technical means to manage risk, can be applied to a residential care home setting with positive outcomes for the quality of residents' lives. Major studies of care in local authority homes have concluded that it does not currently provide older people with an environment in which they can 'maintain a level of control supported by the right to privacy, continuity and security' (Willcocks et al. 1987: 138). This is because concepts such as privacy, respect and choice tend to be regarded as privileges rather than rights (Booth 1985). These attitudes have not been changed by codes of practice or quality of care guidelines. Rather, I would suggest, it is the ideology of care itself which impedes change. A focus on the hospitality model used in hotels rather than on care may be a way to enable older people to retain their adult status while receiving the support they need.

REFERENCES

Adams, R. 1996. *The Personal Social Services*. Longman, London and New York.
Booth, T. 1985. *Home Truths*. Gower, Aldershot.
Davies, B.P. and Knapp, M.R.J. 1981. *Old People's Homes and the Production of Welfare*. Routledge and Kegan Paul, London.

DHSS 1977. *Residential Homes for the Elderly: Arrangements for Health Care*, a memorandum of guidance, Department of Health and Social Security. HMSO, London.

DoH/SSI 1989. *Homes are for Living in*, Department of Health/Social Services Inspectorate, HMSO, London.

Dixon, S.R. 1991. *Autonomy and Dependence in Residential Care*. Age Concern Institute of Gerontology Research Paper No. 5, Age Concern, London.

Mars, G. and Nicod, M. 1984. *The World of Waiters*, George Allen and Unwin, London.

Means, R. and Smith, R. 1983. From public assistance institutions to 'sunshine hotels': changing state perceptions about residential care for elderly people, 1939–48. *Ageing and Society*, 3, 2, 157–81.

Morris, J. 1993. *Community Care or Independent Living*. Joseph Rowntree Foundation, York.

National Institute for Social Work 1988. *Residential Care for Elderly People: Using Research to Improve Practice*. Practice and Development Exchange, National Institute for Social Work: London.

Phillips, J. 1992. *Private Residential Care: the Admissions Process and Reactions of the Public Sector*. Avebury, Aldershot.

Sinclair, I. (ed.), 1988. *Residential Care, the Research Reviewed*. HMSO, London.

Townsend, P. 1962. *The Last Refuge: a Survey of Residential Institutions and Homes for the Aged in England and Wales*. Routledge and Kegan Paul, London.

Wagner Development Group 1992. Wagner Development Group Conference Report. *Elders: the Journal of Care and Practice*, 1, 1.

Willcocks, D., Peace, S. and Kellaher, L. 1987. *Private Lives in Public Places*. Tavistock Publications, London.

Wood, R.C. 1994. Hotel culture and social control. *Annals of Tourism Research*, 21, 65–80.

CHAPTER 26

MALIGNANT SOCIAL PSYCHOLOGY

Tom Kitwood

Here, in outline, is an account of the process of dementia in an older woman, covering a period of eight or so years in all. . . .

Margaret B. died in March 1995, at the age of eighty-nine, in Bank Top Nursing Home. The first episode that really convinced her husband Brian that something was seriously wrong occurred in the summer of 1987, while they were on holiday in Spain, staying in a large hotel. One morning when she was collecting her breakfast in the dining room she got completely lost; she could not find Brian, or their table. When he found her she was very upset and frightened, and apparently had no idea where she was. She seemed to lose confidence from this point forward, becoming increasingly anxious and confused. Margaret had shown some signs of forgetfulness before this time; for example, she had difficulty remembering the names of their six grandchildren. She had also made a few odd mistakes, such as coming home from the supermarket with cat food, despite the fact that their last cat had died several years before. Brian had simply passed off these things as part of growing older; after all, he and his wife were both approaching 80.

Margaret had always been a very conscientious person, loyal to her husband and family. She had worked part-time for a while, but mainly her life had centred on the home. Brian was a strong and upright man,

Source: *Dementia Reconsidered: the Person Comes First*, Open University Press, Buckingham, 1997, pp. 38–42, 45–9.

highly efficient and organised. He was respected in the community, although few people knew him well. He had been a very strict father to their three children, and he had always had a rather formal manner with his wife. As a couple, Margaret and Brian 'kept themselves to themselves'. They had no close friends. Their daughter Susan had emigrated, and both of their two sons had settled in distant places.

After the episode in Spain, life for Brian and Margaret became more and more difficult, although neither of them understood what was happening. Brian found himself resenting Margaret's unreliability, and to his shame he became openly critical of her mistakes. When she showed signs of anxiety or sadness, he often told her to 'pull herself together'. Sometimes she came close to him, pleading with him to hold her and help her to feel safe; usually he pushed her away, or suggested that she go and sit down while he got on with his various jobs. On a few occasions he became really angry with her, which was very unlike how he had usually been. One afternoon she wandered away from home, and when Brian returned she was nowhere to be found. The police picked her up in a distant part of town. He was furious about this, telling her it was a disgrace to the family and all they stood for. From this point forward he felt it was necessary to lock her in the house whenever he went out.

Although Brian knew a little about Alzheimer's disease from television, and things he had read, he did not consciously connect this knowledge with Margaret's behaviour. It was only in 1990, when Susan came on a visit from Australia, that the realisation dawned. Susan was a nurse. She immediately recognised the signs of dementia, and insisted that her mother was taken to the doctor. Margaret was given a provisional diagnosis of Alzheimer's disease, and the doctor suggested that Brian should do the best he could to look after Margaret at home.

Brian's response was dramatic. He quickly absorbed all the information about Alzheimer's disease he could lay his hands on, and set about looking after Margaret in the most efficient way. He took over all the housework and cooking. If she hovered around him while he was doing his tasks, he made her return to the sitting room. When he went shopping, he went alone. As soon as Margaret began to have problems with continence, he obtained help from the advisory service, and did all that was necessary to avoid unpleasant accidents. When she developed problems with sleeping, he took her to the doctor, who prescribed some night sedation. Although the task of looking after Margaret was extremely tiring, Brian was determined to play his part well.

By late 1991 Brian knew that it was all getting too much for him. He was becoming increasingly tired and irritable; Margaret was more and more bewildered and tearful. Brian called in the social services.

After Margaret's assessment it was decided that she should go to a day centre. This gave Brian some relief, although Margaret was often very upset before going, and sometimes seemed extremely confused on her return. He never went with her to the centre, but kept in touch with the manager by telephone.

A new crisis developed in mid-1992. Brian's health was deteriorating; he had developed angina. Margaret was extremely confused and agitated; her medication was increased. The day centre manager stated that Margaret was no longer an appropriate client because her dementia was too severe. The district nurses who came in to help get Margaret to bed were usually in a hurry, and they talked to each other continually while they gave her a bath and put her to bed. This seemed to make Margaret very upset. One evening she bit one of the nurses on the arm, which caused great distress. For Brian, this was the last straw. After talking things through with the social worker, he came to the conclusion that Margaret would have to go into full-time residential care. He felt extremely guilty and uneasy at the prospect.

Brian had heard that The Gables was a good home. He rang the manager, who immediately offered a place for Margaret. One day in November Brian told Margaret that they were going out for a ride in the car, although he did not say where they were going. This was how she entered residential care. As Margaret was very anxious and tearful, the manager suggested that Brian should not visit for several days, to give time for her to get used to her new home.

Unfortunately, Margaret did not settle in The Gables. Her distress and agitation caused great annoyance to other residents; she would not stay in bed at night. Brian usually visited her three times each week, but soon she appeared not to recognise him and often ignored him. One evening one of the residents shouted very abusively at Margaret, and Margaret hit her in the face, causing severe bruises. The family of this resident immediately lodged a complaint, and insisted on an inquiry.

Two days later Margaret was taken to a psychiatric assessment ward, where she spent six weeks. She was given heavy tranquillising medication. After this she was placed in Bank Top Nursing Home, which had a wing entirely for people with dementia.

At Bank Top, Margaret remained under sedation. Her life consisted of being got up in the morning, having her breakfast, and then being put in a chair. Here she sat for hours on end, half awake, half asleep, and occasionally wandering around. Around 8.00 p.m. each day she was put to bed. Within four months she had lost the use of her legs. She was becoming very thin, and often left her food. Only one member of staff realised that Margaret was often eager to eat, but needed prompting about actually doing it. Brian's visits became less and less frequent; he saw little point in coming. The two sons did not come at all. For the very last part of her life Margaret spent longer and longer periods lying on her bed. She was fed, mainly with liquid food. One morning it was found that she had died.

Although this narrative taken as a whole is a fiction, each element of it is based on events that have actually happened. Also, while The Gables and Bank Top Nursing Home have no existence in reality, they both epitomise the poorer quality kind of place where people are taken in for residential care. The story of Margaret and Brian is typical of how dementia has been lived out in recent years in Britain, and it has close parallels in other industrialised countries. Several people have said to me, after I have used it in training work, that it almost exactly describes a case they know, or even what has happened in their own family.

If we follow the development of any person's dementing condition closely, again and again we will come to see how social and interpersonal factors come into play, either adding to the difficulties directly arising from neurological impairment, or helping to lessen their effects. In the light of this it is extremely difficult to hold to the view suggested by the standard paradigm: that the mental and emotional symptoms are a direct result of a catastrophic series of changes in the brain that lead to the death of brain cells – and nothing more than that. This narrow conception of the ill-being that dementia often entails can easily divert attention away from the inadequacy of our social arrangements, and it has led to a gross imbalance in research. Insofar as it has done this, it might be regarded as a 'neuropathic ideology' – a body of opinion that systematically distorts the truth.

In moral terms, it is clear even from the brief account given here that there were many points at which Margaret was not treated fully as a person. She needed comfort in her anxiety, but Brian was unable to give it. She pleaded for encouragement and reassurance when her self-confidence was failing, but she met criticism or anger. She wanted a 'way of life', a continuity with her past, but her role as the homemaker was totally stripped away. The day centre was unable to provide her with occupation within her range of capability, and it failed to offer her the kind of company with which she could feel at ease. Neither The Gables nor Bank Top had developed the skills among staff that would enable them to provide effective psychological care for residents with dementia. Margaret's 'behaviour problems' were never explored in a sympathetic way, or traced back to their roots; eventually they were controlled by medication, but at the cost of suppressing much of what enabled her still to be a person, and possibly of adding further damage to her nervous system.

In a case such as this one might be tempted to blame the main carer, but it would be both psychologically inept and morally blind to do so. Those who have this role take on, almost single-handed, a colossal task. The weight of evidence from anthropology is that no individual was ever 'designed' for such an onerous commitment; human beings emerged through evolution as a highly social species, where burdens are carried by a group. Even in those rare instances in industrial societies where the care is genuinely shared by several members of the family, the situation is far less fraught and strained.

Brian, in the story, was left to live out the consequence of the tendency of our kind of society to force into isolation people who are under pressure. Furthermore, he had received no preparation, practical or psychological, for his new role. He was the product of his own upbringing, with its many limitations, and of his own attempts to measure up to the common standards of how to be a man. At many points his own needs were not met, and when the situation became really difficult he received no support. Where 'community care' was available, it consisted mainly of *ad hoc* interventions, and when the situation became really difficult it proved completely inadequate. Some of the things Brian did to Margaret fell far short of true respect for her personhood, but what about his personhood too? Locking his wife in the house when he went out might be considered deeply immoral, but perhaps it was the 'least bad' thing that he could do in the circumstances. As Margaret's dementia grew worse, no one helped Brian with his feelings of anger, inadequacy and guilt; no one enabled him to come to terms with his own tragic predicament.

So this story of one person's dementia is much more than that of an advancing neurological illness. It is absurdly reductionistic to suggest, as some have done, that 'everything in the end comes down to what is going on in individual brain cells'. In very many cases, we find that the process of dementia is also the story of a tragic inadequacy in our culture, our economy, our traditional views about gender, our medical system and our general way of life. In engaging with people who are in Brian's position we should take great care not to be judgemental; it is probable that they already carry a very heavy burden of guilt feelings. The fault lies in the context, and at a systemic level; it is the culmination of a long historical process. That whole context needs radical improvement – through a change in the culture of care. But that is a task that has, until very recently, been almost totally neglected.

If the story of Margaret and Brian is typical, it points to a disastrous incompetence within contemporary societies. At this point in history it is certainly not convenient for any government to take the 'rising tide' of dementia seriously; it has such momentous implications for health services and social care, and it points to an immense educational deficit. In broad cultural terms also, we are still largely unprepared for the new situation, where there is a vast new field of moral responsibility. This general ineptitude at a societal level goes back for many centuries; Europe never had a golden age of compassion and enlightenment.

[. . .]

Depersonalising elements

Care practice, then, whether in institutions or in 'the community', contains the residues of at least four depersonalising traditions: bestialisation, the attribution of moral deficit, warehousing, and the unnecessary use of a medical model. Among all fields, provision for people who have dementia is perhaps the most affected, because gross under-resourcing is compounded by fear, defence and a pervasive ageism.
[. . .]

Almost as soon as I became involved with dementia, I was strongly aware of these depersonalising tendencies; I decided to make them a topic of research. My method involved a simple form of critical incident technique; essentially, making brief notes on episodes as soon as possible after they had been observed, and then attempting to classify them (Kitwood 1990). The term which I gave for these episodes was 'malignant social psychology'. The strong word 'malignant' signifies something very harmful, symptomatic of a care environment that is deeply damaging to personhood, possibly even undermining physical well-being. The effect of the psychosocial environment on health is just beginning to be understood, particularly with the study of stress and the genesis of conditions such as cancer. The term malignant does not, however, imply evil intent on the part of caregivers; most of their work is done with kindness and good intent. The malignancy is part of our cultural inheritance.

My original list contained ten elements:

1. *Treachery* – using forms of deception in order to distract or manipulate a person, or force them into compliance.
2. *Disempowerment* – not allowing a person to use the abilities that they do have; failing to help them to complete actions that they have initiated.
3. *Infantilisation* – treating a person very patronisingly (or 'matronisingly'), as an insensitive parent might treat a very young child.
4. *Intimidation* – inducing fear in a person, through the use of threats or physical power.
5. *Labelling* – using a category such as dementia, or 'organic mental disorder' as the main basis for interacting with a person and for explaining their behaviour.
6. *Stigmatisation* – treating a person as if they were a diseased object, an alien or an outcast.
7. *Outpacing* – providing information, presenting choices, etc., at a rate too fast for a person to understand; putting them under pressure to do things more rapidly than they can bear.
8. *Invalidation* – failing to acknowledge the subjective reality of a person's experience, and especially what they are feeling.

9. *Banishment* – sending a person away, or excluding them – physically or psychologically.

10. *Objectification* – treating a person as if they were a lump of dead matter: to be pushed, lifted, filled, pumped or drained, without proper reference to the fact that they are sentient beings.

Since the time of my first study of malignant social psychology I have added seven further elements to the list:

11. *Ignoring* – carrying on (in conversation or action) in the presence of a person as if they were not there.

12. *Imposition* – forcing a person to do something, overriding desire or denying the possibility of choice on their part.

13. *Withholding* – Refusing to give asked-for attention, or to meet an evident need.

14. *Accusation* – blaming a person for actions or failures of action that arise from their lack of ability, or their misunderstanding of the situation.

15. *Disruption* – intruding suddenly or disturbingly upon a person's action or reflection; crudely breaking their frame of reference.

16. *Mockery* – making fun of a person's 'strange' actions or remarks; teasing, humiliating, making jokes at their expense.

17. *Disparagement* – telling a person that they are incompetent, useless, worthless, etc., giving them messages that are damaging to their self-esteem.

[. . .]

Malignant social psychology is, perhaps, the most glaringly bad part of the care traditions that we have inherited. Fortunately, it is relatively easy to sensitise staff in formal care settings to its presence, and to reduce it greatly through a series of short training sessions.

REFERENCE

Kitwood, T. 1990. The dialectics of dementia: with particular reference to Alzheimer's disease. *Ageing and Society* 10: 177–96.

CHAPTER 27

EXPOSING ABUSE IN CARE HOMES

John Burton

Noreen's younger sister, Brenda, who lived in a neighbouring local authority area, worked for six months as a part-time care assistant in a small voluntary home for older people. Although she had never before been a
residential care worker, she didn't find it difficult to get a job in this home,
ten minutes' walk from her own house. She asked about work there one
day and she was told to come back the next day to start. To begin with,
she was paid in cash by the 'matron', and after a couple of weeks, when
she was deemed satisfactory, she was put on the payroll. There were very
few staff and nearly all of them had been recruited in the same way. Poor
as the conditions and pay were, Brenda liked the residents and found a lot
of the work very satisfying. Within days of starting, she could see that the
way she chose to work was making quite a difference to residents' lives: at
the same time she realised that the general standard of care was very poor.
It was several weeks though, before she began to understand that the care
was worse than poor – it was abusive and cruel.

As a newcomer she was not at first 'initiated' into the regular abuse that
was going on. She did not immediately understand that the screams she
heard from the 'confused' residents were in fact screams of pain, because
other staff told her not to worry and said that 'they' were always like that
when they got up in the morning, or when they were taken to the toilet.
Later she was shown what 'had to be done' with 'confused' residents. If
they were dirty in the morning – and they usually were – they were first
wiped with the wet sheets and then pulled from the bed, stripped of their
night clothes and sat on the commode. The bedclothes were removed and

Source: *Managing Residential Care*, Routledge, London, 1998, pp. 222–31.

the bed made up. The residents were then washed roughly and their first set of day clothes (from a common stock) were put on. Brenda was told that if you didn't force them you would never get them out of bed and dressed, and, since there were only two people working in the mornings with fourteen residents, most of whom were incontinent, you couldn't hang around. If the residents were to be got up and taken down to breakfast by 8 a.m. you had to 'pull them around a bit'.

Brenda also discovered that some of the screams coming from the toilets were caused by something even more horrific. The 'deputy matron' took it on herself to 'manually evacuate' residents who were constipated. This involved putting on rubber gloves (which were otherwise in very short supply) and inserting her fingers into the resident's anus to pull out impacted faeces.

The residents were short of food and were sometimes begging for drinks. After putting Brenda on the payroll, the 'matron' explained to her that, although staff were not well paid, the low pay could be compensated for by perks. These included taking the pick of the deliveries of food which a large, high-class supermarket sent to the Home each week with the intention and reasonable expectation that the relatively expensive items would provide welcome treats for the residents; but the smoked salmon, joints of meat, ice cream, cheese cake, fresh juices and exotic fruit and vegetables all went home with staff. The residents sometimes had the bread or the plain biscuits, if there were some left over after staff had taken what they wanted, but what the residents ate was not extra for them; it simply reduced the expenditure on essential provisions.

Residents who had no relatives visiting were completely at the mercy of the abusive regime. Brenda was increasingly disturbed by what she was seeing, and with each new revelation she became unhappier but more determined to stay. At first she just blamed the individual workers who did these things, but as she too found herself tempted to hurry the residents because time was so short, she understood how difficult it was to work in any other way. After a few weeks she spoke to the 'matron' about her concerns. She was told that the Home was no different from any other and that there was nothing to be done about it. 'In the old days', said the 'matron', 'none of these residents would have been in a home, they would have all been in hospital. We just get sent the dross now. They're all incontinent and senile, and the committee haven't given us any more staff.'

Brenda was perplexed by many things – by the drunken doctor who visited weekly but hardly ever saw residents; by where the residents' money went to; by who was really in charge – but she became so anxious about the welfare of the residents that she came into the Home on her days off to check that they were all right. Other staff thought that she was odd and warned her against 'over-involvement'. Far from being the 'nice little part-time job' which Brenda had been looking for when she took it on, the work was becoming a more than full-time obsession, and while her family sympathised and tried to support her, they could see it was making her ill. She could talk about nothing else at home and was often in floods of tears.

Of course, the obvious person to talk with about her worries was Noreen, but though she loved her dearly, Brenda had wanted to do this job without the advice and instruction of her big sister. Noreen was the oldest in a family of six and Brenda the youngest. Fifteen years her senior, Noreen had been a bit like a mother to her when she was a child, and Brenda just knew that her sister would tell her exactly what to do.

On one of her days off, Brenda called at the Home early in the morning before going out to do some shopping for herself. She went straight upstairs to see a resident who was 'difficult' but of whom she was very fond. In spite of everything, the old woman still retained her spirit. She would fight and swear and shout, but sometimes she was quietly appreciative of Brenda's gentle care. As Brenda approached the resident's room, she heard her screaming and she heard the 'deputy matron' shouting, 'Don't you think you can scratch me, you filthy old bitch. I'll teach you a fucking lesson.' Brenda also heard a smacking sound. She burst into the room to see the worker standing over the naked resident beating her with her urine-soaked rolled-up nightdress. Brenda snatched the nightdress from the 'deputy matron', and, only just managing to restrain herself from attacking her, growled, 'How could you? Get out.' The woman left the room, protesting that the resident had attacked her and showing a long scratch on her arm.

Staying with the resident, Brenda rang the call bell repeatedly until the other member of staff on duty came to the room. She explained what she had seen and told her colleague that she was going to do something about the situation, and that the 'deputy matron' was not to come near the resident. 'If she so much as touches her again, I'll kill her.'

Not having a clue what to do, she rushed home and rang Noreen, who told her to write down everything she had witnessed that morning, then to ring the police, the chair of the committee, and the inspection unit and tell each of them exactly what had happened. Brenda had never heard of the inspection unit but it sounded to her as if this was exactly the sort of problem inspectors should be there to solve, and so she rang them first. She was put through to an inspector who said that it wasn't his home but that what she had told him was indeed very serious and he would pass the information on to the right person who would ring Brenda at home as soon as possible. Next she rang the chair of the committee, who didn't sound at all surprised and said he thought things might have got a little bit out of hand. He was calm and unruffled, and he strongly advised Brenda against ringing the police because, he said, they would not understand and probably wouldn't be interested. He told her to meet him at the Home straight away.

Brenda returned to the Home. The committee chair had not arrived but she discovered that he had phoned immediately after he had spoken to

Brenda to instruct the 'deputy matron' to go home, and he had asked the 'matron' to come in. Brenda spent an anxious hour waiting for him to arrive. When he and the 'matron' arrived at almost the same time, he told Brenda to meet with them both in the office. She began to feel as if it was she who was in the wrong. The chair said that he had already spoken with the inspector, who agreed with him that the 'deputy matron' had obviously momentarily lost her temper, but that 'it happens'. Because Brenda had chosen to 'make a mountain out of a molehill', the deputy would have to be suspended for the moment, 'until the fuss dies down'. He said that the inspection unit would not be investigating the incident and would be quite happy for him to do so, and to send them his report. Had she got anything more to say than she had already said on the phone?

Brenda was shocked. She felt completely alone and unaccountably ashamed of herself. Near to tears and panic, she remained silent. The 'matron' said that after all she was a new and inexperienced member of staff, and that unfortunate things do happen in the work, but that she would just have to get used to it. She mustn't take it on herself to contact anyone outside, particularly the inspection unit, without consulting the 'chairman' or her first. Fortunately, she said, he had been able to sort out the inspector before the whole thing got completely out of control. Frightened, angry but still silent, Brenda got up and walked straight out of the Home to her own home.

Even before she reached her own door ten minutes' walk away from the Home, she had already begun to doubt that she had really seen and heard what had been done to the resident. The more she went over it, the more she wondered if she had exaggerated it and if she had been altogether mistaken. There was no one at home and she rang Noreen again. When she heard her sister's voice she broke down and began to sob that she had made a fool of herself, and berated Noreen for giving her such bad advice. It had got her nowhere, she said. Gradually Noreen encouraged her to tell her what had been said at the meeting with the committee chair and the 'matron'. 'Did you write down what you saw this morning, as I told you to?' 'Yes.' 'Well, read it to me then.' Brenda read it and began to believe herself again.

Although Noreen had little faith in inspectors herself, she knew that in this sort of situation they *should* be able to investigate and take action. She advised Brenda to ring them again because, as she pointed out, the inspector for the Home had not yet heard Brenda's story for himself, and Noreen was inclined to doubt that an inspector would agree to the cover-up which the committee chair seemed to be proposing. She also told Brenda that she should still ring the police because what she had witnessed was a violent assault.

Brenda was trembling as she rang the inspection unit again and managed to get through to the right person. He sounded most understanding but he said that the chief inspector had discussed the situation with the committee chair and he had been told that there was no need to get involved at this stage. Brenda began to panic. She could not accept this. She demanded to see the inspector. 'I thought you were meant to protect residents. That woman will be back to work tomorrow and she'll do it again. You have got to do something.' The inspector agreed to see her, first saying he had no time until the next week, but then, at Brenda's insistence, he arranged to meet her late in the afternoon of the same day.

Brenda spent three hours with the inspector and the chief inspector. She tried to tell them everything – about the incident in the morning but also about all the other abuse as well. They took pages of notes and thanked her for having the courage to come to them.

With her heart in her mouth, Brenda went in to work the next day. The 'deputy matron' was not there. The other staff and the 'matron' were coldly hostile to Brenda; she felt as if she had been sent to Coventry. She got on with her work and took her breaks with the residents rather than the staff.

The day after, she went in to work to find two inspectors doing a surprise inspection. The 'matron' called in another care assistant to boost the staffing and it was all smiles and second helpings throughout the time they were there. The chair of the committee happened to drop in midway through the morning and spent a long time with the inspectors in the office.

Brenda felt immense relief. At last something was being done. It seemed that the 'deputy matron' had been suspended and that a proper investigation was taking place. The inspectors took copious notes and wanted to look into every nook and cranny of the place.

Without the 'deputy matron' around Brenda was less anxious about the immediate safety of residents, but some things got worse because it became apparent that she had been the organising force behind the conduct of the Home, such as it was. Quite quickly, the vestiges of discipline, which had just about kept call bells answered and staff following some sort of procedure in their work, disappeared. Staff spent more time together in the staff room, office or kitchen talking and smoking, and Brenda, always keen to be with residents, became more isolated. She found she was doing nearly all the work when she was on duty, and even when she was just visiting, she felt she had to respond to residents who needed attention but weren't getting it from the staff on duty.

Having had high hopes of change for the better after the inspection, Brenda once more began to despair. After two weeks she rang the inspector to find out what was happening. He told her that they were writing the report and a draft would go to the 'matron' and committee chair within the next two weeks. Brenda was exasperated when the inspector explained that there would be a lengthy process of consultation and amendment to the draft report before a 'public' report was finalised and Brenda could see what the results of the inspection were.

Initially she had expected so much of the inspection but now she began to wonder if she should ever have said anything about the incident or the Home. The 'deputy matron' was not working at the Home any more but Brenda had seen her there a couple of times. The other staff continued to be hostile; even so, two of them had come to her privately and said that they thought she was right, but added hopelessly, 'What can you do?' Brenda had received several anonymous threatening phone calls at home and her new coat, hanging in the changing room at work, had been cut from top to bottom. She kept getting the feeling that it was all her fault, and that the more experienced staff were probably right – 'What can you do?'

Brenda hung on somehow until, four months after the incident, the inspection report was published. She wouldn't have known it was available if she hadn't been pestering the inspection unit to tell her. As it was, none of the staff in the Home got to see the report, and Brenda had to collect it from the unit.

It was fourteen pages long. Brenda found it difficult to understand but scoured it to find references to the incident. Although it was critical of many of the practices and procedures of the Home, and listed ten requirements and twenty-two recommendations at the end, there was no mention of what had happened. Most extraordinary of all, the final paragraphs of the report said that the Home 'continued to operate within the requirements of the *Registered Homes Act*'.

Noreen had been trying to keep in touch with Brenda throughout this period. Brenda was reluctant to talk and felt ashamed of how little she had achieved. She thought that Noreen would have handled it much better – she, Noreen, wouldn't have let them get away with it. Nagging at the back of her mind too was her failure to get in touch with the police.

Soon after she had read the inspection report, another care worker told Brenda that the 'deputy matron' was now working in a nearby Home. Brenda was seething with anger. As far as she could see, no changes were being made at the Home as a result of the report; care was even worse than when the 'deputy matron' had been there; and now she'd gone elsewhere to abuse more defenceless old people.

On the day the inspection report was published, the old woman who had been beaten was sent to hospital with pneumonia. Brenda went to visit her and sat holding her hand, crying and whispering over and over again, 'I'm sorry.' Three days after admission, the old woman died. When Brenda heard the news she handed in her notice and went home that evening and rang the police.

Again Brenda was interviewed for several hours and she signed a statement about what had happened more than four months before. The detective who interviewed her said that such cases were very difficult, especially since it was now so long after the event, and anyway the alleged victim had died. Even if she had still been alive, he added, she would probably have been unable to give evidence. Also it didn't look good that Brenda had given in her notice and that she was so critical of the Home. He said that it was unlikely he would be able to find sufficient evidence for a prosecution if the social services inspection unit had already investigated the matter. However, he would certainly look into it and let her know what the outcome was. As the detective was going, he began to ask Brenda questions about her family both in England and in Ireland. Brenda's husband worked for a motorway maintenance firm and they had three grown-up sons. The policeman wanted to know what they did and where they lived. 'Just a chat.' Brenda had been subjected to 'chats' like that before. As he left, she knew her allegation had no hope of proper investigation.

What Brenda didn't know

Brenda had no inkling of the power of the 'players' in this awful experience or of the connections between them – why should she have?

The chair of the committee was previously a prominent local politician who retained his contacts with and influence in the ruling party. As leader of the council he had fixed many deals and covered up many scams. The other members of the committee which ran the Homes were under his thumb and left him to make all the decisions. He employed his niece as the administrator of the charity in spite of the fact that she could barely add up, took three hours to type a letter, and was unable to take minutes at meetings. He was effectively in sole control of a £2 million business and awarded contracts to friends, bought and sold assets (Homes), and was free to organise the finances to suit himself. He had even set up schemes whereby small amounts of residents' personal allowances were taken in cash by his daughter.

The 'chairman' (as he was always known) had a direct line to the director of social services and to the leading members of the party in power. To him, the introduction of inspection had been no more than a nuisance since he could always 'fix' any inconvenient problems which arose. He was also a prominent member of his local Masonic lodge, so it was not surprising when his fellow member – the detective – readily accepted his explanation of the unfortunate incident involving the 'deputy matron'. They had also agreed that Brenda was a somewhat suspect witness.

Although he could not stop Brenda eventually telling her story to the inspection unit, on reflection he reckoned it was better that she had done or she might have been tempted to go to the press or some 'left-wing organisation of busybodies'. As soon as he had received Brenda's first call, he got on to the director of social services to make sure that the inspection unit didn't come sticking their noses in. The director immediately contacted the chief inspector to tell her to keep well out of it, and she in turn instructed the inspector to listen sympathetically but to do nothing until it had blown over. An unannounced inspection would certainly give the impression of taking appropriate action, but she knew that it would in fact delay any comment for several months. The 'chairman' readily agreed to 'letting the deputy matron go' and providing her with a good reference as the best way of preventing any further similar problems occurring in the Home.

The inspectors and chief inspector resented the way in which they were pushed around and their reports were censored, but they had allowed it to start in a small way when they were first established, and now they were so deeply implicated in cover-ups and collusions that they could see no way of reversing the position other than by leaving the unit altogether.

On receipt of the draft report, the 'chairman' had removed all direct and indirect references to the incident. He was quite happy to let the requirements and recommendations pass because he had seen most of them before anyway, and had no intention of doing anything about more than a very few. [. . .]

CHAPTER 28

REGULATING INFORMALITY: SMALL HOMES AND THE INSPECTORS

Caroline Holland and Sheila Peace

Fifty years ago, most older people who were unable to take complete care of themselves were either looked after in their own homes, or moved into an institution under the care of professionals. Unless something went horribly wrong, the state had little business with what went on in people's own homes and did not attempt to regulate either the homes or the caregivers. Arrangements now, however, tend to be more complex, with professional and voluntary carers going into people's homes to supplement self-care and family care, and people going out of their homes for day care or respite care.

The range of possible care settings has also increased in type (e.g. adult foster care, extra-care sheltered housing, specialist care homes) and in size, from homes with more than sixty beds to single placements. They cover what have been both 'domestic' and 'non-domestic' environments. Regulation has gradually encroached on most of these situations and the White Paper *Modernising Social Services* extended some aspects of regulation to include for the first time domiciliary care (DoH 1998a).

Over the past few years we have been researching the most domestic in type of currently regulated care settings: small residential homes for older people. These are homes where one, two, or three adults reside and receive accommodation and personal care from a non-relative. After the implementation in 1993 of the Registered Homes (Amendment) Act 1991, any such home had to register with the local authority (although small homes for children were exempt at this time) and this responsibility fell to the inspectors based in local authority Registration and Inspection (R&I)

Units. There are around 7,000 small homes for adults in England: about half are registered for people with learning disabilities and a third for older people, but there are also homes for people with mental illnesses and for people with addiction problems (DoH 1998b). However, they form a much smaller percentage of residential provision for older people than for people with learning disabilities and mental illness.

The histories of small residential homes for older people are varied. Many started out offering adult placements in family homes, and some of them still function within placement schemes. Occasionally care workers or nurses have set up a small home as a result of the closure of a local hospital, maybe with specific residents in mind. Some were set up as small businesses, often within the owner's own home – what is known in the USA as 'mom and pop homes' (Morgan *et al.* 1995) – whereas others appear to be more purely commercial, with the owner living elsewhere and employing a manager. Some are run by voluntary organisations and charities. Many of the most recent registrations have been 'small homes' within nursing homes: i.e. two or three beds registered as a 'residential home' in order to avoid dual registration. Although the total numbers of small homes have been generally increasing, including those run by voluntary organisations and charities, it looks as though some businesses are short-lived.

Our research has taken two directions. In 1997/98, pilot work carried out in Bedfordshire, Buckinghamshire and Hertfordshire included a survey of all small homes and an in-depth analysis of the quality of life experienced in six of these homes (Holland and Peace 1998). In 1999, a national survey of R&I Units in England was undertaken to learn more about this emerging regulatory work (Holland and Peace 2001).

Small homes

Data from the pilot survey in the three authorities showed that a wide range of building types, sizes and locations are being used for small home businesses, but a typical home would be a five-bedroomed detached domestic house, with a built extension or some aids or adaptations installed. The six small homes selected for further study, however, revealed something of the diversity of these small residential homes:

■ a large seven-bedroomed, sixteenth-century listed building in extensive grounds,
■ a 1940s town bungalow with a garage converted into staff accommodation,
■ a three-bedroomed ex-council house attached to the owner's home, on a 1970s council estate,
■ a five-bedroomed 1940s house, on a long urban street of mixed properties,

■ a modern-styled 1970s five-bedroomed house in a large garden, over-looking countryside,

■ a 1950s bungalow with an extension loft conversion and an extension into the rear garden.

The detailed study utilised observation and interview techniques. We found people fiercely defending the essential domesticity of their homes. Four of the houses had been the owners' own home before they took in residents, and they continued to be the family home. The owners wanted their home to be as comfortable as possible, so they placed much emphasis on the quality of decorations and furnishings, keeping the place smelling nice, and avoiding any appearance of an institution. Some of the owners had opened their small homes in reaction to what they saw as the 'regimentation' of larger residential homes.

From the outside the owners had kept their houses looking ordinary and unmarked as 'Homes', and inside they resisted having noticeboards or lists of rules in the hallway. They tried to make medicine cupboards and paperwork unobtrusive, for example keeping files in a kitchen cupboard. They were already worried about regulation issues such as whether they would need to log the contents of fridges, whether residents could use the kitchen under health and safety rules, and the provision of sinks in rooms or en-suite bathrooms. All these were felt to be problematic given the size of these houses. Sometimes the boundaries between the domestic and the regulated were difficult to determine as this comment shows:

> We can't allow them (the residents) into the kitchen because of the health and safety regulations. I had great battles with the inspecting officer, who said they should not be allowed into the kitchen because of the contamination. Although our staff have been on the food hygiene course, residents obviously haven't. I said that it was a small home, and if they wanted to go in and take their relatives in to make a coffee, or to do baking under supervision, my residents weren't going to be stopped from doing that. He's not happy with it but he allowed it. They go in once a week, wash their hands, wear an apron, fasten their hair back or wear a hat, so they are supervised under basic hygiene rules by members of staff. None of them just pop in, because one is very confused and another is too frail. (He) possibly could, but he's not safe. He is registered partially blind, and I wouldn't like him to start using the geyser in case he burns himself.
>
> *(Interview with homeowner)*

Residents had their own small bedrooms, but they shared lounges and dining rooms with other residents or the rest of the household. The whole household might be five to eight people, including in some the owners' children. The residents normally ate main meals together, but not usually with the family. The rest of the time they did their own thing in their bed-rooms, the living areas or the garden. They liked being in a small group (although this presents its own problems) better than being in a larger home. They liked knowing the owner and staff very well, and being around in the 'ebb and flow' of family life: visitors, shopping trips, gossip, and so on. They thought their situation was superior to an 'old people's home'. Other members of the household had time to talk to them about their lives and knew them as individuals. Generally they felt that their pref-erences and tastes were taken into account. One resident said that the home was most like 'a comfortable private hotel'.

However, it is true that running a small home demands a level of flexi-bility between public and private lives. For the home is also the work-place and all life must go on. One homeowner said:

> *We decided that we couldn't have anybody round for dinner because you had residents in. We didn't have parties and things that you used to have. But then I decided that yes, OK, it's their home, but at the end of the day it's also my home, so we decided that we would carry on as normal ... I think you have to do that. If you can't do that, when you've got children, then you can't have a residential home because it's not fair to your family.*

Regulation and inspection

Flexibility may be needed but regulators had some problems with the notion of small homes. Ninety-nine of the 107 (93 per cent) local authority R&I Units attached to social services responded to the survey. There was a wide range in the provision of small homes for older people in their areas, ranging from none to 448. Those with the largest numbers of small home registrations were generally counties: twelve of those which responded had more than 100 small homes each and two had more than 400 small homes each. As shown in Table 28.1, metropolitan areas had the smallest number, although differences did exist between cities and districts.

Table 28.1 Average number of registered small homes for older people by type of area.

	Number of authorities	Average number of small homes
County Councils	30	123
Metropolitan Borough Councils	27	29
London Borough Councils	21	23
Unitary authorities	15	31

Source: Holland and Peace, 2001.

In 1993 existing small homes were obliged to register with the local authority, and since then almost all new registrations have involved an initial visit from the Inspectorate and an interview with the owner. However, inspections have not been mandatory and there has been much variation between authorities in the frequency and detail of inspections after the initial registration. The essential instruction to Inspectors was that they should use a 'lighter touch' with regard to small homes:

> *Ministers intend that a lighter touch should be applied to small homes. Following consultation, some provisions applying to larger homes have not been applied to small homes in an attempt to keep, in particular, specific additional requirements on those providing care to a necessary minimum. Authorities are not expected to check routinely on compliance with the remaining part of regulation 10 or on any other requirements about the situation in the home e.g. record keeping. If they do, they should bear the need for a lighter touch in mind.*
>
> *(DoH 1992)*

But how has this 'lighter touch' been interpreted? Many do not like the vagueness of the phrase. In the survey some authorities had decided not to inspect small homes unless they received a complaint. Many of those that did, frequently aimed to make what at most was an annual announced formal inspection, or at least one every two or three years. Only a small number of authorities made regular informal visits, or unannounced inspections. Inspections were often reported to be less formal than those of larger homes, and to require less paperwork. Reports were less likely to be publicly accessible than those for larger residential homes.

There appeared to be a tension between the desire of authorities to carry out an adequate inspection programme for small homes and their ability to do so given limited available resources. They were also very mindful of the differences within the sector:

> *The premises are expected to be domestic in nature. An inspection would be looking for services and arrangements that would normally be regarded as adequate for family living to be an accepted standard. In assessing a 'fit person' we would be looking for a basic understanding of the needs of people being cared for and a respect for their privacy, dignity, independence, choice, rights and fulfilment. Homes not run by 'the family' will be expected to demonstrate a commitment to good employment practices and staff training. A manager would need to be registered.*
>
> *(Response to open question in survey)*

The lighter touch was also interpreted by some authorities in relation to the inspection process itself and issues of record-keeping. For example, shorter forms were used for some small homes inspections and, in some areas, the homes might be required to keep fewer records than larger homes. Nevertheless, in most authorities they were required to keep the following:

- a record of medicines,
- a statement of the aims of the home,
- a record of residents' money and valuables deposited,
- details of employed staff,
- a daily register of residents,
- details of other people providing personal care,
- an occurrence book,
- records of incidents, accidents, complaints or abuse allegations.

The homes are required by official regulations to produce their own complaints procedure and to provide residents with information about how to contact R&I Units. Indeed the R&I Units tended to rely on this procedure as a means for accessing complaints. Given that monitoring has been irregular in some cases, this may have increased the vulnerability of some residents.

The regulators tended to keep records about the buildings that were used as small homes, about staffing, and about other people who were resident. But few had a record of the fees charged to privately funded residents or of the personal details and care requirements of existing residents. In 1999, when this research was undertaken, small homes residents were a very neglected group and some R&I Units were concerned that, once registered, small homes may be virtually free from scrutiny. Many R&I Units now take the view that small homes should be treated in exactly the same way as larger homes, and indeed the White Paper introduces a requirement that annual inspections are undertaken. In future the regulatory practice for small residential homes and adult foster care will be developed by the Care Standards Commissioners as a consequence of the Care Standards Act 2000, and the development of National Minimum Standards and Regulations.

Thus the basic question is: how can small homes be adequately regulated without squashing their best asset, their informality? Many of these small businesses are first and foremost family homes: some of the owners said they would rather stop taking residents than turn their homes into 'little institutions'. Increasing the formality of small homes in terms of regulatory procedures and requirements, would not necessarily address particular weaknesses in terms of support and appropriate methods of inspection. Some initiatives, which have already been taken in a minority of areas, include advocacy services for residents, training sessions for staff, owner support groups, and inspection schedules that have been adapted for small homes. But these measures can take more time and thought than 'tick box' approaches, and it remains to be seen along which route national and local policies on regulation will be taken.

REFERENCES

Department of Health (1998a) *Modernising Social Services*, CM4169, London: The Stationery Office.

Department of Health (1998b) *Personal Social Service. Residential Accommodation. Detailed Statistics on residential care homes and local authority supported residents, England*, London: Government Statistical Service.

Department of Health (1992) Local Authority Circular LAC (92) 10.

Holland, C.A. and Peace, S.M. (1998) *Homely Residential Care: The Report of the Pilot Study of Small Homes for Older People*, School of Health and Social Welfare, The Open University.

Holland, C.A. and Peace, S.M. (2001) *The Small Homes for Older People Survey, 1999*, Research Report, School of Health and Social Welfare, The Open University.

Morgan, L.A., Eckert, K. and Lyon, S.M. (1995) *Small Board-and-Care Homes. Residential Care in Transition*, Baltimore: The John Hopkins University Press.

CHAPTER 29

COMMUNITY CARE LAW AND THE HUMAN RIGHTS ACT 1998

Luke Clements

The classification of the European Convention on Human Rights as a 'negative rights'[1] instrument, focusing on hard, civil and political rights would, at first blush, appear to exclude the soft rights one generally associates with community care. On the face of it, these are 'comfort' issues – such as extra help in the home, hot meals and residential accommodation.

The dearth of European Court of Human Rights decisions in relation to the rights of frail elderly people, physically disabled people and people with learning difficulties might be seen as supporting this contention. This is not, however, the case. Whatever the intentions were of those who drafted the Convention over fifty years ago, today it is of central relevance to community care law.

The issue of access

At the heart of the Convention is the 'universally recognised fundamental principle' that all individuals must have access to the civil justice process.[2] Access to the civil justice process is, however, precisely what is denied to the vast majority of community care service users – many of whom are unassertive, poorly informed and have impaired communication or mental capacity skills.

An impaired ability to self-advocate is not in itself a problem, where there is ready access to advocacy services. Thus, in relation to detention and treatment decisions under the Mental Health Act 1983 the procedures that ensure access to legal representation have resulted in a substantial volume of court complaints. A similar argument may also be advanced in relation to children taken into public care.

Article 6: the right to a fair and independent hearing

In *Airey v Ireland* (1979) the European Court of Human Rights held that effective access to a fair civil justice process (under Article 6) required, in appropriate circumstances, the availability of legal aid. Effective access for persons under physical and mental incapacity difficulties must require the development of an entitlement to advocacy of the type envisaged by the Disabled Persons (Services, Consultation and Representation) Act 1986.[3] That there is scope within the common law for such a development is unquestionable given its accommodation of the MacKenzie[4] friend. The Human Rights Act 1998 is likely therefore to hasten the inevitable and necessary development of the 'advocacy movement' for disabled people.

The problem of 'access' to justice goes beyond the mere question of the absence of a right to an independent advocate: our domestic law creates procedural barriers that restrict certain disabled people's access to the court. The most fundamental obstacle is the absence of clear legal principles relating to the making of decisions on behalf of people who lack sufficient mental capacity. The failure of successive governments to implement the Law Commission's Paper on this issue constitutes perhaps the most serious discrimination against disabled people in the United Kingdom.[5]

Enormous practical difficulties are created by the Civil Procedure Rules that oblige people with limited mental capacity to act through a third party (known as a 'litigation friend'). How, for instance, can the financial exploitation of an incapacitated adult by their main carer come to the notice of anyone able to intervene? How can a young woman with similar impairments in the care of protective parents assert her right to a private sexual life?

Aside from the lack of any clear 'rule of law' in relation to the rights of persons lacking the necessary mental capacity, they face severe procedural problems in litigating violations of their rights. The court rules stipulate that 'litigation friends' can only commence proceedings if they give the court a personal undertaking to be responsible for the costs of the proceedings.[6] Such a blanket requirement constitutes unreasonable discrimination against disabled people: if a costs guarantee is appropriate, why then is it not required for all litigants?

Before proceedings (or any other process to enforce their rights) can be initiated on behalf of persons lacking sufficient capacity, evidence must be obtained. Access to files, indeed to virtually any information, is effectively barred in relation to adults lacking capacity. Confidentiality is used as a trump card; because the incapacitated person is unable to make an informed request to access the information, no one is entitled as a matter of law to do this on his or her behalf. A lacuna in the Data Protection Act 1998 remains, notwithstanding that its contravention of Articles 8 and 14 of the Convention has been repeatedly drawn to the attention of the UK Government and the Data Protection Commissioner.[7]

The third way and the recasting of 'public'

Whilst community care law bears the indelible stamp of its poor law origins,[8] its present shape still predominately reflects Beveridge's vision of the welfare state: the all-powerful (postwar) state that could slay the giants of want as it had slain the giant evil of fascism. For him, society was a very real thing, albeit inseparable from the state. Margaret Thatcher, of course, famously questioned the existence of 'society' and, via the NHS and Community Care Act 1990, sought to extend the privatisation agenda into health and community care via the creation of NHS trusts, the greater use of independent residential and nursing homes and the general promotion of the 'mixed economy of care'.[9] Hitherto public functions were devolved to private and independent providers with the state fulfilling the rump role of 'purchaser'.

Section 6 of the Human Rights Act 1998[10] constitutes a dynamic third stage in the shifting approach to the public/private divide. Rather than re-nationalise the provision of community care services, it recasts the definition of a public authority, 'to embrace any person some of whose functions are of a public nature. The expansive nature of this concept was explained by the Lord Chancellor who stated that the key question is whether the body in question has 'functions of a public nature. If it has any functions of a public nature, it qualifies as a public authority.'[11] On this basis, private community care providers (such as residential care home proprietors or voluntary sector service providers such as Age Concern, MIND or housing associations[12]) are 'public authorities' in relation to anyone for whom they provide publicly funded care. Such providers now shoulder public responsibilities for their vulnerable clients and are accountable in public law for their actions. The Department of Health has accordingly emphasised the need for English social services departments to 'ensure that contractors and independent providers are made aware of their new duties'.[13]

Article 2: the right to life

Article 2 requires states to take reasonable measures to protect life.[14] Evidence suggests that relocating institutionalised elderly people to a new residence may have a dramatic effect on their mental health and life expectancy,[15] some research studies suggesting that the increase in mortality rates might be as high as 35 per cent.[16] In recognition of this danger, guidance on the 'transfer of frail elderly patients to other long stay settings' (HSC 1998/048) was issued on 2 April 1998.

Many residential home closures involve the relocation of extremely frail elderly people who have spent very many years in a particular home. In addition, in *R v North & East Devon Health Authority ex p Coughlan* (1999)[17] the Court of Appeal held that a closure of the NHS facility in question amounted to an interference with the applicant's right to enjoy her home under Article 8. The Human Rights Act 1998 will accordingly require public authorities to justify closures, not merely by the 'due process' standard of having carried out appropriate consultations but also by the standard of being satisfied that its substantial obligations under Article 2 have been met.

Article 3: the right not to be subjected to degrading treatment

There is widespread physical, financial and sexual abuse of disabled adults.[18] Article 3 places a positive obligation on the state to take action to ensure that no one suffers from degrading treatment. In *Z & others v UK*, 10/9/99, the European Commission of Human Rights considered (unanimously) that Bedfordshire social services department had violated Article 3 by failing to take action to protect a number of vulnerable children whom it knew to be the victims of ill-treatment and neglect. Without referring to this opinion, the Court of Appeal in *re F (Adult: Court's jurisdiction)* (2000)[19] acknowledged the 'obvious gap in the framework for [protecting] mentally incapacitated adults' from abuse. The case concerned a young woman with profound learning disabilities, who had been sexually abused. The Court stated that, unless domestic law enabled courts to intervene, 'this vulnerable young woman would be left at serious risk without recourse to protection'. Having regard to the new environment consequent upon the Human Rights Act 1998, the court unashamedly developed the common law principle of 'necessity' to provide the protection required by the convention (essentially a new adult wardship jurisdiction); as Sedley LJ put it, to 'speak where Parliament . . . was silent'.

The Strasbourg court has additionally held that there is a positive duty on states to conduct independent investigations where credible evidence exists that a person has been subjected to abuse. Although the case concerned brutality in a police station (*Assenov v Bulgaria* (1998)) it applies with equal force to allegations that (for instance) a person has been abused whilst in a residential care home. A failure to conduct a properly independent and rigorous investigation will itself constitute a violation of Article 3.

Article 8: the right to a private and family life

Article 8 inevitably raises a large number of questions in relation to the rights of disabled people to a family life; not least the extent to which siblings of a profoundly disabled child have the right to a 'family life' which is only practically available if adequate services are provided to the disabled child; the right of disabled children to live with their families, when a disproportionate number face an institutionalised childhood,[20] and the rights of married people to live together in care homes.

Article 8 is also concerned with the right to a private life; and one of the most private aspects of this is a right to a sexual life.[21] Whilst the European Court of Human Rights has considered a large number of cases concerning the rights of homosexuals and transsexuals under Article 8, it has not had the opportunity to consider any cases concerning the rights of disabled people to a sexual life. As noted above, this is hardly surprising given the taboo nature of disability in general within Western European society and in particular the issue of disabled people's sexuality. Who is going to be able or willing to bring such a case to the court on behalf of a mentally incapacitated person?

The issue appears simple; to what extent does the positive obligation underlying Article 8 extend to the provision by the state of the means for a person with profound physical impairments to have a sexual life – by way of sexual aids and assistance – and to what extent do our criminal laws unreasonably discriminate against people with a learning disability? The Sexual Offences Act 1956 criminalises sexual activity involving 'mental defectives'. Whilst the present review of the legislation[22] makes certain proposals in this respect, it remains to be seen if they are adequate or if there is the political will to ensure that such change occurs.

In X and Y v Netherlands (1985), the Court held that 'private life' includes a person's physical and moral integrity. Y, a person with learning difficulties, complained (assisted by her father, X) that she had been unable to begin criminal proceedings against the man who had sexually assaulted her because she lacked the necessary competence under Dutch law. The Court held that there had been a violation of Article 8 as the State had failed to secure respect for her private life, by ensuring that her abuser was prosecuted.

Article 10: freedom of expression

The Article 10 right includes, not only the right to freedom of expression, but also the right to 'receive and impart information'.

The widespread failure of the health services, as well as education and social services to ascertain the wishes and feelings of disabled people, and particularly disabled children with profound impairments, is well documented.[23] All too frequently this occurs (in part) due to a shortage of therapists.[24]

Arguably the right of a disabled person to therapies which enable him/her to communicate engages the obligation under Article 10[25] (and possibly Article 6(1) in enabling him/her to self-advocate). At the very least, therefore, health authorities must positively consider this obligation when deciding what level of therapy/advocacy services it funds in this area.

Article 1, protocol 1: the right to peacefully enjoy possessions

The convention requires that interferences with a person's peaceful enjoyment of his/her possessions should be in accordance with the law and proportionate. Where the interference concerns a social security benefit,[26] then additionally there should be a right to challenge the interference before an independent and impartial tribunal under Article 6(1).

Appointeeships under Regulation 33 Social Security (Claims and Payments) Regulations 1987, enable the Secretary of State to pay an individual's social security benefits to a third party where s/he believes that a person lacks the necessary capacity to handle his or her own affairs. The decision is not amenable to any appeal process which conforms with the requirements of Article 6(1), and accordingly the process appears to violate the convention.

Resource issues

In *R v Gloucestershire County Council ex p Barry* (1997)[27] the House of Lords approved in principle the right of local authorities to reduce community care service provision where they faced severe financial resource shortages. In the first instance decision[28] McCowan LJ had emphasised that this principle was subject to a number of constraints not least where the disabled person 'would be at severe physical risk' if the services were not provided. In such cases he held that services must be provided regardless of resources.

In the human rights context one might rephrase this principle by stating that local authorities cannot use resource shortages as a reason for refusing services where, as a consequence, there 'would be a risk that the disabled person's rights under Article 3 (degrading treatment) or Article 2 (right to life) would be violated'. Indeed it might be argued that the correct principle is now that resource constraints are irrelevant if the service is required in order to satisfy any of the disabled person's rights under the

Convention (i.e. right to a private and family life under Article 8, or to the means of expression under Article 10, etc).

Conclusion

The European Convention on Human Rights protects many rights that are of fundamental relevance to disabled people. The fact that they have not accessed these rights (and the convention process) constitutes the most pressing human rights issue affecting disabled people. This difficulty was well expressed by the distinguished judge, Sir Stephen Sedley, writing prior to the coming into force of the Human Rights Act 1998. The challenge to us all, he suggested, was to ensure that society's (then) losers and winners did not merely become the same losers and winners under a Human Rights Act.[29]

The powerful will always find ways of asserting their rights. For a human rights culture to flourish, however, the civil justice system must be structured (or re-structured) to ensure that the weak have an equal opportunity to enjoy their rights. At present they demonstrably do not.

NOTES

1 Negative human rights are those which require the state to refrain from action which defeats individual rights (i.e. not to torture or interfere in private life or restrict expression). In contrast positive rights place obligations on the state to take action, for instance to provide a homeless person with a house, or an unemployed person with a job. The European Convention on Human Rights was drafted primarily with a view to protecting negative, not positive rights.

2 *Golder v UK* (1979).

3 Sections 1 and 2 of which put advocates ('authorised representatives') on a statutory footing. These sections have not however been brought into effect because of 'their resource and administrative implications'.

4 *McKenzie v McKenzie* [1970] 3 W.L.R. 472, [1970] 3 All E.R. 1034.

5 'Mental Incapacity' (Law Commission Paper No. 231 (1995); and see also 'Who Decides?' Lord Chancellor's Department Cm 3803, (Dec. 1997) and 'Making Decisions' Lord Chancellor's Department Cm 4465; (Oct 1999).

6 Rule 21.4.3.c, Civil Procedure Rules.

7 See for instance para 2.29 et seq: Clements. L (2000) 'Community Care & the Law', Legal Action.

8 ibid. para 1.5.

9 The White Paper *Caring for People* (1989 Cm 849), para 1.11.

10 Under which it is unlawful for a public authority to act in a way which is incompatible with a Convention right.

11 Hansard 24 Nov 1997: Column 797.

12 Now generally referred to as 'residential social landlords'.

13 LAC (2000)17; but no equivalent guidance has yet been issued in Wales.

14 *Osman v UK* (1998) *The Times*, 5 November.

15 See, for instance, *International Journal of Geriatric Psychiatry*, vol. 8, p. 521 (1993); also see *The Times* (1994) 7 July, 'Elderly patients die within weeks of transfer'.

16 'Relocation of the aged and disabled: A mortality study', *Journal of American Geriatric Society*, 11, 185.

17 *The Times*, 20 July (CA).

18 'Setting the Boundaries: Reforming the law on sex offences', Home Office, July 2000, para 0.17.

19 *The Times*, 25 July.

20 Barnes, C. (1991) *Disabled People in Britain and Discrimination,* London: Hurst and Company/University of Calgary Press, in association with the British Council of Organisations of Disabled People.

21 *Norris v Ireland* (1988).

22 'Setting the Boundaries: Reforming the law on sex offences', op. cit.

23 See *Disabled Children: Directions for Their Future Care*; Department of Health Social Care Group (1998) which noted at para 10.3 that 'Typically, the section of the form headed "child's view" was left blank' or the social worker made comments such as 'She is unable to verbally communicate therefore her view is not available'; and at para 10.4 that many young disabled people did not have access to a communication system which suited their needs.

24 Russell, P. (1988) 'Community approaches to serving children and their families'. In D. Towell (ed.) *An Ordinary Life in Practice*, London: King Edward's Hospital Fund for London.

25 Whilst the jurisprudence of the European Court of Human Rights may not have developed to a stage where it would find that Article 10 created a positive right to a therapist, it is quite possible that domestic courts will make this development. The Department of Health appears to accept such a proposition; it quotes with approval (at para 3.125 'Assessing Children in Need and their Families: practice guidance', Department of Health (2000)) the assertion made by Jenny Morris that 'disabled children have the human right to take part in play and leisure activities and to freely express themselves' (Morris, J. (1998) *Accessing Human Rights: Disabled Children and the Children Act*, The Who Cares? Trust, London, p. 20).

26 *Schuler-Zgraggen v Switzerland* (1993).

27 1 CCLR 40; [1997] 2 All ER 1; [1997] 2 WLR 459.

28 *R v Gloucestershire County Council ex p Mahfood and Others* 1 CCLR 7; 94 LGR 593, DC.

29 First Steps Towards a Constitutional Bill of Rights [1997] EHRLR Issue 2.

CHAPTER 30

SELF-ADVOCACY FOR PEOPLE WITH LEARNING DIFFICULTIES

Simone Aspis

There are many definitions of what self-advocacy is amongst people with learning difficulties, service providers, course tutors and different social movements. For analysis purposes I decided to use the self-advocacy definition which has been adopted by People First. People First is the only organisation run and controlled by people with learning difficulties.

People First Workers (1996a,b) say self-advocacy includes:

■ speaking up for yourself;
■ standing up for your rights;
■ making choices;
■ being independent;
■ taking responsibility for oneself.

Self-advocates (Dawson and Palmer 1993) suggest, in order to advocate, one needs to:

■ resist practices which oppress you, by challenging people in power;
■ have the right to challenge others and be angry;
■ challenge carers when the need arises.

Source: 'Self-advocacy for people with learning difficulties: does it have a future?', *Disability and Society*, 12.4, 1997, pp. 647–54.

Self-advocacy training

In order for people with learning difficulties to advocate they need to learn skills. Service providers, adult training centres, special schools and colleges are now devising courses to teach people about making choices, taking responsibility and how to speak up. [. . .].

The City Lit (Sutcliffe 1990) runs courses which will teach self-advocacy skills to people with learning difficulties; skills acquired will include speaking up for oneself and or supporting others in a group to make choices, decisions and plan for change on an individual or collective level; taking turns in speaking and listening; valuing personal experience and opinions; asking and answering questions; understanding the difference between assertion and aggression; and use of body language.

During the course, self-advocates are taught skills for participating in meetings which includes understanding the format and structure; language (agendas, minutes, apologies); devising rules and roles people play (Sutcliffe 1990).

Self-advocacy is seen as the process of acquiring the confidence to make decisions at varying levels for oneself. This would include making decisions about day-to-day activities such as what to eat or what clothes to wear.

With encouragement and confidence, the person will make decisions which affects his/her own life such as choosing and getting a job; getting married or moving to more independent accommodation (Sutcliffe 1990).

Sutcliffe associates self-advocacy with individual change; recognising life stories, and experiences and skills development.

The problem with running these courses is that people do not gain the confidence to speak up in their own lives outside the course. The courses focus very much on developing communication skills to interact with other people rather than skills and knowledge needed to gain change. This is illustrated by hearing some ideas on how self-advocates negotiate for changes in their lives which are reflected by self-advocates (Dawson and Palmer 1993).

Also, courses do not include teaching students how to gain effective change through challenging policies and the law. There is also no examination of power relationships between self-advocate and institution or government staff or elected members.

Self-advocates getting changes

In all cases, self-advocates believed that they need to negotiate change with a member of staff without recognising the importance of changing the institution's rules. The self-advocate thought it was individual staff members who had the power to make decisions and permanent changes. At the moment the change being enforced is dependent on the goodwill of the staff rather than a protected right provided by the institution. Self-advocates did not appear to have the knowledge to insist on institution's rules and policies to change.

A group of self-advocates were asked at a Kings Fund conference (Wertheimer 1987) about ideas on how they would make changes in their lives. Participants said:

■ There are all sorts of ways of negotiating for change. Some are informal (like going to have a chat with the centre manager) and some are more formal (like going to meetings and putting over your point of view).
■ Self-advocates need to feel comfortable about going to meetings and speaking up.
■ If one sort of negotiation does not work try another way!

Self-advocates did not just talk about methods of negotiating for change by having meetings with staff and bosses, but also achievements they have made. All the self-advocates' achievements have been making changes within existing services.

Below are examples of how and what changes self-advocates have achieved. In all examples, self-advocates thought they were going to be successful in gaining changes within services through asking individual service employees to make the change. Instead they should concentrate on changing the policy so that changes become protected rights and not based on the 'goodwill' of others. In all cases below the method ought to be gaining a policy change.

A *group of self-advocates* were unhappy with the on-going training – on no salary – in their workshop. Self-advocates who went to the same workshop had arranged a meeting with the workshop manager to ask him when does the training stop and the job begin.

One self-advocate managed to negotiate with the workshop manager to receive a wage for his job. Other self-advocates who are in a similar situation will not receive a wage for the jobs they are doing. If all the self-advocates demanded a wage for their jobs then at worst the workshop manager will reverse the decision made giving one self-advocate a wage. The workshop manager may not be in a position to pay all self-advocates a wage because of budget or policy constraints. Even if the workshop manager decided to pay all the self-advocates a wage what happens once she or he leaves? The decision could be reversed once a new workshop manager takes over because she or he will want to work within the institution's policies.

Hillingdon People First decided they wanted to have a coffee machine installed in their Adult Training Centre. They arranged a meeting with the centre manager. The manager agreed with their proposal and the machine was installed.

Hillingdon People First received a coffee machine – there was no indication whether the coffee machine was bought or leased from a company. What happens if the coffee machine breaks down, will there be a budget for repairs or replacement? If the centre manager is replaced then will the new centre manager support the idea for continuing with having a coffee machine?

Ravenswood self-advocacy group had talked about labels which were being used on their mini-buses. The self-advocates had written a letter to the board of trustees and they had agreed to remove the labels on their mini-buses.

Breakaways group in Fairways Day Centre wanted the term changed from 'clients' to students. The group had sent a survey to all the Surrey Day Centres asking them to complete and return the survey with a letter to the Director of Social Services. After discussions with the Director he told the clients that they could be called whatever they liked. Difficulties arose when the staff did not want the change.

Both Breakaways and Ravenswood self-advocacy groups wanted the labels replaced or removed. There have been attempts to work collectively recognising that there are service users with similar concerns and that the strength in numbers will increase the pressure for change. With the Breakaways group the director said that the users can call themselves whatever they wanted. Difficulties arose in the day centre where staff did not want to comply with using the term student rather than client. The Director did not change the policy so that all the staff *have* to use the same term.

Ravenswood self-advocacy group was successful with getting the labels removed from the mini-buses because of the goodwill from the board of trustees. A new board of trustees may choose in the future to label the buses again.

The common theme running through the method of getting change is to negotiate with individual people who are in power rather than changing the policy so that change is much more long term. At anytime changes can easily be reversed as institutions' policies have not been amended in line with the change. Speaking up is confined to making choices or making changes within services, based on the 'goodwill' of service employees.

Self-advocates' achievements are cosmetic. In all instances of labelling, service providers only had to change the label name on the stationery or vehicles. When changes are made they are to do with minor arrangements in a service. Service providers can still treat people with learning difficulties in the same way as people who were previously labelled as mentally handicapped. Throughout the process of self-advocacy there has not been a transfer of power from service provider to the person(s) with learning difficulties.

The changes that people with learning difficulties are seeking such as not being labelled or having better facilities within day centres are not legal rights. There is no piece of legislation to stop charities or any organisations from labelling people. People with learning difficulties will see it as their right not to be labelled. However, in reality people with learning difficulties are labelled all the time in law. Another example of how people with learning difficulties talk about rights is the following extract from *Everything You Ever Wanted to Know About Safe Sex*, a pamphlet issued by People First.

We have the right to:

- *Have information about our bodies and how they work.*
- *Have information on sex and learn about sex.*
- *To be treated like adults.*
- *Have sex with whoever we want to if we both agree.*
- *Have privacy – somewhere to meet, like our bedroom, where nobody will enter.*

These are 'moral rights', a right that a person *should* have. These rights are dependent on the goodwill of others.

In reality a person with learning difficulties does not have the above sexual rights. [. . .] Because the above rights are not legal rights then there is no duty for someone else to take appropriate action or to get redress if the right is being violated.

Explaining about rights within a moral context has the following problems. People with learning difficulties are led to believe:

- they have more rights than they really do;
- they are already equal with other people in society;
- they have the same rights as everyone does;
- there is no redress if the right is not being enforced;
- there is no reason to campaign for enforceable legal rights.

Moral rights can cause inconsistency on enforcement. For example, a woman with severe learning difficulties may have a sexual relationship in group home A, whilst in group home B she could be refused this right. It makes it difficult for individuals to see their mistreatment within a common framework, e.g. lack of legislation. There could be many different reasons why a person is being denied a right by another person within a moral context. For example, Group Home Manager A may say on religious grounds, Group Home Manager B may say because the woman is not able enough, Group Home Manager C may say because of protecting the woman.

Service providers

It is not surprising that service providers are jumping on the band wagon of self-advocacy. Service providers will pay self-advocacy groups to find out what people with learning difficulties want from their services; speaking up about what services they want; for example, where do you want to live (a group home; a residential home; your own flat with support)? Self-advocacy has become a tool to find out what people with learning difficulties think of services, rather than to challenge the philosophy of services and the system that creates them and their inherent limitations. As a consequence, the service provider limits the scope of what self-advocates are able to speak up about. Service providers' existence and power is left unchallenged by people with learning difficulties; associated legislation gives certain people the power to label people and then segregates them, which results in the position of people with learning difficulties in our society being left unchallenged.

Unfortunately, the independent self-advocacy groups have also become a victim of service providers buying them out via providing service agreements if they will offer user expertise. This means that service providers and other agencies (normally run by non-disabled people) are dictating what people with learning difficulties should be speaking up about:

> We expect the system to resist change. If we are not careful, self-advocates will be given all the time they want to speak for themselves, to say what they want, to publish books. And the system may not take a blind bit of notice.
>
> (Simons 1991)

Conclusion

As more and more service providers offer self-advocacy within their services or provide service agreements to independent self-advocacy groups, the greater the control these people have over what people with learning difficulties should speak up about. As a result self-advocates will be forced into only speaking up about choices of services which are provided by the local or health authority.

Self-advocacy courses have heavily concentrated on developing inter-personal and communication skills which are valued and accepted by professionals (service providers) and how to win the goodwill of others. The teaching of rights has been based within a moral context; telling people what (moral) rights they ought to have, rather than what (legal) rights they do and do not have. Moral rights are given by the goodwill of others whilst legal rights must be enforced and upheld by other people.

Due to only having knowledge about rights within a moral context, self-advocates see themselves as only needing to negotiate with staff and managers to get changes within a given service. Service providers have ultimate control, their authority going unchallenged by people with learning difficulties and maintaining full control over services (as policies or legislation will not reflect agreed changes). This leads to people with learning difficulties only being able to see what they want in terms of services and only receiving the benefits of change depending upon the manager or staff on duty in a given service.

Self-advocacy has become very much a tool to support people with learning difficulties to accept their position in society where their participation is dependent on the goodwill of others usually professionals and service providers. This makes people with learning difficulties feel good and accepted by these people who have power.

Self-advocacy facilitators or tutors hesitate to support people to go the full way in gaining change in policy or legislation because they fear that self-advocates may fail and have less confidence to speak up again in the future. However, denying people with learning difficulties this knowledge will stop people from gaining real change: the right to stop people in power labelling people and segregating them from the rest of society. In short, self-advocacy has become a tool to support people with learning difficulties to accept the best out of a bad deal rather than gaining the ideal which could lead to creating something new, whilst challenging society's values which seek to label and stigmatise people.

The accepting of getting the best of a bad deal comes from the internalised oppression of people with learning difficulties. Throughout their lives people with learning difficulties have also been labelled as being stupid, childish or idiots. People with learning difficulties do not like being called names nor do they like the thought of not being able to learn. As a consequence people with learning difficulties have had a poor self-image of themselves. Through the labelling process people with learning difficulties have had their expectations of life limited by other people. They are told to accept what is 'realistic' rather than having the challenge to go for something that is not available.

Also when growing up, people with learning difficulties learn that professionals are helpful and supportive by the one-to-one attention they receive. This intense attention is not given by other people with learning difficulties or disabled people. They will do anything to be accepted by able-bodied people or people who are valued by society like service providers, social workers and professionals. The bare fact that a service provider nods or passively listens to a person with learning difficulties makes him or her feel valued. Current self-advocacy is therefore being modelled on the internalised oppression of people with learning difficulties.

Due to this, self-advocacy has become concerned with supporting individuals to gain individual 'realistic' change within institutions by using inter-personal skills valued by professionals without challenging their status and power.

I conclude to say that self-advocacy cannot be a liberating experience if its process and contents are being managed and controlled by the same people who have the power to oppress those who have been labelled as having learning difficulties.

REFERENCES

Dawson, P. and Palmer, W. (1993) *Taking Self-advocacy Seriously* (EMFEC).

People First Workers (1996a) *Speaking Out For Equal Rights Workbook 2*, Equal People Course Books (Buckingham, Open University, People First, and Mencap).

People First Workers (1996b) *Working Together For Change Workbook 3*, Equal People Course Books (Buckingham, Open University, People First, and Mencap).

Simons, K. (1991) *Sticking Up For Yourself – Self-advocacy and People with Learning Difficulties* (Bristol, Norah Fry Research Centre).

Sutcliffe, J. (1990) *Adults with Learning Difficulties, Education for Choice and Empowerment* (Leicester, National Institute of Adult Continuing Education).

Wertheimer, A. (1987) *Self-advocacy Skills Training* (London, Kings Fund).

PART IV

TERRITORIES AND BOUNDARIES

INTRODUCTION

In adopting the theme of territories and boundaries, our focus is not primarily on actual space or geographical boundaries, lines on maps and fences around buildings (important though these sometimes are in the provision of care and support). Instead we provide the basis for an explanation of how formal and informal, visible and invisible practices and assumptions define responsibilities and roles in social care. By exposing and questioning boundaries and territories, possibilities for new partnerships and collaborations emerge.

The first challenging chapter reminds us that, in regard to coordinated action, patterns of communication are rapidly changing. Expert information, guidance and instruction are increasingly available, literally at the press of a button. As experts and professionals are rapidly discovering, the Internet is no respecter of disciplines and mystiques. So, in Chapter 31, John Hudson helps us think through some of the implications for community care services, of this new 'information age'.

Chapter 32 includes three first-hand accounts of support and care work. First, there is a day in the life of Carol McHugh, a mental health outreach worker. Next Sally French and John Swain describe how one particular local voluntary organisation works to support disabled people. Third, Julia Johnson writes about being a social worker at the time of the Seebohm reorganisation. The question of how care work is organised in the context of public and private spaces in then explored in more depth in Chapter 33. Here Julia Twigg reports on her study of how bathing is provided for people who need assistance, and what this means for those who provide it.

At this point attention reverts to the big picture. In Chapter 34, Caroline Glendinning reviews policies on home care services in various European countries. One of the interesting contrasts that she notes concerns the boundary between social and nursing care, something touched on by Julia Twigg, and this is examined in more detail in the UK context in the next two chapters. Jane Lewis, in Chapter 35, analyses how the boundary between health and social care for older people is managed. She concludes that this has been determined primarily by national policies regarding public expenditure. In Chapter 36, Allison Worth exposes some of the marked differences in how the needs of older people are assessed in practice in Scotland. She found that, although social workers and district nurses approached the task very differently, both groups were concerned about resource constraints and matters of eligibility.

In Chapter 37, Christine Oldman critically examines policy regarding the respective responsibilities of housing and social care services. In her view, the concept of need has been and remains fragmented. The consequence is what she describes as 'woefully inadequate' investment in appropriate and adequate housing for social care recipients.

In the last three chapters, attention turns to the inter-personal relationship between provider and user. Here an important focus is on direct payments and the impact of this on power relations. In Chapter 38, Frances Hasler, of the National Centre for Independent Living, shows how the Direct Payments Act (1996) offers opportunities for new partnership arrangements when disabled people organise their own support. Currently much carework is underpaid and undervalued. Is there a way of increasing job satisfaction and the rewards of such work? Clare Ungerson, in Chapter 39, details some of the policies being developed in different countries, including various payment schemes. She discusses the question of what strategies might both help to empower those in need of support, and raise the status of those providing it. In this context, it is appropriate to turn, finally, in Chapter 40, to three personal testimonies of what is involved in managing support. First, Alice Kadel offers a description of life as a 'Country Cousin': a scheme providing short-term live-in carers. Next we include a short extract from Daphne du Maurier's novel *Rebecca*, in which she describes the experience of being a companion. Finally, we end with Ruth Bailey's vivid description of life supported by a personal assistant in 'It's my party'.

CHAPTER 31

COMMUNITY CARE IN THE INFORMATION AGE

John Hudson

According to Tony Blair, the United Kingdom in the 1990s was entering a 'new age of information [which] offers possibilities for the future limited only by the boundaries of our imaginations' (Cabinet Office 1998: 1). The information age will, he has argued, bring social and economic change 'as fundamental as the shift from agrarian to industrial production' (Blair 1999: viii).

In expressing such views, he was merely bringing to the policy realm ideas much discussed in sociology that a new economic paradigm was emerging, predicated upon knowledge industries and new information and communication technologies (ICTs). While the status of such claims is certainly contestable, the notion that we now live in an information society has gained widespread popular credence. More importantly perhaps, governments throughout the western world are increasingly acting on the basis that such claims are true, most drawing up extensive and explicit plans to adapt their activities for the brave new world of the information age (OECD 1998; Policity.com 2000)

The Blair government has outlined plans that can be roughly divided into three areas. First, it has identified a need to modernise the structure of government services in order to maximise the potential of ICTs. In particular, it has emphasised the importance of using new technology to improve the administrative efficiency of services and to improve and extend access to services. Here, the government has laid down a radical agenda for reform, its *Modernising Government* White Paper setting strict targets for the implementation of 'e-government'(Cabinet Office 1999).

A second area of change is economic policy, the government identifying a need to facilitate structural changes in the economy in order to maximise the benefits of the emerging digital age. In particular, by creating financial incentives for the technology-based industries that it believes will be at the core of the new 'knowledge economy', it has set itself the target of becoming by 2002 'the best place in the world' to conduct 'e-business'.

While this issue might appear to be of limited relevance to community care, it links with the third area of concern: the need to prevent the emergence in this new high-tech, high-skill, high-wage economy, of a 'digital divide' between the 'information haves' and the 'information have-nots' (Cabinet Office 1998). In order to participate in the new age of information, citizens will – at the very least – need access to ICTs in order to consume electronic products. Increasingly, they will require skills in operating ICTs to gain well-paid employment. For this reason, the government was concerned that new technology should not generate new forms of social exclusion (Hudson 2000; UK-Online 2000).

Clearly then, at the end of the second millennium, the government believed that ICTs were likely to bring profound changes to the ways in which it would deliver services in the future. However, information age government at the ground level often seemed to be something that existed a long way into the future (Bellamy and Taylor 1998; Hudson 1999).

Social services agencies

What, then, is the picture of ICT use in local authority social services departments (SSDs) in the year 2001? Just over a decade ago, Griffiths' seminal report highlighted information systems as a key weakness within this sector. In his typically prosaic style, he claimed that 'the present lack of refined information systems . . . would plunge most organisations in the private sector into quick and merciful liquidation' (DoH 1988: 4). Since then, various government reports have confirmed the problematic nature of information systems in the social care field. For example, in 1992, it was noted that the majority of SSDs regarded poor systems as a key barrier to the implementation of the community care reforms. In 1995, the Social Services Inspectorate (SSI) reported the continuing widespread weakness of information systems, concluding that 'SSDs are finding it difficult to implement effective information strategies and systems' (SSI 1995: 2), and two years later it again noted 'the inadequacies of Social Services Departments' systems for collecting, sharing and using information' (SSI 1997: 1). In short, while SSDs had upgraded their systems in the previous decade, the pace of technological change had been such that their use of ICTs was still somewhat dated.

In having problems adopting ICTs, SSDs were by no means unusual as far as the public sector was concerned; the Department of Social Security (DSS) and the National Health Service (NHS) had also been widely criticised. What makes the situation in the social services sector a little more unusual, however, was the fact that the government had charged SSDs with the task of improving their use of ICTs but had done little to help them meet this demand. While the NHS and the DSS had several high profile and high-cost flagship projects pushed forward by central government, cash-strapped SSDs had generally been left to struggle along as best they could. Indeed, in an environment of ever-growing demands, combined as it was with ever-increasing pressures on budgets, it was hardly surprising that SSDs were finding it difficult to carve out resources for ICTs.

It might be argued that this was not in itself a bad thing. Social services are, fundamentally, human services. Increasing resource pressures and changing work roles appeared to be reducing the time social workers had to spend with their clients, not least because of the increasing amount of time spent on collecting information for administrative purposes (Levin and Webb 1997). Significantly, there had been suggestions that such trends were damaging the quality of the service provided to users (NISW 2000). Diverting financial resources from front line services in order to invest in ICTs, and/or making ICT use integral to the social work task, might not be the most sensible way forward. Indeed, for some years a core of theorists had argued that the cold, rational and steely nature of ICTs means that the technology cannot be placed in a complex and human-based service like social work without fundamentally clashing with its values (Bamford 1996). Social work students were deeply suspicious of computer techno-logy, with over a quarter regarding the rising use of ICTs as likely to be damaging to society (Morgan 1996: 7). Others expressed diluted versions of the following view of social workers:

> *In many ways this is the last group of people likely to embrace a tech-nologically-aware, structured decision-making managerial culture. Seeing themselves as the enabling care manager, juggling resources with the aid of a spreadsheet, a database and a word processor is not the image most social work students dream of at night.*
>
> *(Kerslake 1996: 12)*

Irrespective of whether or not ICTs clash with social work values, there were certainly many social workers who resisted the imposition by man-agement of information systems on their work, because they feared that such systems would lead to a fundamental shift in working practices. In some areas, there had even been enough unrest to produce industrial action (Hudson 1999).

Where systems had been implemented, there had often been severe 'Garbage In, Garbage Out' (GIGO) problems. Information systems are only as good as the information held within them, but numerous studies had shown that high levels of data inaccuracy were commonplace and were not always accidental (Glastonbury 1993). Data relating to service activities generally has to be collected by relatively autonomous frontline workers. If they have no real commitment to this task, or if they feel the data will undermine their autonomy, then it is likely that the data they collect will be of a poor quality. This in turn means that the outputs of information systems based on this data is also likely to be 'garbage'. The Social Services Inspectorate had suggested that the emergence of GIGO in some SSDs was serious enough to call into the question the value of computer-based – as against paper-based – information systems (SSI 1995).

None of this might matter, except that the post-Griffiths community care regime is very much predicated on accurate and reliable information systems (Bovell *et al.* 1997; Lewis and Glennerster 1997). In an ideal world, care managers constructing individual care packages for their clients need fast access to accurate and up-to-date information about their client's needs, the service options on offer, the price of individual service options, and details of the budgetary resources available for the client under consideration. Yet, despite implicit government acknowledgement that such data are a prerequisite for a properly functioning market, the vision of information-driven decision-making has not yet emerged. A lack of funds for investment in new systems, combined with problems in using available systems effectively, means that the situation at the start of the 2000s is little different from that which had shocked Griffiths at the end of the 1980s.

If the picture within SSDs is troubled, that within many of the organisations that form part of the new mixed economy of welfare is still worse. When it comes to garnering the resources – financial, political or technical – required to implement ICT-based reforms, local SSDs generally face a comparative disadvantage when compared with the NHS and DSS. Being large and centrally-based, the latter find it easier to gain funding from the Treasury, have better and more established links with industry, and generally command more effective support from Whitehall. Yet, when SSDs are compared with voluntary organisations – particularly the smaller ones – they have a distinct advantage in terms of ICT use. One study, for example, concluded that while voluntary organisations were keen to take advantage of the Internet, in practice many suffered from a lack of technical knowledge and a wariness of incurring significant investment costs without accruing identifiable benefits. In a telling comment of the situation facing many voluntary organisations, one cash-strapped manager expressed feelings of frustration:

> *People have been on at me for years to get a fax. Now I've got a fax they're telling me to get onto the Internet.*
>
> (NISW 1997)

In short, the process of getting technology in place – never mind using it effectively – was also a problem for many voluntary agencies, and this remains one of the key reasons why Griffiths' vision of an information-driven quasi-market is still a long way off. If one takes the social care sector as a whole, notions of an information revolution are clearly way off the mark and, in a very real sense, information systems are acting as a barrier to change rather than driving it forward. As another NISW study pointed out, information systems designed in the 1970s and 1980s were struggling with the organisational changes brought about in the 1990s (NISW 1996: 1).

Yet, while the public sector generally – and the social care sector in particular – was slowly being eased into the 'information age' in the 1990s, the indications were that large sections of the British public were keen to take advantage of new ICTs. Indeed, according to government figures, by the first quarter of 2000, one in four households had access to the Internet, proportionately twice the number who had access for the same period in 1999 and almost three times as many as in 1998 (ONS 2000).

While there are clear social divisions in the use of the new technology – rich households are more likely to have access than poor ones and lone parent families or retired households are the least likely to have access – the evidence clearly shows that the image of the Internet user as single, young, white and male is a stereotype; indeed, households containing two adults and two or more children are the most likely to have access. Internet use across the social spectrum has grown – and is predicted to continue to grow – exponentially. What is more, interactive digital television is predicted to have a still wider reach in the near future (Cabinet Office 1999). Significantly, some commentators have argued that, as we become familiar with new forms of communication, radical changes in the way we seek social support may have started to emerge (Burrows *et al.* 2000).

Might, then, the real changes to community care in the information age come from outside, rather than within, government?

Virtual community care

Even if government has lagged behind in the technology stakes, service users with a need for social support have not. The increasing number of households 'wired up' to the Internet has been accompanied by an explosion in websites and Internet-based discussion groups concerned with social or health related issues. Burrows *et al.* (2000) have examined the growing phenomenon of on-line self-help and social support – what they term 'virtual community care' – and have suggested that there are far-reaching implications for social policy.

While the Internet is often thought of as an arena for commercial or entertainment activities, the fact that significant numbers of people use the Internet to discuss, research and explore health and social issues has often been overlooked. By mid-1999 the thirteen social or health related newsgroups of the uk.people.* usenet hierarchy (a set of e-mail based discussion groups) were generating an average of 600 messages per day. These groups form just a small proportion of the already large number of groups based in the UK that are active on the Web and that deal with such diverse health and social issues as living with HIV+, caring for dependent relatives, coping with alcoholism, and living with a disability. It is estimated that, in mid-1999, some 18,000 people with epilepsy, at least 35,000 who were drug or alcohol dependent, 246,000 with diabetes, 317,000 with sight problems and 352,000 with hearing problems were Internet users and many of these people will use it to gather, exchange and provide information relevant to these problems (Burrows *et al.* 2000).

What is particularly interesting, however, is how the Internet has facilitated the creation of self-organised, bottom-up fora. Numerous electronic self-help groups have emerged that are by-passing government altogether; indeed, in many cases, such groups are international. Many who have joined these groups are searching for information or advice from similarly placed individuals – rather than from welfare professionals – on ways in which to tackle their own health problems or those in their families. While the advice they receive is often based on experience rather than scientific evidence, it would be wrong to characterise the exchanges as ill-informed. Indeed, the quality of the discussions is generally very high, with departures from the 'accepted wisdom' robustly defended with experiential knowledge from group members (Muncer *et al.* 2000a). Following Giddens (1994), it is suggested that this interweaving of lay and professional expertise will be a key feature of information society and, significantly, that it is likely to act as a challenge to professional power and knowledge (Muncer *et al.* 2000b).

At the turn of the century, 'virtual community care' is still in its infancy. In the long run, however, it is likely to have profound consequences for social policy:

> *In its potential at least, we suggest that it could represent an as yet little understood challenge to dominant postwar models of social policy; as an embryonic cyberspatial social form it could represent one element of a shift away from a conception of welfare based upon rationally administered state provision coupled with paternalistic professionally determined needs and bureaucratic organisational delivery systems towards one more characterised by fragmentation, diversity and a range of individualisation processes.*
>
> *(Burrows et al. 2000)*

Conclusion

Whatever the future holds, it is clear that 'the information age' will present significant challenges for the social care sector. All agencies in the mixed economy of care have traditionally struggled to keep pace with technological change and this situation is unlikely to change in the foreseeable future. Unfortunately, the rate at which new technologies penetrate society has apparently increased dramatically in recent times; while it took thirty-eight years for the radio to achieve 50 million users worldwide, and thirteen years for the television to reach the same level, the corresponding figure for the World Wide Web has been a mere four years (UNDP 1999: 58). So, while social care organisations have made significant progress, the continual shifting of the technological goalposts has meant that they still lag behind.

What this means for community care in the future is unclear. The Blair government believes that greater use of ICTs holds the key to the modernisation of public services, and successive governments have believed that ICTs can help to improve the efficiency of services. Nevertheless, in practice, employing the technology has been much easier said than done. Like any set of policies, ICT plans have to be steered through a complex set of interests before they can be implemented. In the public sector, much technological change has been successfully resisted by front line workers – particularly professional workers – and, even without this, policies have often lacked the necessary resources for successful implementation (Hudson 1999). The aim of delivering all services electronically by 2005 means little when there is a very real absence of internal – never mind external – information systems. What is more, the question needs to be asked as to whether electronic access is necessarily a particularly useful policy objective in community care.

Whatever, it is clear that technological change will continue apace. As this brief review of some of the issues facing the social care sector demonstrates, ICTs have presented – and will continue to present – significant challenges to those responsible for the delivery of services. At the same time, ICTs open up important new opportunities both for service providers and for service users. As developments unfold, it is vital that all those involved in community care and welfare remain alert to this technological dimension. In the words of Dale Spender (1995: 251), 'What social policies now need is a cyber-dimension.'

REFERENCES

Bamford, T. (1996) 'Information Driven Decision Making: Fact or Fantasy?' in A. Kerslake and N. Gould (eds) *Information Management in Social Services*. Aldershot: Avebury.

Bellamy, C. and J. Taylor (1998) *Governing in the Information Age*. Buckingham: Open University Press.

Blair, T. (1999) 'Foreword' in A. Leer (ed.) *Masters of the Wired World: Cyberspace Speaks Out*. Pearson: London.

Bovell, V., J. Lewis and F. Wookey (1997) 'The Implication for Social Service Departments of the Information Task in the Social Care Market', *Health and Social Care in the Community*, 5, 94–105.

Burrows, R., S. Nettleton, N. Pleace, B. Loader and S. Muncer (2000) 'Virtual Community Care? Social Policy and the Emergence of Computer Mediated Social Support', *Information, Communication & Society*, 3(1), http://www.infosoc.co.uk/00109/feature.htm

Cabinet Office (1998) *Our Information Age: The Government's Version*. Cabinet Office: London.

Cabinet Office (1999) *Modernising Government*. Cabinet Office: London.

Department of Health (1988) *Community Care: Agenda for Action (Griffiths' Report)*. HMSO: London.

Giddens, A. (1994) 'Living in a Post-Traditional Society' in U. Beck, A. Giddens and S. Lash (eds) *The Politics of Risk Society*. Oxford: Polity.

Glastonbury, B. (1993) 'The Implications of Information Technology in Social Care' in J. Bornat, C. Pereira, D. Pilgrim and F. Williams (eds) *Community Care: A Reader*. Basingstoke: Macmillan.

Hudson, J. (1999) 'Informatization and Public Administration: A Political Science Perspective', *Information, Communication & Society*, 2(3), 318–339.

Hudson, J. (2000) 'The Prospects for Information Age Government' in R. Burrows and N. Pleace (eds) *Wired Welfare? Essays on the Rhetoric and the Reality of e-Social Policy*. Centre for Housing Policy Discussion Paper Series, York: Centre for Housing Policy.

Kerslake, A. (1996) 'Information Management: Beyond Information Technology' in A. Kerslake and N. Gould (eds) *Information Management in Social Services*. Aldershot: Avebury.

Levin, E. and S. Webb (1997) *Social Work and Community Care: Changing Roles and Tasks*. NISW: London.

Lewis, J. and H. Glennerster (1997) *Implementing Community Care*. Buckingham: Open University Press.

Morgan, A. (1996) 'First Year Social Work Students and the Impact of Information Technology: a Pilot Study', 9(4), 2–11.

Muncer, S., R. Burrows, N. Pleace, B. Loader and S. Nettleton (2000a) 'Births, Deaths, Sex and Marriage … But Very Few Presents? A Case Study of Social Support in Cyberspace', *Critical Public Health*, 18(1), 1–18.

Muncer, S., B. Loader, S. Nettleton, N. Pleace and R. Burrows (2000b) 'Heterogeneity in Systems of Social Support: A Systematic Qualitative Comparison of Two On-line Self-help Groups' in R. Burrows and N. Pleace (eds) *Wired Welfare? Essays on the Rhetoric and the Reality of e-Social Policy*. Centre for Housing Policy Discussion Paper Series, York: Centre for Housing Policy.

NISW (1996) 'The Social Services Information Agenda', *NISW Briefing*, 17, http://www.nisw.org.uk/pold/fulltext/niswb17.html

NISW (1997) 'The Voluntary Sector and the Internet', *NISW Briefing*, 23, http://www.nisw.org.uk/publications/briefing23.html

NISW (2000) 'Modernising Social Work', *NISW Briefing*, 29, http://www.nisw.org.uk/publications/briefing29.html

OECD (1998) *Information Technology as an Instrument of Public Management Reform: A Study of Five OECD Countries*. PUMA 98(14). Paris: OECD.

ONS (2000) 'Internet Access: First Quarter 2000', July 2000, http://www.statistics.gov.uk/pdfdir/inter0700.pdf

Policity.com (2000) 'Electronic Service Delivery Clearinghouse', http://www.policity.com/ESD/index.html

Spender, D. (1995) *Nattering on the Net: Women, Power and Cyberspace*. Victoria: Spinifex Press.

SSI (1995) *Social Services Department Information Strategies and Systems (with Reference to Community Care): Inspection Overview*. London: DoH/SSI.

SSI (1997) *Informing Care: Inspection of Social Services Department Information Strategies and Systems (with Reference to Community Care)*. London: DoH/SSI.

UK-Online (2000) 'Brown Sets Out Multi-Million Pound Programme to Bridge the Digital Divide', http://www.ukonline.gov.uk/news/news18.htm, 11th October.

UNDP (1999) *Globalization with a Human Face*. New York: United Nations.

CHAPTER 32

PROVIDING SUPPORT

32.1 HOUSE CALLS

Carole McHugh

Source: *The Guardian: Society*, 13 October 1999, p. 3.

Wednesday, 13 October 1999

I went to see Jenny on my way in to work today. She's forgetful about taking her medication, and without it her behaviour appears unusual to other people – she talks to herself constantly and sometimes shouts in the street. I don't force her to take her pills, but sometimes a quick cup of tea and gentle reminder works really well. When I first met her, Jenny would frequently harm herself and was in and out of hospital, but she's much better now.

I get to the office at about 9 a.m. and one of my colleagues tells me Marie has rung. Marie has recently moved into a shared house with two other people and she's going through a bad patch. Her previous medication seemed to make her hallucinations worse and she's still not totally comfortable being on her own. Although her housemates have only gone to the local shop, Marie is scared. I decided to go and see her.

I check my diary, plan my visits and go through my messages, prioritising as I go. Then I get in the car to go and see Marie and, hopefully, visit George, an elderly man who lives near her.

Marie's mood is low. We make some tea together and talk about her trip to the dentist yesterday – she went out on her own for the first time in six weeks. She tells me she doesn't want any fillings and we swap notes on dental fears. It's important to see Marie when she feels like this. There was a time when she wouldn't communicate how she felt, but she's now able to talk to her housemates and ring us if things bother her.

Over 80 per cent of the people we support have been in hospital, repeatedly caught up in what psychiatrists call the revolving door syndrome. They get well enough to leave hospital but don't have the support they need to remain healthy in the community. United Response, the organisation I work for, gives them individual support to help break the cycle. It's really rewarding working with people who don't want to be re-admitted, but want to help themselves.

Marie and I have put a date in the communal house diary that I will come and see her on Wednesday. If it's nice weather we might sit in the garden and she wants to buy me some tasty biscuits to go with my tea.

I pop in to see if George is OK and eating properly. He's eighty, has little sight and severe depression. George is lonely and needs more company; it's hard for him to visit his friends now his eyesight is deteriorating. I set off for my meeting with the CMHT (community mental health team): local psychiatrists, social workers and community psychiatric nurses. I talk about Marie's progress. We all feel that shared accommodation suits her and that there has been a marked improvement. I let her key worker know about her mood today and she decides to visit her more frequently to make sure Marie's medication is still suitable.

The CMHT ask me to support someone new to us. Jill is thirty-six and has had a schizophrenic-type illness since she was twenty-one. Most of the time she's so ill she doesn't feel like getting out of bed and she's reluctant to cook, clean or dress herself. Her elderly parents help her to do all of this, but they're worried about what will happen to her when they die.

We will try to help Jill become more independent and start doing things for herself again. Unless we start helping now she'll go into hospital. It's a situation thousands of parents across the country face. We plan to work towards getting her to go to our local drop-in centre. There she will meet other people and be given the opportunity to make links with her local community. We can also help her with more practical things.

I nip into the office. All of my team are out visiting people, but there's a message on my desk that Marie has rung. She feels fine and thanks me for going to visit her.

I start to think about my last visit of the day. I'm off to see Anne, who's moved back into the area. She was found sleeping rough last night. She will need my help to move her belongings from a homeless hostel to a mental health housing scheme.

I'm apprehensive about seeing her as I know she has no money until her benefits come through tomorrow. I know she'll be hungry. Do I resist the urge to buy her some fish and chips on my way round to her?

32.2 ORGANISING VOLUNTARY SUPPORT

John Swain and Sally French

Source: J. Swain, M. Gillman and S. French (eds) *Confronting Disabling Barriers: Towards Making Organisations Accessible*, Venture Press, Birmingham, 1988.

'Herefordshire Lifestyles' was founded in 1985 in the city of Hereford, and in 1999 it became a registered charity. Disabled and non-disabled people work as equal partners within the organisation and on the board of trustees.

The aim of 'Herefordshire Lifestyles' is to enable every disabled person in Hereford to live a life of his or her choice. In its 1996 Annual Report, it states:

all people are entitled to the means to achieve a good quality of life, with opportunities unhindered by barriers and inadequacies due to ignorance, prejudice and discrimination.

'Herefordshire Lifestyles' is dedicated to enabling individual disabled people to fulfil their aims and ambitions in any area of their lives, whether it be a trip to the local shop or embarking on a new career. One-to-one support, mainly by volunteers, is provided where the person seeking assistance is always in control. The organisation promotes what is called 'a blank sheet of paper' approach where people listen and respond to the aspirations of disabled individuals and provide one-to-one assistance:

From the outset the principal activity has been to encourage, enable and, if appropriate, arrange the necessary training for disabled people to achieve the personal goals they have set themselves, sometimes against formidable odds.

'Herefordshire Lifestyles' has a national reputation for its innovative, pioneering approach. In recent years Lifestyle organisations have been established in twelve other British cities and interest is spreading in continental Europe. Part of the work of 'Herefordshire Lifestyles' is to support this expansion.

'Herefordshire Lifestyles' is committed to responding to requests for assistance from individual disabled people. These requests might concern accommodation, education, finance, health, mobility and transport, personal care, sport, social and leisure activities, training and employment. Joan, a participant we interviewed, explained:

> I was introduced to Jenny, my volunteer, and when I came out of hospital I went to the technical college and did a computer course. I think the most important thing is that anything I've wanted to know they've found out for me, and it's not always a case of doing it for you but enabling you to do it for yourself. When I found out that I would have to use the wheelchair I thought, 'Well, that's it, I'm just going to have to sit at home now and do nothing', but they raised my confidence a lot. I thought, 'Yes, I can do these things.' The biggest difference I've noticed is that my children could always find me at home, Mum was always in. Now they say, 'This is ridiculous, I'll have to make an appointment with you.'

The help is provided in accordance with the wishes of the disabled person. Veronica, who works for the organisation, explained:

> The main philosophy is that people are in charge of their own destiny. It's the disabled person that we are concerned with. It's what they want to do and where they want to go, and sometimes when they come here it's the first time that somebody has really concentrated on them and what they want.

Paid workers and volunteers can accompany disabled people, on a one-to-one basis, to any local venue or event of the disabled person's choice; for example the pub, an evening class, the local shop or a hospital department. This assistance may be reduced as the disabled person becomes more confident. Joyce, who has received support from 'Herefordshire Lifestyles' and now works as a volunteer and trustee, explained:

> I talked about how I used to love dancing and they said to me, 'Well, why don't you go again?' So they found me a volunteer who took me to a dance club and the first night I was there I met somebody who I used to know forty years ago and she picks me up every week and I've been going ever since ... I also took up swimming lessons. These are things I'd never done ... I really thought my life was finished when I became disabled. It raises your self-esteem and your confidence ... You tend to feel that the world belongs to the able-bodied people and you have to take a back seat all the time and it makes you get up and go.

It is recognised that people's goals and ambitions are varied and change over time. The organisation aims to be flexible enough to respond appropriately. This is achieved by very flexible working hours and allowing staff to respond to needs as they arise. Heather, who works for the organisation, said:

> *We work a given number of hours and we decide what is the most appropriate use of that time and that's guided by what people want ... It works in our favour too because we can be flexible, as long as we cover the hours by the end of the week, it doesn't matter.*

'Herefordshire Lifestyles' liaises closely with over seventy organisations and is dependent on co-operative partnerships with them. These include statutory bodies, such as social services and the health service, voluntary organisations of and for disabled people, and commercial organisations. Rather than providing services directly, 'Herefordshire Lifestyles' assists disabled people to access services which are available to the community.

The funding of the organisation is always precarious. It is raised from Trusts, the National Lottery Charities Board and from individual donors. In 2000, only 67 per cent of the budget came from social services.

'Herefordshire Lifestyles' operates within a framework underpinned by the social model of disability. It is recognised that the barriers disabled people face lie within society and that these barriers must be dismantled if disabled people are to live the lives of their choice and to secure their full citizenship rights. The organisation aims to help disabled people gain the knowledge and find the strength to dismantle barriers themselves.

Joyce said:

> *When you've done something that you've never done before it's a wonderful feeling of achievement ... I used to think, 'There's nothing I can do, I can't sew, I can't read, I can't go out.' You get to the stage where you think there is nothing at all that you can do. But there are plenty of things you can do and do well. I do more now than I've ever done before and that's what keeps you alive really, isn't it? – the stimulation and the interest.*

Disabled people, whether participants, volunteers or employees, are treated equally. Joyce explained:

I was amazed when Len asked if I would be a trustee because I didn't think that people like me sat on boards. I really thought that it was a big joke and said, 'Are you serious?' I always thought it was business people, smart people with loads of money and power.

Some of the environmental barriers disabled people commonly face have been removed in the offices of 'Herefordshire Lifestyles'. Information produced by the organisation is, for example, put on audiotape, and Joyce, who is visually impaired, has adapted computer equipment to use in the office. Access to the building is not, however, ideal for people with motor impairments. Heather said:

The main entrance in the front is pretty hard for anyone who is a wheelchair user to get through and then there's another door. It's not the easiest of buildings to get into. I think if our office was anywhere but at the front of the building it would be a problem but we generally see somebody who is trying to get in . . . but it's not ideal.

A compromise has been reached over access as the building is ideally suited on the High Street and is rent free. It is, however, impossible for many people with motor impairments to get upstairs, which can lead to a lack of privacy as the downstairs office is busy.

The organisation has been criticised for not campaigning for the rights of disabled people. Heather believes this is through:

a lack of understanding of where our viewpoint is with the individual, if they want us to do something we will help them to do it. If they want to campaign and go on a demonstration we will help them to do it, but it is not our role to make these decisions, particularly as I am not disabled. I need to be guided by individuals to do what they want me to do. We will do anything provided it is not illegal.

The ethos and philosophy of the organisation, the large number of disabled people in positions of control, and the working arrangement within the organisation, have all contributed to appropriate attitudes and behaviour towards disabled people. Joan explained:

They're always there but they don't force you into things, they don't push. There is no 'You've got to do this' or 'You ought to do this'.

Joyce agreed:

> *They don't tell you what you need. They talk to you and then they might make suggestions, and they might come up with things that you've never thought of that you feel really keen to do.*

32.3 BEING REORGANISED

Julia Johnson

I particularly remember the interview. It was in February 1970 and it was snowing. I got the train there and as it came into the station, I thought, 'This looks like the bleakest place on earth'. It was an industrial city in the Midlands of England. I came out of the station, it was cold and windy and I walked down to the Children's Department. It was a pokey little building and there was brown lino on the staircase. I reported for my interview and felt very nervous. There did not appear to be any other interviewees. I later realised that I was one of the first graduates that they had ever interviewed for a job as a child care officer. I suppose I was part of that new army of graduates coming out of university at the end of the 1960s, social science graduates who began to move into social work. During the interview I felt that they were just praying that I was going to say the right things, they seemed so keen to appoint me.

Working in the Children's Department

I got the job and started work in the summer. I was only twenty-three and it was a totally new experience in every respect. I remember the very first family that I got involved with, virtually on my first day, was a woman from Scotland and her little daughter. She had just arrived in the city. She had found a flat but had no furniture and no money and was in a pretty desperate situation. By the weekend I was driving round with bags of old clothes that I had collected up from friends and family and various other things to try to help them out. Very soon, many people in such circumstances were to become my 'cases' and part of my 'caseload'.

Initially, I accompanied one of the senior child care officers on visits to learn the ropes. But soon I had a caseload put on my desk – this was literally a pile of about twenty or so brown buff folders with people's case notes in. I was told that what I should do was to get round, visit each one and 'build up a relationship' with them. I hadn't had any kind of training for the job. I really had no idea what I was doing. But I was given a booklet which had been published in 1946 by the Pacifist Service Unit called 'The Problem Family', and this was my guidebook as to how to go about working with children and families.

I remember one of the 'cases' was a little boy who was in the local isolation hospital. He was two-and-a-half years old, and he had been there since he was six weeks old. He had been taken away from his (young, single) mother when he was only a few days old and the local authority had assumed 'parental rights'. He had been placed in the Children's Department baby nursery where he had contracted e-coli infection and this led to his admission to the isolation hospital. And he was literally in isolation in one room. The only human contact he had was with a handful of nurses. He couldn't be sent back to the nursery until he produced three clear stool samples and by the age of two and a half, that still hadn't happened. Another 'case' in my pile was a young teenager who was living, and had been living for a very long time, in what was then called a 'sub-normality' hospital. She hadn't been visited by anybody for years. I think it was the first time I had ever been in a sub-normality hospital and when I walked into the ward I found it to be full of very severely learning disabled children. The nurses carried my charge into the office and sat her cross-legged on a chair and I was sat opposite. No one offered to interpret the sounds and signs she was making and I simply didn't know how to communicate with her. I felt very humiliated and very useless and I think the nurses enjoyed every minute of it. It was awful to see and then become part of such destruction to children's lives.

Within a very short space of time I was giving evidence in court for care proceedings, interviewing potential foster or adoptive parents, taking children into care, battling with social security, the housing department, the gas and electricity boards (as they then were) about Benefits, rent arrears and disconnections. I was visiting parents in prisons and young people in remand centres and what had been Approved Schools. The 1969 Children and Young Persons Act had just been implemented: 'Approved Schools' and 'Approved School Orders' had been replaced by 'Community Homes' and 'Care Orders'. Radical changes to child care policy were in the air.

As I recall there were about fifteen of us in the Children's Department, which was ultimately accountable to the Home Office. The Children's Officer, who headed up the Department, was just down the corridor and readily accessible. We were in no sense a team. Rather we were a group of people with a diverse range of statutory responsibilities, each working with our individual 'caseloads'. We worked closely with probation officers, health visitors and the NSPCC inspector, many of whom we shared cases with.

There were two other local authority departments in the city at that time, also working in the field of personal social services, but accountable to the Ministry of Health. The Welfare Department worked with older people, disabled people and homeless people, and the Mental Welfare Department worked with people with mental health problems and learning difficulties. The Welfare Department, as I subsequently discovered, employed just two unqualified social workers, who, like myself, were newly-appointed graduates. Between them they covered the whole city, one the south and the other the north. Their job in the main was to arrange residential care for older people, emergency accommodation for homeless people and day care and holidays for disabled people. Home helps were supplied by the local health department and were not part of their remit and meals on wheels were supplied by the WRVS. The Mental Welfare Department was larger but its work was primarily linked to hospitals – undertaking emergency admissions, servicing psychiatric outpatient clinics and, in the case of people with learning difficulties, working in conjunction with Adult Training Centres. In addition to these three departments, there were medical social workers working at the general hospital who were employed by the health service. Their job was to ensure that people discharged from hospital, particularly older people and disabled people, were fixed up with suitable support systems.

This fragmentation of the personal social services was about to change. Following the Seebohm report, and the subsequent Local Authority Social Services Act (1970), the three Departments were to be merged to form the Social Services Department. The city was to be divided up into five areas and we would each be allocated to one of them. We were to become 'generic' social workers, which meant that I would no longer specialise in child care but would undertake work in all areas of the personal social services. The home help service was also to come under our wing and later, following the reorganisation of the health service, medical social workers became local authority employees too. I don't remember having had an awful lot of guidance or training in preparation for this radical transition.

The switch to social services

One Friday, in September 1971, we finished work as child care officers in the Children's Department and, on the following Monday morning, we reported as generic social workers to our new offices in the newly-formed Social Services Department. The team I joined was based in an office in what had been the Welfare Department, which was not far away from the old Children's Department. I duly turned up on the Monday morning and met my new colleagues. There were three of us from the Children's Department, one the Welfare Department and two from the Mental Welfare Department. In the first few weeks, possibly for the first couple of months, it was all pretty chaotic. The area officer hadn't been appointed. So, in charge of us were two senior social workers, one from the Children's Department and one from the Mental Welfare Department. Basically they were responsible for allocating work to us. Right from the start, however, we were a team. We were all in one room and we had regular meetings. Every one of us had an enormous amount to learn about areas of work we had never been involved in before.

To start with, we didn't seem to have any 'cases' anymore, just a few that we had each brought with us, who already lived in the area that we were now working in. It must have been an awful upheaval for service users who were being transferred from one area office to another and from one social worker to another. I remember managing to 'hang on' to a couple of cases that weren't in our area, one was the Scottish family I met in my first week as a child care officer. So we seemed to have plenty of time to go out with each other and to start acquiring new knowledge and skills and to get to know the area, the local homes and day-centres that we were going to be working with. For the first three months we did much more learning than actually working. I particularly remember the journeys out to the local psychiatric hospital, eleven miles away. I used to drive out there with the senior social worker, previously in the Mental Welfare Department, and learned a huge amount from him on those car journeys. This was important because I too had now become a 'Duly Authorised Officer' under the 1959 Mental Health Act.

It was quite a shock when the newly-appointed area officer arrived who was extremely enthusiastic and rather aggressively managerial. We didn't quite know what had hit us. We were moved to another office, still in the city centre, while we awaited the building of our new locally-based area office. A community worker was appointed to our team and the Department appointed a research officer. A home help organiser and occupational therapist were appointed. We started mapping out our area. We had a huge map on the wall, we marked all the local facilities, the phone boxes, particular kinds of shops, and we got a lot of encouragement to work in a creative, preventive sort of way. We started having meetings with local people and set up a good neighbour scheme for older people in our area.

Of course it was not just service users who were being chopped and changed around. Long established working relationships with other professionals such as probation officers, health visitors and community psychiatric nurses were disrupted and new relationships had to be forged. This created considerable anger and frustration initially. At the same time, however, we were developing closer links with professionals who were area based, such as GPs and district nurses.

Those early days were a new adventure. Most of us were very young. It was an exciting time. Now, as well as children and families, I was working with people with mental health problems, people with learning difficulties, older people and disabled people, who all lived in the area which I was now allocated to. We were still working with individuals in the end but in a very different way. We were working with people within a local community context. And we did have a feeling of team solidarity.

Whilst all this was going on, training opportunities were being expanded and many of us were encouraged to take these up. So, in January 1973, I embarked upon a new generic training course at the local university. It was two years full time and I was seconded on full pay. When I returned, I went back to the same team but now in a purpose-built area office in the area of the city that we were covering. Now, with local authority reorganisation in 1974, we were part of a new county council with a headquarters forty miles away. It was all a far cry from the Children's Department where I had started my social work career only four years previously.

CHAPTER 33

CAREWORK AND BODYWORK

Julia Twigg

The ideology of home is almost universally recognised and endorsed within British culture, and its principal features – the ethic of privacy, the power to exclude and the embodiment of identity – are significant in structuring the care encounter from both sides. These central values are as much endorsed by the careworkers as by the older and disabled people. Workers regard their own homes in the same way, so that rules of behaviour that attach to these values are part of the taken-for-granted reality of their own social lives. The 'power' of these structures is thus deeply embedded socially, and does not have to rest solely on an internalisation of 'good practice'. This is important in explaining the degree of power that home gives to recipients.

Home

Careworkers, in entering the home, enter space that they recognise as private; and some described the uncertainty of the first visit, waiting on the doorstep wondering who and what lay behind the front door: 'The first time is always a bit, I mean I can feel, it's not my territory. And it's theirs, and I feel really not at ease.' Coming into the home of someone is an odd and unsettling experience, one that can make careworkers feel vulnerable. As [one careworker] explained:

Source: *Bathing – the Body and Community Care*, Routledge, London, 2001, pp. 42, 79–83, 88–9, 137–49.

I think you feel a little bit humble as well, because you're going into a strange person's home, and even if they ask you to make a cup of tea, it's like going into your friend's house and your friend says, go and make a cup of tea, unless you've been in that friend's house before, you don't know where the cups are and you don't know where the sugar's kept, and it's sort of like you're in there in somebody's house as a worker ... it's a very, very weird experience.

Although they come to do a job of work, they accept that they are in some measure bound by the norms of being a guest. These mean that you have to ask permission both to enter and to do certain things. Some clients were very guarded about their space; others less so. As one careworker commented:

You can walk into a place that's like a palace and somebody will be very free with it and just let you wander around. You walk in somewhere that is in squalor and they'll be very precious about everything you touch.

Workers are bound by the general social norms of not being over-inquisitive or looking openly around and not going beyond limited permissions, particularly in the early stages of the relationship: 'You don't take anything for granted. I mean I wouldn't just go and get towels or anything.' Care staff were explicitly instructed not to wander about or look in drawers in case there were accusations about theft.

From the perspective of the clients, receiving help means having to accept people coming into the home. Responses to this varied, and class and gender were both relevant. Those with middle and upper-middle class backgrounds, accustomed in the past to having domestic help, in some cases servants, were unsurprisingly the least concerned about the potential intrusion of careworkers. Sir Peter, a retired senior naval officer, interpreted the experience positively:

INTERVIEWER: Do you ever mind all these people coming into your house?
SIR PETER: Not in the least.
INTERVIEWER: So you never feel it's a bit of an invasion of your –
SIR PETER: No, I was delighted.

Others did feel it an intrusion, though one that they simply had to accept as part of the cost of staying at home. For some the presence of any careworker in the home, particularly if unfamiliar, created a sense of unease. Mrs Sheils, living with her partner Mr Hedges, commented: 'You have to sit and, you know, there's a stranger in the house, and you feel, well, good, they'll soon be finished, and that will be it.' The ease of home had been disturbed by the presence of a stranger, it could not be restored until they had gone.

For Mrs Bucknell it was more a sense that her life itself was now on view, open to public scrutiny and comment. Accepting careworkers for her meant that her home had become part of the wider public world outside. Though she could no longer get out, she remained very conscious of local reputation, and she was concerned that one of the careworkers was a gossip and felt that the whole world now knew her business: 'They come in, you see, they know everything ... and they know my business, and everything – so I don't like it.'

Responses to the intrusion of care tended to reflect gender. The sense was more strongly expressed by women, unsurprisingly since women are more closely associated with the territory of home, and more accustomed to controlling and ordering it. Mr O'Brien, by contrast, an Irish working class man caring for a wife with dementia, was happy to hand over the space of the flat to the careworkers when they came to give his wife a bath and clean the flat.

MR O'BRIEN: I get to know them very well, yes. Of course, when they come here they're in charge of the flat, they're in charge of the kitchen, they can help themselves to whatever they want. I make it quite clear to them that the kitchen's there for them.
INTERVIEWER: So you hand it over to them, as it were?
MR O'BRIEN: Yes, entirely, yes, yes – oh yes, yes.
INTERVIEWER: And that's OK, you don't feel they kind of come bustling in and –
MR O'BRIEN: No, no, no, no – no, they're quite, quite good [used here as a positive emphasis].

For him, domestic territory was naturally female, and receiving help there in tune with normal gender expectations.

For Mr Colegate, however, the coming of help was experienced as an intrusion. He cared for a wife with multiple sclerosis and the steady progress of her disease meant that more and more of the space of the home was dominated by her care needs. Careworkers came and went all day. He sometimes had no sense of who would be in the house.

INTERVIEWER: Do you ever feel that your house is a bit taken over by all sorts of people from all these agencies I mean?
MR COLEGATE: Well sometimes, I hate it, it doesn't feel like me own house, I've never really settled here to be honest.

As a defence he had instituted an informal reordering of the house, recasting the kitchen, where his wife no longer went, as an office-cum-sitting-room for himself. There at least he was able to establish some control over the space which was otherwise dominated by her care needs and the activities of careworkers.

The ideology of home plays an important part in the power dynamics of care, endowing older and disabled people with an element of control, and making it possible in some degree to resist the dominance of careworkers and professionals. Home is space that belongs to the occupant, and this social norm is underwritten legally. Older people can refuse admission to professionals and shut the door in their face. Social services have no general powers of entry (even in the case of children), and short of 'sectioning' the individual, or making them subject to an order under the Public Assistance Act 1948 (something only done rarely when the conditions of the individual are so extreme as to threaten life), they cannot force their presence or their care on reluctant recipients. The strength of the legal position may not always be understood by clients, but the social norm on which it rests is. There were examples in the study where older and disabled people had exerted control over the situation and effectively 'dismissed' a careworker, asking that they should not be sent again. Though I would not want to exaggerate this element of control, it does ultimately rest on the capacity to exclude, that material and ideological feature of home. It is impossible to believe that older and disabled people would be able to exercise this kind of preference or control over staff employed in institutional settings.

The second source of power derives from the home as the embodiment of identity. This puts a limit on the degree to which an individual can be depersonalised. To be depersonalised is at worst to lose your name, your history, your identity; it is to be literally and metaphorically stripped, made subject to anonymous and collective regimes, the process classically described by Goffman (1961) in his account of the Total Institution. But at home, surrounded by your possessions – family photographs, pictures of yourself when young, holiday mementoes, books – it is not possible to be wholly reduced to anonymity. In this setting, it is hard for someone to be treated like a cypher, an object simply to be cleaned and ordered. The surroundings of home are therefore an important buttress of the individual. Mrs Ostrovski was a large powerful woman with a vigorous mind who had worked as a translator, but who was now confined to her bed, camped out in the corner of a rambling flat filled with books, pictures and itinerant lodgers. She explained how personal possessions establish social status. This is important because being dependent is depressing, and possessions help you to maintain a sense of self. She contrasted this with what went on in hospital:

MRS OSTROVSKI: Because maybe at home, when you are at home and around all sorts of rubbish of yours so they don't think you are exactly, you know, bad you know, but in hospital you are just coming out of the crowd, you are aged seventy five – 'Yes dearie, yes darling, good show, jolly good.' [mimicking a silly patronising tone]

INTERVIEWER: Right, so do you think having home around you makes a difference?

MRS OSTROVSKI: Well yes I think it gives you that – it gives you, because to need somebody's help, it's already – you need to concentrate your strength not to go down, not to become depressed.

Later we returned to the theme:

INTERVIEWER: You said something about all the things around you, and as I sit here I can see, you know, all these books and pictures and things.

MRS OSTROVSKI: That gives you identity, as I say, and *you* are not at a disadvantage. I think in hospital you are at a disadvantage. You are just a nonentity who came from the street, you know, and you are treated as they please.... Here you are not the one lost. The other person is coming from outside.... If we are talking of who is up and who is down, you are up. You are on your own ground.

This aspect of power and control was endorsed by the careworkers also. As Zara commented, again drawing on the contrast between home and residential care:

Them being at home, they feel more confident. In their own surroundings. And it's like, not saying that I am an intruder, but it does, like I am a bit of an intruder so I have to do things the way they want it done.... If they're in the residential home I have to do for them what should *be done and what I think is good enough for them.*

Disability and its consequences threaten the traditional ordering of the home, in some cases imposing a radical reordering. [...] Mrs Elster is totally confined to her bed. She lives, sleeps, washes, dresses there. As she says: 'I've been sitting here like this for six years.' By the bed she has an elaborate set of tables on which are arranged all her needs: books, papers, pills, cushions. She has a stick to reach objects, and she also uses this to haul her legs up and manoeuvre them on to the bed when she wants to lie down. She has a chemical toilet next to the bed, and careworkers bring basins and cloths, so that the bathroom is brought to her and arranged around her body.

Her life has become condensed around the bed, and from this vantage point she commands the flat. Her control extends even to cooking and gardening. She has food and plants brought to her and she chops and sorts them on a table, replanting pots and dicing vegetables:

I have the girls bring in on a large tray what is left in the fridge, not milk and that kind of thing, but food, eatables, perishables and then I pick over that. Well now, I would say to them, oh yes do this you see and also I will have a, what's the name, bread board and a small saucepan please.

She looks out into the basement space at the front of the high Victorian Italiante house and sees the plants and flowers. Social life is limited but she can wave at those neighbours who see her, though this only happens at twilight when her lights are on and the curtains are not drawn.

Maintaining this regime requires considerable mental effort. She has a complicated set of practices, and she orders herself and the flat closely: 'Because my routine is a little bit like a plan you know, general's plan of his army, got to do that, so we can do this, and if we don't do that, then we can't do that.'

She constantly thinks ahead. By dint of this and her determination and courage she has been able to remain at home for six years in difficult circumstances. But to do this she requires the help of careworkers, and they have to follow her directions closely. This can be a source of difficulty as they tend to resent such close ordering of their work:

They don't like it, being told, although I try and do it as nicely as I can. Like today I, somebody doing something and I, what did I say, oh no not that, and she said [imitates someone making squealy niggly reluctant sounds].

Her immobility however enables them to escape, and they can use the space against her. She described how they hid in the kitchen, pretending to be working, while they called their friends on their mobile phones. They thus establish their own private territory in her flat, out of sight of her managing gaze.

We now turn to the opposite extreme, where the traditional ordering of public and private was fully maintained and careworkers closely restricted where they could go. This is most characteristic of situations where there was another family member living in the house and Mr Hedges and Mrs Sheils were the clearest example. Mr Hedges was disabled and lived in a rather dark housing association basement flat. A former hospital porter, he had come to Britain from the Caribbean in the 1950s. His partner, Mrs Sheils, was white. They both had a strong sense of the territoriality of the flat and of the parts of it that were private. As Mr Hedges commented: 'This lady [Mrs Sheils] has two places don't let nobody go – in the bathroom and her kitchen.'

This ordering of space even applied to close family like grandchildren. He did not mind a stranger coming in to help, provided they did not attempt to go anywhere they liked: 'There's certain place they can go, but certain place nobody, where I don't like – in our bedroom or our kitchen or anything – no way – not even our own children do it.'

When the careworker came to give him a bath, the clean clothes were laid out in the bathroom, so there was no need for the careworker to wander about looking for things in the bedroom, and he did not go into that space:

> *My clothes is out,... hung on the door inside the bathroom – when I bath he can just take them up. So we have no problem there. Anybody want to come here can come, but they must know what their place is, because if they don't, then they know where the door is.*

Unusually in the sample, Mr Hedges was always dressed when the careworker arrived – most people wait in their night clothes – again part of maintaining normal life and its proprieties. It was notable that this pattern even applied to Joshua, the careworker with whom Mr Hedges was close. They had a lot in common, including the experience of being 'black' and coming to Britain as young men. Mr Hedges spoke of him warmly 'like a son', one of the few people in the study to use a familial model for the relationship. Even this closeness, however, did not erode the structures of privacy, and Joshua did not move freely about the flat.

Much of the strength of these structures related to the fact that Mr Hedges and Mrs Sheils were a couple. The spatial ordering of the house in linked to the structural intimacy of the couple. The capacity of couples to assert their privacy against helpers and professionals is an added dimension of the power of home. Home is a power base for older disabled people containing both ideological and material resources that can underpin their independence and power of self determination. This is strengthened in the case of couples who are better able to assert their privacy against the intruding eyes and judgements of workers and professionals. (This barrier applies also to the process of research itself. It proved hard to ask questions about intimate care in the presence of the other member of the couple. To do so became a violation of their own privacy and the partner typically put up a barrier that was not present when the disabled person was interviewed alone.) This is one of the reasons why couples pose difficulties for institutional care. A number of studies have noted the way institutions discourage the development of any physical relationships between residents (Wilkin and Hughes 1987). In large part this arises from negative attitudes to sexuality among the old. But it also reflects a recognition that the existence of a sexual, marital relationship creates a territory of privacy in which workers feel it awkward to intrude. The bedroom of a couple is private in a way that no other residents' can be. Although in theory single residents have their own private space, this is in practice constantly trespassed upon. In the case of a couple, however, the dominant norm is sufficiently strong to create unease and embarrassment even among care staff.

Bodywork

Carework has traditionally been presented in ways that downplay its character as bodywork. [. . .] All cultures have patterns of belief and practice which govern and proscribe behaviour relating to the body. In the west, our way of dealing with the body, sexuality and dirt is to take them into a privatised context that makes them relatively inaccessible to us as a subject for social enquiry (Lawler 1991). There is little or no public discourse of the body and its functioning. It is rarely referred to directly, beyond the world of childhood, intense intimacy or crude jokes. This chimes with the form of analysis presented by Elias (1978). The body occupies a territory where language itself is problematic, awkwardly polarised between the medical-clinical and the vulgar-demotic. Lawler (1991) notes how nursing texts are coy about what the basic work of nursing entails. It is regarded as 'obvious', and the actual embodied reality, either glossed over or fragmented into a series of what are termed 'personal care deficits'. In this way the body and its embarrassments are rendered safe, abstract, subdivided and scientific.

The body in care is, if anything, more silenced. As we noted in relation to touch, there is no comparable discourse to that of nursing theory with which to describe the processes of care. These practices remain in a zone of silence. As a result careworkers receive little help in dealing with them from their managers or their organisations. [. . .] Careworkers are on their own in these areas, they either learn by catching sight of others or developing techniques of their own. Either way, their practice is rendered invisible, something beyond the limits of official discourse.

To some degree careworkers concur in this implicit valuation of their work. In describing it they tend to play down the aspect of bodywork, and emphasise 'care' instead. Though it is the body element that marks personal care off from mere domestic cleaning (something that careworkers feel they have moved above in terms of status), it is not the element that they stress. Rather they emphasise the emotional and interpersonal aspects, and the skills required to negotiate and maintain these. These are the most enjoyable and personally rewarding elements; and the parts they want to foreground.

As part of this, careworkers were sometimes circumspect when exposing the realities of their work to public view, as the following exchange
illustrates:

INTERVIEWER: How do you find dealing with that [faeces], is it difficult?
JAY: *Interesting* (laughter) – it depends where they put it!

Her use of 'interesting' was partly irony but also contained a sense of
guarded constraint in exposing these aspects of the work. As a colleague
added:

PAT: They all guess, they all know the sort of job you do, don't they –
JAY: That's right.
PAT: I mean you don't go into details, but they just – I mean different
   people say: 'Oh, I couldn't do that.'

Bates and Lee-Treweek report a similar reticence among careworkers in
exposing the realities of their work to the wider world (Bates 1993; Lee-
Treweek 1998). [. . .]

Coping

Mostly careworkers accept that dealing with human waste is part of the
job, and that they have to buckle to and suppress any sense of disgust:

> *When Mrs Jones isn't quite so well one day, and you've got diarrhoea
> from the toilet to the front door, you know. You've got to be able to
> have a bit of a stomach for the job to actually be able to clear that up.*

Some workers internalised the situation and managed their feelings by
thinking themselves into the position of a recipient of care. Others consciously reordered the client as a baby – sweet, innocent of intent in
making a mess, and vulnerable. Though such techniques could help the
worker, they underlie the general infantilisation of older people. Some
workers saw dealing with dirt as part of women's inevitable role in life,
linking it back to motherhood: 'true there is some dirty aspect of it, but as
a woman, you know, you don't bother.'
   Stella, the New Age-influenced worker, struggled with the essential
ambiguities of bodywork in her sense of revulsion mixed with a wish never
to reject the client as a person:

> *I think . . . there's a part of me that just if something is difficult to look
> at, difficult to touch I almost feel like I want to embrace it just so that,*

just because I rejected it so fully you know. It's just the person ... I don't want to feel that revulsion for another human being.

Avoiding direct language is one of the techniques deployed by careworkers in negotiating the body taboos. Careworkers described how they chatted away on the surface while getting over the more difficult or embarrassing aspects in silence. In this way naming the unnameable could be avoided; and language was used to distract and ease rather than to express. Jokes were also a useful distraction.

SUSIE: If you have a joke with them.
MOIRA: You get things done.
SUSIE: You're getting it done before they realise because they're busy laughing.

Humour was a means of coping, both for themselves and the client:

We joke – I joke, specially if you're actually washing them and they start having a motion and, you know, you say: 'Oh, we've got a surprise here – one minute!' You know, but you just, you can't do it any other way really.

The body and humour are closely linked: dirty jokes, sexual innuendo, 'lavatory' humour – the body is the focus of all these. Mulkay sees discordance and incongruity as at the heart of humour; jokes occur where the single vision of the serious, official account is disrupted by the intrusion of other parallel interpretations and realities (Mulkay 1988). Douglas similarly sees jokes as generated by ambiguity in the social system (Douglas 1975). The body is a ripe source of this, partly because in Douglas's system, it is the symbolic embodiment of the social order generally, and partly because there is an inevitable discordance between the aspirations of formal social life and the desires and failings of the body. The more formal the occasion, the more embarrassing or humorous the body's lapse. In the case of carework, joking was largely used as a means of easing situations that were otherwise embarrassing.

Sometimes, however, the joking was less kindly. In one or two of the group interviews where respondents were more at ease and less concerned to present an idealised account, a different, harsher tone emerged, one of sardonic humour in which 'horror stories' were shared as part of a collective release of feeling in which the solidarity of the workgroup was asserted. Mostly these related to sexual incidents, but the disgusting habits of clients were also recounted. Desiree joked how some of her clients were obsessed with their bowel function, demanding that workers give them suppositories: 'one morning he had two and it wasn't working and he wanted me to put my hands up there and help it along. I told him no way, I'm not doing that.' The group, continuing the vein recounted other cases:

DESIREE: And Mr Jones he takes medicine every single night, to go, so in the morning you sit him on the commode and he has to, you have to be there 'til he's done something.

TONI: Yeah and he must have a look at it.

DESIREE: Yeah, you have to show it to him. Honestly! If you throw it away without him knowing, there's a big argument. He'll say, half, quarter or a full load. Every morning, that's what I'm faced with at nine o'clock in the morning, every single morning.

Workers do not necessarily lose their sense of disgust or their underlying feelings of resentment and anger at what they are required to do. These were predominantly black workers caring for upper middle class white people, and the interview was shot through with tensions in relation to 'race' and class that were reworked into bodily expression. In these more transgressive interviews elements of disgust were not hidden but used against clients. [. . .]

Carework is about dealing with human waste: shit, pee, vomit, sputum; and as such involves managing dirt and disgust. Miller (1997) in his analysis of disgust argues that it is the most visceral of emotions. The idiom of disgust evokes the sensory experience. Taste is the core sensation, mouth the core location and rejection via spitting and vomiting the core actions – actions repeated in our facial expression of disgust. Disgust is rooted in fear of contamination, whether directly through oral incorporation or touching, or more remotely through visual images or moral pollution. [. . .] Disgust, Miller argues, is rooted in the organic, and above all in the bodily. Disgusting things are slimey, oozing, slithering, moist, clinging; not dry, cold or hard. Disgust is also closely related to other people. Our capacity for self pollution is limited, and it is other people's dirt that concerns us most strongly. [. . .] Disgust is also closely related to other people. Our capacity for self pollution is limited, and it is other people's dirt that concerns us most strongly. [. . .]

If we explore the aspects the workers found hardest to cope with, they clearly reflect the category systems described above. Dealing with incontinence was recurringly identified as the most difficult thing to manage. Smell was also hard to bear, and for reasons that echo Lawton's (1998) analysis; it had an all-pervasive, stomach-turning quality that lingered about the person:

SUSAN: Someone in a mucky bed, you know, you just – you can put all the protective clothing on, gloves, your plastic apron and everything, but you sometimes feel unclean.

VICKY: The smell stays with you.

Beyond that, individuals varied in what they found difficult. Sharon could not cope with teeth: 'Give me a dirty bum any day than teeth.' Other respondents chimed in:

PETRA: Toenails is mine. I don't like them.
(All speak at once)
VAL: Washing feet and legs when the skin is flaking off, that always gets to me.
TRACEY: What gets to me is when they're coughing up phlegm and put it in a bowl.
(Groans all round.)

Other interviews expanded on the list: 'one thing I can't do is if they need their noses blowing'; 'false teeth'; 'when you hear somebody being sick, you never get used to it, I don't think, anyway'. All share a common source of disgust in the category system recounted by Miller (1997) and Douglas (1966, 1970). It is other people's bodies and especially the by-products of bodies, or the parts of bodies that are anomalously connected, that are the main focus of revulsion. [...]

Odours by their nature cannot be easily contained; they escape and cross boundaries. This boundary transgressing quality acts 'to threaten the abstract and impersonal regime of modernity' (Classen *et al.* 1994: 5). It runs counter to our modern world view with its emphasis on discrete, defined divisions and on individual privacy. Smell and disintegration undermine current individualistic constructions of the person as stable, bounded and autonomous. [...]

Hidden work

So far we have treated carework as dirty work in the obvious way. But carework is so in a second, more sociological sense, also. The term was developed by Hughes and others to cover degrading tasks that are integral to society, but that society does not want to acknowledge, and are by common consent hidden. Emerson and Pollner (1976) extended the terms to cover breaches of the moral order at work, encompassing aspects of the job that are shameful, disliked and counter to the self image of the worker. Psychiatric work they argue abounds with dirty work because its day-to-day realities are in conflict with the therapeutic ideal, and they cite getting rid of drunks and derelicts from the psychiatric clinic as part of the dirty work of mental health nursing, something that has to be done, but no one wants to be seen doing.

Dirty work is managed by society through a variety of strategies: by delegating distasteful tasks to lower level staff; by hiding the activity from view; and by otherwise bracketing off the work mentally and socially. Carework illustrates all these. As we noted, the basic bed and bodywork of nursing is commonly delegated to the most junior staff, and dirty work transferred down the occupational hierarchy from nurses to careworkers. Dirty work is also hidden from view. Much bodywork takes place behind the screens and in the back bedrooms of institutions. We owe to Lawler and her path-breaking analysis in *Behind the Screens* (1991), the important perception that this work is obscured not only to protect the privacy of the patient, but also the status and public esteem of the worker. Bodywork is potentially demeaning work, and nurses go off stage to perform it. It may involve inflicting embarrassing or painful procedures; and this needs to be hidden if the image of the nurse is to be maintained. In a similar way Lee-Treweek's account of careworkers in a residential home, shows how aspects of the work that are at odds with the caring image are managed spatially by being confined to the privacy of the bedrooms (Lee-Treweek 1994). It is here that the basic work of washing, ordering and at times disciplining residents takes place. This 'dirty work' of care is hidden in order that the institution can display the 'product' of its caring regime in the form of the 'lounge standard' patient. Carework in people's own homes requires less in the way of such spatial stratagems since it is by its nature more hidden.

Fundamentally, carework is 'dirty work' because it deals with aspects of life that society, especially modern secular society with its ethic of material success and its emphasis on youth and glamour, does not want to think about: decay, dirt, death, decline, failure. Careworkers manage these aspects of life on behalf of the wider society, ensuring they remain hidden, tidied away into the obscurity of institutions or private homes.

REFERENCES

Bates, I. (1993) 'A job which is "right for me"?: social class, gender and individual-isation', in I. Bates and G. Riseborough (eds) *Youth and Inequality*, Bucking-ham: Open University Press.

Classen, C., Howes, D. and Synnott, A. (1994) *Aroma: The Cultural History of Smell*, London: Routledge.

Douglas, M. (1966) *Purity and Danger: An Analysis of the Concepts of Pollution and Taboo*, London: Routledge and Kegan Paul.

Douglas, M. (1970) *Natural Symbols*, Harmondsworth: Penguin.

Douglas, M. (1975) 'Jokes', in *Implicit Meanings: Essays in Anthropology*, London: Routledge and Kegan Paul.

Elias, N. (1978) *The Civilizing Process: The History of Manners*, Oxford: Black-well.

Emerson, R.M. and Pollner, M. (1976) 'Dirty work designations: their features and consequences in a psychiatric setting', *Social Problems*, 23, 243–54.

Goffman, E. (1961) *Asylums: Essay on the Social Situations of Mental Patients and Other Inmates*, New York: Doubleday.

Lawler, J. (1991) *Behind the Screens: Nursing, Somology and the Problem of the Body*, Melbourne: Churchill Livingstone.

Lawton, J. (1998) 'Contemporary hospice care: the sequestration of the unbounded body and "dirty dying"', *Sociology of Health and Illness*, 20, 2, 121–43.

Lee-Treweek, G. (1994) 'Bedroom abuse: the hidden work in a nursing home', *Generations Review*, 4, 1, 2–4.

Lee-Treweek, G. (1998) 'Women, resistance and care: an ethnographic study of nursing auxiliary work', *Work, Employment and Society*, 11, 1, 47–63.

Miller, W.I. (1997) *The Anatomy of Disgust*, Cambridge, Mass.: Harvard University Press.

Mulkay, M. (1988) *On Humour: Its Nature and Its Place in Modern Society*, Cambridge: Polity.

CHAPTER 34

EUROPEAN POLICIES ON HOME CARE SERVICES COMPARED[1]

Caroline Glendinning

Studying how welfare services are funded and provided in other countries can help us think about policy in the UK in a number of ways.

- Because we are familiar with the policies and services here, we often take them for granted. It may be difficult to recognise the assumptions and beliefs which underpin particular services or arrangements, simply because we are so familiar with them. For example, exactly what assumptions do we make about the responsibilities of families and individuals? Looking at services and policies in other countries can help to throw into perspective the things we take for granted, to ask questions we might not otherwise have thought of, and to reach a better understanding of some of the more subtle factors which shape our own welfare state.
- Examining welfare arrangements in other countries can help to identify similarities as well as differences. For example, welfare states in Scandinavian countries are often regarded as sharing many common features. These similarities can help us understand the common social, political, cultural and economic factors which affect such countries, now and in the past.
- Comparisons can provide a basis for judgements – for example, about whether services in one country are more or less generous, or more or less effective, in some countries than in others. The European Union has supported the establishment of Observatories – networks of independent experts – to gather information and compare provision across the EU in policy areas such as family policy, ageing and social protection. Such comparisons can provide evidence for arguments for better provision in less generous countries.

This chapter describes the funding and organisation of home care services in the UK, Denmark, the Netherlands and Germany. These countries have been selected because they all experience the pressures of an ageing population, coupled with financial constraints on welfare spending. Each country has a more or less explicit policy of encouraging older people to remain in their own homes for as long as possible, despite physical or mental frailty (a policy which is sometimes called 'ageing in place'). This opposition to institutional care is also apparent in policies in each country for younger disabled people as well, although in many instances the actual services received by working-age disabled people tend to be more generous than those received by older people.

In many countries home help services traditionally provided help with domestic household tasks – cleaning, laundry, shopping, food preparation and other household chores, while nurses dealt with personal care – washing, dressing and toileting, as well as giving medication and treatments. However, as the chapter will show, the boundaries between these different activities have become blurred, with former home help services increasingly focused on providing personal, rather than domestic, assistance. It is therefore more appropriate to use the term 'home care' rather than 'home help' services, to reflect this change. It also throws into question the boundaries between health and social services; between the roles of different professionals; and between the responsibilities of welfare professionals, individuals and families. Have tasks which were formerly carried out as part of 'health' provision been redefined as 'social' care and, if so, what are the consequences of this? If home care services no longer help with housework whose responsibility is this?

United Kingdom

Since the early 1980s, there has been a major shift away from long-term care in hospitals; patients are now also discharged much more quickly from hospital after illness or surgery. Older people are now encouraged to stay in their own homes as long as possible, with local authority social services departments responsible for funding and arranging both home care services and, when this is no longer possible, placements in residential and nursing homes. There is also growing pressure on the NHS and local authorities to work together to provide intensive support and rehabilitation services at home, to prevent older people being admitted to hospital for acute care and to support them at home after early discharge.

Successive governments since the early 1980s have emphasised that primary responsibility for supporting older people lies with their families; statutory services are increasingly intended only to supplement family care, or support older people without close kin. The responsibilities and needs of 'informal' carers have therefore become increasingly visible; carers can request an assessment of their needs for services and may be able to claim grants and social security payments to support their caring role. Demographic changes mean that an increasing proportion of these carers are the spouses of frail older people and therefore also elderly themselves.

Funding and organisation

Home care services are funded from a combination of central and local taxation. Older people can refer themselves for home care as well as being referred by a professional. Following referral, local authority social workers or 'care managers' are responsible for assessing an older person's needs for home care and other 'community care services'. Assessment arrangements and eligibility criteria are decided locally; there are no national guidelines on the levels of home care services which should be provided or who should receive them. Consequently there are wide variations between local authorities in the availability of home care services and the ease with which older people in different areas can obtain them.

Local authorities are encouraged to purchase home care services from private agencies on behalf of older users. However, the development of the private home care market has been relatively slow – only about half of all home help contact hours are purchased from private agencies – and many older people themselves prefer services provided by the local authority itself. In many areas, therefore, services consist of a mixture of in-house and external private provision (the latter particularly during evenings and weekends, with local authorities' own services providing weekday cover only). National standards and inspection arrangements governing the quality of both public and private home care services have been slow to develop.

Levels of spending on all local authority social services are tightly controlled by central government. Since the early 1980s, older people have increasingly been charged for home care services; 94 per cent of local authorities charge some or all of their users. Major differences have emerged between local authorities both in the levels of these charges and how users' contributions are assessed; these differences are expected to be harmonised by 2005.

Pressures and trends

The amount of help which older people need at home has increased substantially and home care services now have to cope with much higher levels of disability and frailty among older people. This is the result of:

- demographic factors (increased longevity and, therefore, increased risks of infirmity and disability);
- changes in NHS services (closure of long-stay wards and earlier discharge after illness or surgery); and

■ increased pressure on local authority social services departments to enable older people to remain at home and prevent admissions to residential and nursing homes.

Home nursing services have also changed, with a greater emphasis on treating acutely ill people at home rather than in hospital and much less on routine personal care – washing, dressing, toileting, supervision and routine medication. Local authority home care services therefore increasingly fill the personal care gap and are therefore less able to undertake traditional home help tasks such as cleaning the home and laundry.

Consequently, local authority home care services now perform many activities which would previously have been the responsibility of the NHS, whether through hospital or community nursing services. Because of the charges made for home care services, many older people therefore now pay for services which they had expected to be provided free of charge by the NHS, in return for the tax and insurance contributions paid during their working lives.

> *I am 80 and for years I and my ... [employer] paid our contributions in the belief that I was providing, as Beveridge had stated, for all necessary care from cradle to grave ... Only recently have the rules been changed. I regard this as a blatant breach of contract by the Government who took my money promising care, then reneged on the contract after I had paid all my dues.*
>
> (Letter to Royal Commission on Long-Term Care)

However, the boundaries between home nursing (health) and home care (social) services are still unclear and coordination between the two services can be poor. Increasingly, therefore, home care and home nursing services are under pressure to work more closely together. For example:

■ joint assessments of an older person, covering medical, nursing and home care needs, are encouraged;
■ in some areas, services are based in the same building, to improve access;
■ many areas are trying to integrate their home care and home nursing services, using new flexibilities introduced in the 1999 Health Act.

Funding and service constraints mean home care services are targeted on older people with the most severe disabilities. Even so, average levels of provision are low, with older people receiving on average only two and a half to three hours of home care services each week. Only about 20 per cent of those needing help with household tasks (some 600,000 people aged 65 or over) receive any home care service at all. A much larger number purchase home care services privately or rely entirely on family or friends. Traditional home help services are now rare, although a government grant has been available to local authorities since 1999 to develop preventive services – these include low level domestic and practical tasks around the home.

Although choice over service provision is promoted as an ideal, in practice this is restricted for all but the most affluent older people who can afford to buy their own home care. For everyone else, local authorities act as 'purchasers' of services on their behalf. Only since February 2000 have older people been able to receive direct cash payments instead of home care services from their local social services departments, with which they can purchase services to suit their particular needs and preferences. From April 2001 family carers have also been able to receive such payments. It is likely that these options will spread very slowly.

Although current policy promotes the development of home care services as an alternative to institutional care, this has been only partially successful. It is often cheaper to fund a nursing or residential home placement than intensive support services at home. Older people without nearby relatives are particularly at risk of admission to an institution, while others may find their discharge from hospital is delayed by a lack of appropriate support at home. In addition, in some parts of the UK, labour shortages constrain the expansion of home care services. However, local authorities are under pressure to work closely with NHS partners to develop a range of 'intermediate' care services, including rapid response teams and intensive, 24-hour home care services, to prevent admission to hospital or another institution.

Denmark

Like other Scandinavian welfare states, Danish services are shaped by two key commitments:

- ■ to comprehensive welfare services, funded out of general taxation and available to everyone who needs them, regardless of ability to pay. If an older person needs home care, it is underwritten by legislation that the state takes responsibility for that care. Families are not expected to have primary responsibility for older relatives; any help from relatives is on top of that given by the state, not a substitute for it.
- ■ to local democracy. Local councils have considerable freedom to decide how much money to allocate to home care services, how many people they will provide these services for, the number of hours of help each receives, and what the eligibility criteria are.

Funding and organisation

Local municipalities (councils) are responsible for both home nursing and home help services. Municipalities have a statutory duty to offer home care services to anyone unable to perform normal activities of daily living, and must provide home care or home nursing services during the night as well as the day. Both home care and home nursing services are provided free of charge to users, and home care as well as nursing staff are fully trained.

Home nursing tends to be relatively short term, providing treatment and care while older people are ill. Home care services provide domestic help – cleaning, laundry, shopping – and personal care such as personal hygiene and dressing. Older people can refer themselves for home care services, as well as being referred by another professional. Home care services are allocated after an assessment of the older person's (in)ability to carry out domestic and personal care tasks. Assessments and decisions about how much help to provide are usually carried out by a nurse, home carer or team manager. The assessment does not take account of any help which relatives do or could provide. Since 1996, contracts between the home help service and users have been required, so that older people know exactly what services they can expect to receive.

Housing forms an important part of Danish community care provision. However, housing and care are separated; even when older people live in specially adapted accommodation, their care needs are still met by the municipality's home care service.

Pressures and trends

Denmark has a determined policy of enabling older people to remain in their own homes as long as possible; all new investment in residential and nursing homes has ceased and their use is discouraged. Instead, innovative and intensive home care services have been developed. All municipalities provide 24-hour home care services; these usually include an emergency service which can be called at any time, as well as pre-arranged visits throughout the day or night. However, because of the Danish tradition of local municipal autonomy, there are wide variations in the coverage of home help services.

Because home care and home nursing services (and other services like occupational therapy) are all organised by local municipalities, it has been easy to create locally integrated services. Most Danish municipalities have integrated teams of eight to ten home helps and home nurses who together are responsible for the care of all the older people in the area. Some integrated teams also work across the community/institutional boundary, providing care to older people in nursing homes as well as in their own homes.

There has been concern about whether Danish home care services can keep pace with increasing demand, caused by rising numbers of older people and the halt on investment in residential and nursing homes. However, there is no evidence that home care services have become more difficult to obtain and virtually all municipalities provide 24-hour services. Indeed, more people received home help services in 1994 than in 1988; between 1987 and 1996 the proportion of over-80s receiving home care increased from 36 per cent to 49 per cent. Nevertheless, there has been a drastic reduction in the number of hours of home care which most people receive. In addition, cleaning, shopping and cooking is given less priority than personal care; older people now receive domestic help only if their particular circumstances justify this, no longer on a routine basis. There is considerable dissatisfaction among older people about these changes, particularly the withdrawal of cleaning and other household services (satisfaction with personal care services remains high).

Although home care services are free of charge, some municipalities have responded to the continuing demand for domestic help by introducing extra services for which users must pay. These services include cleaning, laundry and delivery of meals to the home. These services can be purchased alongside the free home care service, as substitutes for the tasks which home carers no longer carry out.

Some municipalities have started to contract out services to private agencies – particularly the additional domestic services for which users must pay. However, the privatisation of these services has been highly controversial, because of:

■ political opposition to the notion of profit-making from welfare services; and
■ threats to the integrated home care and home nursing services, and possible loss of quality and continuity of provision.

In the municipalities where private services are available, between 30 and 50 per cent of users opt to receive domestic and practical help from a private provider. However, personal care is still almost always provided by the municipal home help service.

The provision of round-the-clock home care services offers older people in Denmark a real choice between remaining in their own homes or entering institutional care. Even where the cost of intensive home care services exceeds the cost of a place in a home, older people can still choose to remain at home. In addition, the 1998 Social Services Act allows municipalities, in exceptional circumstances, to employ a close relative to provide home care, subject to the normal assessment. The relative is paid the same rate, and enjoys the same employment rights as other municipal home carers.

Since 1998, municipalities have been required to publish quality standards for their home care services. An assessment for home care services must specify what help will be provided and the date when the arrangement will be reviewed (at least every six months if personal care is required). The home carer is required to sign after each visit to show s/he has provided the help as stipulated in the care plan. While safeguarding quality, this does reduce the ability of the carer to respond to sudden changes in an older person's needs.

Germany

Both income maintenance and healthcare services in Germany are funded through state-regulated national insurance schemes, which traditionally covered retirement, accident, unemployment and sickness. These were joined by a new care insurance scheme, which was phased in between 1994 and 1997.

Before 1994, growing numbers of older people needing long-term support and services were not covered by the sickness insurance scheme, which covered only short-term needs associated with acute illness. Older people therefore had to 'spend down' their lifetime savings, purchasing home care services privately and eventually becoming eligible for home care services or residential care funded through means-tested local social assistance schemes. However, because of the widespread coverage of German social insurance schemes, the close relationship between insurance entitlements and citizenship, and the stigma associated with means-tested social assistance, this was considered unacceptable and discriminatory.

Funding and organisation

The new care insurance scheme is funded by contributions from employers and employees. Participation in the scheme (or a private equivalent) is compulsory for everyone who is a member of a sickness insurance scheme, and social assistance claimants are also covered; only three per cent of the population is uninsured. Current cohorts of older people became eligible immediately the scheme was introduced, with their benefits funded from the contributions of current employees and employers.

Eligibility for care insurance benefits is decided by an independent medical board, which is financed jointly by the sickness and care insurance funds. Older people are assessed according to standard guidelines, which set out different levels of 'care dependency'. These guidelines cover the entire country, so all applicants are assessed according to the same criteria, wherever they live. Assessments cover the help needed with personal care, mobility and eating; help with domestic or household chores has low priority. The severity of an older person's care dependency – the frequency and length of time for which s/he needs help with these tasks – in turn determines the level of benefits, which are paid at one of three grades.

Once eligible, older people can choose between a cash benefit, home help and day care services in kind, or a combination of the two. The cash benefit option is worth about half of the value of services which are provided in kind. For example, someone assessed as 'medium care dependent' (needing help at least three times during the day, several times a week) can choose between a monthly cash benefit of £246, or home care and/or nursing services in kind to the value of £534 (2000 benefit rates). Eligibility for care insurance also entitles older people to day care (including costs of transport to day care) and respite care so that a family carer can have a break, and help with costs of special equipment or house adaptations. Care insurance also pays the pension and accident insurance contributions of family carers and for institutional care for the most severely 'care dependent' older people.

There is no history of local authority home help services in Germany. Home care services are poorly developed, partly because of the lack of funding before the introduction of care insurance. Traditionally, home care services have been provided by a cartel of non-profit organisations, each with its own particular religious, social or political affiliation. These organisations dominated local service provision, services were often duplicated and there were few financial or other incentives to develop innovative new services.

The care insurance legislation ended this monopoly, as it allowed new, non-profit and commercial organisations to compete for contracts with care insurance funding bodies on the same terms as the traditional provider organisations. All these organisations now have priority over public sector organisations in competing for contracts from care insurance funds.

Pressures and trends

By 1998, about 1.8 million people received care insurance benefits, the majority living in their own homes rather than institutions. Although the value of the cash benefit is around only half that of the service in kind option, the vast majority of recipients choose the cash benefit. In 1998, 76 per cent of care insurance beneficiaries in private households chose the cash benefit; 11 per cent chose services in kind; and 13 per cent chose a combination of the two (the number of people choosing the combination is increasing).

The unpopularity of the service in kind option reflects the attitudes of older people towards the traditional provider organisations, which have historically played a very limited role in the provision of home care and are therefore still felt to constitute an unacceptable intrusion into the private world of family care-giving. This cultural legacy also helps explain the overwhelming preference for the cash benefit option, which is frequently used to pay close relatives to provide care. The popularity of the cash benefit option in turn reduces pressure on service provider organisations to develop a wider range of flexible, responsive services. The cash benefit option therefore represents a major incentive for home-based family care and as long as it continues to be so popular, there will be little pressure for new home care services to be developed.

Even where older people do opt to receive home care services in kind, these are restricted to the types of help which the care insurance funds will pay for and there remains little choice over the range of services on offer. There are also very few information, advice or brokerage services to help older people optimise the limited choices which are available; such services are provided at the discretion of individual municipalities and counties. Isolated or confused older people are at a particular disadvantage here.

Because the qualifying threshold for even the lowest level of 'care dependency' is quite high, people who might benefit from early intervention or preventive services are likely to be excluded from care insurance benefits. Again, this lack of funding also inhibits provider organisations from developing such services.

The care insurance laws allow older people to choose the cash benefit option only if the necessary care can be secured. Everyone choosing the cash benefit must therefore have regular visits from a professional service provider organisation to check the quality of the care they are receiving. However, family members providing care have no entitlement to any payment of their own; it is the older person who is entitled to care insurance and the transfer of the cash benefit to relatives is entirely at her or his discretion.

The Netherlands

Dutch home care services reflect:

- a continuing commitment to universalist principles that similar levels of services should be available to everyone with similar needs, regardless of where they live; and
- a long tradition of provision by independent, non-profit organisations (rather than local authorities or municipalities).

Dutch welfare funding makes a clear distinction between cure and care services. Cure – medical – services are financed through health insurance schemes. Long-term care services are funded from a special national care fund, set up by the 1968 General Act on Exceptional Medical Expenses and financed by tax-related contributions from all citizens supplemented with central government funding. Each year, central government decides the overall size of the national care fund and its distribution between the regions. Regional authorities for long-term care then contract with registered home care provider organisations to provide services. Local government's role is to ensure that different services (including home care and housing) are coordinated locally.

Funding and organisation

Home care services are provided by independent, regional, non-profit foundations. Because the services they provide are publicly funded, they must comply with national quality standards. Traditionally, these organisations provided either specialised home nursing or personal and domestic home help services. However, during the 1990s many foundations merged together, reducing the numbers from 300 in 1989 to 105. Most foundations now employ integrated teams, in which community nurses, auxiliary nurses and qualified home helps work together. Auxiliary nurses mostly provide personal care and home helps provide both personal and domestic care. In addition, teams of unqualified home helps ('alpha helpers') carry out domestic tasks; they work part-time and are not formal employees of the home care provider organisation (and are therefore not covered by labour and employment laws). Most foundations also provide residential homes and intermediate care ('hospital at home') services.

The mergers between foundations lowered overheads and duplication and therefore increased efficiency, but at the same time reduced competition and choice for the regional funding authorities. An average healthcare region, containing around 500,000 people, will now contain only one or two provider foundations. However, central government has begun to resist these developing monopolies, by introducing benchmarks against which outputs, service quality and costs are assessed.

There are very few commercial, for-profit organisations providing home care services; these cater for a minority of very affluent older people. However, more commercial organisations may develop in future, as new cohorts of older people with higher pensions and higher expectations emerge.

Assessments for home care are carried out by an independent team, separate from the organisations which provide home care services. Because budgets for home care services are capped both nationally and regionally, demand often exceeds supply and waiting lists for assessments and the allocation of services following an assessment are common.

Older people are expected to contribute towards the costs of both home care and home nursing services. However, charges are relatively low; even older people with high incomes do not pay the full economic rate. Nevertheless, the introduction of charges has encouraged some older people to switch to one of the new private commercial companies. The pressures on the publicly funded service foundations means that people needing home care in an emergency sometimes also have to purchase this from a commercial, for-profit provider, regardless of whether they can afford it.

Pressures and trends

There have been major pressures to improve the coordination of services for older people in the Netherlands. Regional networks have been established to plan services, allocate resources and regulate service quality. For individual users, joint assessments and care management have been introduced to reduce duplication and gaps. In some areas, all community care and nursing services (including residential and nursing homes) have been brought together into local district teams. Evaluation of these coordination initiatives has shown them to result in more responsive and flexible services and reduce the risk of admission to residential institutions.

Since 1995, a small minority of older (and younger, physically disabled) people have been able to opt for a personal budget – a cash payment to purchase their own services. Eligibility for a personal budget depends on an assessment of care needs (over and above what can be met by relatives) and the amount is calculated according to the hourly rate for the types of help needed. Users are charged on the same basis as they would be for services in kind. Many personal budget holders purchase their home care services from the new commercial provider organisations, while continuing to purchase home nursing from the traditional non-profit foundations. In 1998, 76 per cent of personal budget holders purchased domestic help, 54 per cent purchased personal care and 21 per cent used it for home nursing. Many also used a combination of providers: 23 per cent used non-profit foundations; 27 per cent used new commercial organisations; 44 per cent hired domestic help privately; and 21 per cent paid relatives to provide care. Evaluations of personal budgets have shown the choice and control they offer are popular with users:

> *I have a better grip on the care provided to me and they don't treat me as a number. When I received help from a regular home care organisation, I felt as if I was just a number to them … [Now] the workers I hire, based on my personal budget, usually come in time and the agency no longer sends so many different ones.*
>
> *(Quoted in Weekers and Pijl 1998: 171)*

The personal budget scheme is currently restricted to only five per cent of the total national care budget. This has reduced the threat to the established home care provider foundations, by restricting the amount of public funding available for older people to purchase services from private, for-profit agencies.

Since the 1980s, extended sheltered housing schemes have been developed in the Netherlands. These bring together public housing associations, home care providers and local residential and nursing homes, and involve services which can respond quickly and flexibly to changes in an older person's health. They have been shown to be cost-effective, offering the same quality of care as in institutional settings but at lower cost; and they reduce admission to residential homes among older people with chronic health problems.

Conclusion

Although these four European countries experience common pressures, they have responded in very different ways, which reflect fundamental differences in the underpinning values, funding arrangements and institutional structures of their welfare states. They also reflect differences in the positions of older people within the wider society in each country, their status as citizens and entitlement to services regardless of the help provided by family and friends.

The trend in the UK has been for care responsibilities to be shifted progressively from NHS hospitals to community services, local authorities and families. As a result, older people and their families are meeting increasing proportions of the costs of care, on top of their lifetime tax and national insurance contributions. Although local authorities no longer have a monopoly on home care services, choice remains very limited for most older people and services are rarely flexible or extensive enough for the frailest older people to stay in their own homes. Denmark continues to invest heavily in integrated home care and nursing services. Costs are contained by refocusing municipal services on the provision of personal care; reducing the amounts of help provided; and charging for or 'privatising' traditional domestic and household services. Germany's care insurance scheme has restored significant citizenship rights to frail older people and reduced the power of the well-established cartel of home service providers. However, the qualifying threshold for care insurance is high, choice is limited and most recipients prefer informal care to direct services in kind. In the Netherlands, home care and nursing services are integrated at local level; there is widespread commitment to providing publicly funded care services (albeit with contributions from users) and clear local responsibilities for regulating care.

Overall these countries illustrate major differences in:

■ the responsibilities of the state (at local, regional and national levels) and individual older people (and their families) for funding and providing care;
■ shifts in the boundaries between acute health and social welfare services;
■ levels of coordination and integration of health and social welfare services; and
■ the rights and entitlements accorded to older people as citizens.

NOTE

[1] This chapter has been compiled with the help of Lone Lund Pederson, Michaela Schunk, Sylvia Weekers and Merete Platz.

REFERENCE

Weekers, S. and Pijl, M. (1998) *Home Care and Care Allowances in the European Union*, Utrecht, Netherlands Institute of Care and Welfare.

CHAPTER 35

THE BOUNDARY BETWEEN HEALTH AND SOCIAL CARE FOR OLDER PEOPLE[1]

Jane Lewis

The problem of the boundary between health and social care is not new. It was in large measure a deliberate creation of the postwar welfare settlement. Health and local authorities have always battled over their responsibilities, and the battles have been fuelled by the financial implications of admitting responsibility and by professional ideas as to what health and social care are all about. Loud exhortations by successive governments to practitioners to collaborate have accompanied a neglect of service development. Older people, in particular, have experienced a poor deal, caught between the twin limitations of provision by local authorities and the NHS.

The dimensions of the boundary

The health/social care boundary has three main dimensions: financial, administrative and professional, and these dimensions are intertwined. In regard to the *financial* dimension, the UK is unlike most other European countries in funding health and social care differently – health care being funded through taxation and free at the point of use, social care being provided on a means-tested basis. Some commentators have suggested that it is this funding separation, together with the fact that resources have often been severely limited, that has above all encouraged both local authorities and health authorities to minimise their responsibilities (Glennerster *et al.* 1983). In the case of local authorities, this temptation has been increased by the fact that the government grant for social care has not been ring-fenced. Local politicians have often considered other priorities to be more pressing.

The *administrative* divide was created at the end of the Second World War, when local authorities were left with the responsibility for providing residential accommodation under Part III of the 1948 National Assistance Act, together with a range of domiciliary services, including home nursing and home helps. The 1946 NHS Act made the health service responsible for both acute and 'continuing' care. In 1974, when the NHS underwent its first major reorganisation, home nursing was transferred to the health authorities, and the administrative boundary was thus drawn more tightly. Administrative responsibilities and hence the definition as to what constitutes health and social care has therefore shifted over time. Since the late 1960s, hospital doctors have repeatedly complained that their acute beds are 'blocked' by elderly patients, whom they suggest require social rather than health care. Local authorities, on the other hand, have protested that they are expected to care for individuals with ever greater degrees of infirmity.

Professional rivalries, the third element comprising the boundary, have always seemed the most obtuse to outsiders, as in the case of the seemingly arcane disputes over 'the health versus the social care bath' (Twigg 1997) – free if given by the nurse, paid for if carried out by a home carer. Under the 1946 NHS Act, hospitals were instructed to provide long-term care services for any elderly person in need of constant nursing *and* medical attention. It was a definition that proved distasteful both for the Department of Health concerned about costs, and for hospital doctors imbued with the 'acute ideology' (Hall and Bytheway 1982). And while social workers, having fought to free themselves of medical control within the local authorities, continued to be wary of the influence of 'the medical model', care of older people did not commend itself to them or to their political masters in the local authorities. The question of what should actually be provided has tended to take a back seat, subordinated to these inter-related boundary issues.

Struggling over responsibilities, the 1950s–1980s

The public records reveal that there has been a struggle over the respective responsibilities of health and local authorities from as early as the 1950s. From the late 1950s, central government favoured the view of the Department (then Ministry) of Health's hospital division and medical department, as well as that of many hospital doctors, that the number of geriatric beds should be limited. Ministry officials decided that the boundary should be drawn in terms of the need for different types of institutional care: between those in need of constant care and attention (the responsibility of local authorities) and those in need of constant medical and nursing attention (the responsibility of the health authorities).[2] Decisions about admission to hospital were to be made only by hospital medical staff. Disputes swiftly followed. There was, after all, a large number of elderly people who needed constant nursing care but not constant medical attention, or who needed both on a regular basis, but not all the time.

From the early 1950s, the Ministry of Health sought to contain the number of beds for the 'chronic sick'. An influential Ministerial Committee concluded that no expansion was needed (Ministry of Health 1957). The Ministry followed this up by setting a bed norm slightly below the level of existing provision. George Godber, the Chief Medical Officer, opposed any parallel attempt to increase the nursing responsibilities of local authority homes for fear of recreating the poor law practice of putting the chronic sick into institutions with inadequate medical and nursing care, a position firmly supported by the local authorities themselves.[3] Godber assumed that rehabilitation services would be strengthened and that there would be better liaison. Privately, civil servants accepted that setting a lower bed norm would amount to a reduction in the non-acute role of the hospitals. As the Assistant Secretary in the Local Authority Division of the Ministry of Health observed in 1962: 'we are coming up increasingly against this view that hospitals only have a duty to *treat* the infirm ill. They also have a duty to care for those who need prolonged nursing'.[4] However, this was never made public. Nor was there acknowledgement that the local authorities would have to make provision for more infirm people, or any firm plan at central or local level to develop rehabilitation or domiciliary care services. The attempt to produce a Local Health and Welfare Plan in 1963 offered no real way forward (Cmnd. 1973, 1963).

In short, both health and local authorities endeavoured to avoid responsibility for what was, in the context of demographic change, a growing 'intermediate group' of people who were in need of nursing and/or medical attention on a very regular but not constant basis. Central government was determined to reduce the number of geriatric hospital beds, but not prepared publicly to admit that this would reduce the role of the hospitals in the continuing care of the elderly. There was a genuine hope that advances in rehabilitative medicine in particular would allow more people to be cared for with fewer geriatric beds, but the evidence that such advances were being put into practice was conspicuously lacking (HAS 1972: 25).

On their side, local authorities had their own priorities, which focused on upgrading the old Poor Law institutions and relieving their waiting lists for residential care. Local authorities were more than willing to increase their residential accommodation, but what they did not want to see was an influx of elderly people from the NHS. Thus, they were suspicious of any attempt to get them to do more in order to relieve the hospitals. This explains in large part the very slow development of domiciliary care

(Means and Smith 1985). Local authorities clearly expressed to Ministry officials their fear of doing anything that would enable infirm patients to be discharged from hospitals earlier.[5] From the 1950s the priority was saving money in the hospital sector (Webster 1988: 257), hence the emphasis on short-stay provision and the encouragement of a freeze on geriatric beds. However, any public acknowledgement that this policy involved an increase in local authorities' responsibilities in respect of more infirm elderly people would have provoked immediate demands for a transfer of resources far in excess of anything that was proposed. In addition, any public acknowledgement of a shift in responsibilities would have led to accusations that the scope of NHS care had been reduced and that elderly people were being forced to pay for their care (just such an accusation was to come later, as we shall see later in the chapter). The struggle over responsibilities between the two sets of authorities was extremely detrimental to service development for elderly people, but the failure of central government to acknowledge and deal with the shifts that were taking place was the key issue.

In face of these intractable disputes about responsibilities, central government relied heavily on solutions that addressed only the professional divide between the two services, first exhorting professionals to cooperate and, by the 1970s, imposing new joint planning structures that would encourage cooperation (DHSS 1976). Exhortations to plan jointly were conspicuously unsuccessful in the face of mutual suspicion between health and social services (Sumner and Smith 1969). The litany of differences in funding structures, planning cycles, decision-making processes, work cultures, and (after 1982) geographical boundaries, first identified in the 1970s, have been repeated with depressing regularity since (Glennerster *et al.* 1983; Wistow 1990; Lewis and Glennerster 1996; House of Commons Health Committee 1998). Both health and local authorities had every incentive to limit what they did to address the needs of what was a growing 'intermediate' group of elderly people needing rehabilitation services and non-institutionally based community care.

Giving responsibility to social services: the new community care

By the end of the 1970s the difficulties inherent in a policy designed to shift more responsibility for the care of elderly people to the local authorities, without formally acknowledging any change in the role of either the health or local authorities, were severe. They temporarily disappeared in the 1980s as a result of the massive, unintended injection of funds from the social security budget into private residential care. However, government could not let this way of solving the problem of the 'intermediate group' of elderly people needing care continue. With the introduction of the 1990 NHS and Community Care Act, the struggle over the respective responsibilities of health and local authorities was back on the agenda. Indeed the new transparency of the quasi-market intensified disputes and the responsibilities of the different authorities began to be tested in the courts.

The solution of a unitary authority with a single budget for elderly people, proposed in an influential Audit Commission report (1986), proved unattractive to the Government. The 1988 Griffiths Report suggested that a hospital's responsibility, 'in broad terms' involved 'investigation, diagnosis, treatment and rehabilitation undertaken by a doctor or by other professional staff to whom a doctor has referred the patient'. Elderly people should only be in hospital if they needed '*both* medical supervision and nursing care to be available throughout twenty-four hours' (DHSS 1988, para. 6.12. In this, Griffiths was very much in sympathy with the long-standing demand of many in the medical profession that hospitals should concentrate solely on acute care). Following through the logic of his position, Griffiths recommended that all services other than hospital provision (including nursing and residential homes and domiciliary services) should be commissioned by local authorities. They would receive a specific grant and would be treated as the lead authority. The grant would only be supplied once local authorities had submitted community care plans judged by central government to provide evidence of collaborative planning and the promotion of a mixed economy of care. This amounted to an acceptance of the *ad hoc* developments during the early 1980s. But, whereas hospitals had been able to reduce their responsibilities for long-term care by using the loophole in the social security system, in future the shift of patients out of the hospital would occur in a more controlled fashion as financial responsibility was transferred to local authorities. This constituted a major departure.

The Department of Health had repeatedly refused to amend the definition of responsibilities for care of older people arrived at in the immediate postwar years. It had continued to claim that the policy of limiting hospital geriatric provision did not mean a change in hospitals' responsibilities for long-term care. Its response to the Griffiths Report revealed that this was still the case. Rather than accepting Griffiths' move towards defining the role of the hospitals in terms of acute care, the DHSS maintained the position it had held for the previous thirty years. Thus, in *Caring for People,* the Department's 1989 White Paper on community care, it stated that: 'the key functions and responsibilities of the health service as a whole remain essentially unaltered by the proposals in this White Paper' (Cm. 849, 1989, para. 4.2). It further stated categorically that where people require continuous care for reasons of ill-health, 'it will remain the responsibility of health authorities to provide this' (ibid., para. 4.20). Yet no attempt was made to give this any material substance by reversing the decline in hospitals' long-term care provision that had taken place in the 1980s.

The Department of Health did not attempt to define what it meant by health care and social care. It accepted that in some individual cases there might be difficulties, but once again placed faith in collaboration, suggesting that it was 'critically important for responsible authorities to work together' (Cm. 849, para. 4.2). And, unlike the Griffiths' report which had attempted to link joint planning to resource allocation through the provision of a specific grant, the 1990 Act merely obliged local authorities to 'consult' other authorities. The House of Commons Social Services Committee (1990) was not alone in remaining unconvinced that this would prove sufficient.

The 1990 NHS and Community Care Act had thus conceptualised social care in relation to the problems of social security on the one hand, and of the NHS on the other. There was now a more pronounced shift towards increasing the responsibility of local authorities. It was the product of a 'pincer movement' led by the new-found concern to curb social security spending and the old ambition of drawing a tighter line around the NHS as an acute care service (exacerbated by the sharp increase in the number of people aged over eighty-five, which nearly doubled between 1981 and the end of the 1990s). Service delivery in and of itself was not at the forefront of government thinking.

Conflicts in the open

Lewis and Glennerster (1996: 16) have suggested that NHS officers regarded the 1990 Act 'as good grounds for getting rid of their long-term care responsibilities as soon as possible'. Some health authorities stopped providing any continuing care beds at all (Richards 1996). Eventually, these developments forced the Department of Health publicly to accept that the 1990 Act had led to a reduction in the responsibility of hospitals for long-term care, notwithstanding its earlier claims to the contrary. The immediate catalyst was a 1994 report by the Health Service Commissioner into the case of a seriously brain-damaged patient, for whom the local health authority had refused to accept responsibility. The Commissioner found that, in refusing to spend resources 'on patients of this type', the health authority was failing to fulfil its duties (Health Service Commissioner 1994).

In response to the widespread publicity this case created, the DoH released new guidance on NHS responsibilities, its first detailed statement on this matter for almost forty years (DoH 1995). 'Continuing in-patient care' was identified as one of the range of services which the NHS *should* provide. However, four eligibility criteria were set out, significantly restricting the role of the NHS in comparison with the definitions of responsibility provided by health officials in the 1940s and 1950s (ibid.: 15). An emphasis placed on 'specialist' care was a new departure which, as one commentator suggested, indicated 'that basic nursing care for chronically, but not acutely ill patients, is no longer to be regarded as part of a "comprehensive" national health service' (Richards 1996). To a large extent, however, the guidance merely represented a retrospective acceptance of a situation that had been developing steadily since the mid-1950s. It took almost forty years for health officials to acknowledge publicly that a major implication of their policy was that the role of the hospitals would be restricted.[6]

Pearson and Wistow (1995) have argued that this policy has been 'silent, if not surreptitious', but the historical evidence shows that health officials privately acknowledged that such a change was taking place for much of the intervening period. Their failure to openly confront it served to impede the development of rehabilitation and other services for the intermediate group.

The Labour Government of 1997 showed every sign of continuing to address the professional divide, calling for collaboration and joint working in its White Paper on the NHS (Cm. 3807) and in a subsequent consultative document (DoH 1998). The administrative divide was altered at the margins, the financial divide, barely at all – despite the recommendations (Cmnd. 4192-I) of the Royal Commission on Long Term Care (which was received favourably only in Scotland). With the publication of the NHS Plan (Cm. 4818-I), a new direction began to emerge. Care Trusts, a further development of primary care groups, came onto the scene – amidst much questioning from those in the local authority sector. There were some ring-fenced monies together with an acknowledgement of unmet needs among the 'intermediate group' of elderly people.

What emerges from this analysis is that, if attempts to address the administrative and professional dimensions (and thereby to develop services) are to be successful, the financial dimensions of the health/social care boundary must be tackled first. Taking a long view, however, it is hard to be optimistic about the shift towards primary care.

NOTES

1   An extended version of this argument can be found in 'The Health/Social Care Boundary and Older People: is the NHS Plan the answer?', *Journal of Social Policy and Administration*, (forthcoming).
2   PRO MH 80/47, Undated memorandum on the abolition of the Poor Law.
3   PRO MH 130/266, Sixth meeting of the Boucher Committee, 15/2/54.
4   PRO MH 130/303, Note by Halliday on a letter from Yate to Paget, 22/11/62 (his emphasis).
5   PRO MH 134/41, CCA to Dodds, 12 October 1961.
6   Further interim guidance was introduced in 1999 (DH (99) HSC 1999/180) after another legal case involving a physically disabled woman moved from an NHS nursing home to a local authority home, where she was charged for her nursing care.

REFERENCES

Audit Commission (1986) *Making a Reality of Community Care*. London: HMSO.

Cm. 849 (1989) *Caring for People: Community Care in the Next Decade and Beyond*. London: HMSO.

Cm. 3807 (1997) *The New NHS. Modern. Dependable*. London: the Stationery Office.

Cm. 4818-I (2000) *The NHS Plan*. London: Stationery Office.

Cmnd. 1973 (1963) Health and Welfare. *The Development of Community Care*. London: HMSO.

Cmnd. 4192-I (1999) Report of the Royal Commission on Long Term Care. *With Respect to Old Age: Long Term Care – Rights and Responsibilities*. London: Stationery Office.

Department of Health (1995) Circulars HSG (95) 8 and LAC (95) 5.

Department of Health (1998) *Partnership in Action. New Opportunities for Joint Working Between Health and Social Services*. London: Department of Health.

Department of Health and Social Security (1976) *The NHS Planning System*. London: DHSS.

Department of Health and Social Security (1988) *Community Care: An Agenda for Action*. London: HMSO.

Glennerster, H., with N. Korman and F. Marsden-Wilson (1983) *Planning for Priority Groups*. Oxford: Martin Robertson.

Hall, D. and Bytheway, B. (1982) The Blocked Bed: Definition of the Problem. *Social Science and Medicine* 16: 1985–1991.

HAS (Hospital Advisory Service) (1972) *Report of the Hospital Advisory Service*. London: DHSS.

Health Service Commissioner (1994) Failure to Provide Long Term HNS Care for a Brain Damaged Patient. *Second Report for Session 1993–4*. London: HMSO.

House of Commons Health Committee (1998) *First Report. The Relationship Between Health and Social Services*. Vol. I. London: Stationery Office.

House of Commons Social Services Committee (1990) (580–1) *Eighth Report. Community Care Planning and Cooperation*. London: HMSO.

Lewis, J. and Glennerster, H. (1996) *Implementing the New Community Care*. Buckingham: Open University Press.

Means, R. and Smith, R. (1985) *The Development of Welfare Services for the Elderly*. London: Croom Helm.

Ministry of Health (1957) *Survey of Services Available to the Chronic Sick and Elderly, 1954–5*. London: HMSO.

Pearson, M. and Wistow, G. (1995) The Boundary Between Health and Social Care. *British Medical Journal* 311 (22 July): 208.

Richards, M. (1996) *Community Care for Older People*. Bristol: Jordans.

Sumner, G. and Smith, R. (1969) *Planning Local Authority Services for the Elderly*. London: Allen and Unwin.

Twigg, J. (1997) Deconstructing the 'Social Bath': Help with Bathing at Home for Older and Disabled People. *Journal of Social Policy* 26 (2): 211–32.

Webster, C. (1988) *The Health Services Since the War*. Vol. I. London: HMSO.

Wistow, G. (1990) *Community Care Planning. A Review of Past Experience and Future Imperatives*, CCI 3. London: DH.

CHAPTER 36

HEALTH AND SOCIAL CARE ASSESSMENT IN ACTION

Allison Worth

Assessment is the means by which practitioners ascertain the needs of clients in order to determine the most appropriate location for care and to match services to needs. Assessment involves the collection of information, but that alone is of little value. The process must include the interpretation of information, the planning of interventions, the implementation of strategies designed to meet needs and the evaluation of these strategies (Caldock 1994; Thompson 1995). Information is derived from a number of sources, usually the potential client, carer and relatives or friends and neighbours, and other professionals and service providers. Observation of the person and environment adds further information. The practitioner draws on all this to develop a body of evidence to justify why that person's needs must be met. Risk, needs, resources, the client's views and the views of other parties consulted must all be weighed and balanced. These competing perspectives can create uncomfortable tensions for practitioners involved in complex judgements in assessment practice (Ellis 1993).

District nurses and social workers are key practitioner groups assessing the health and social needs of older people in the community. The overlap between such needs means that skilled assessment, effective consultation and cooperation between health and social work personnel are essential if needs are to be adequately addressed.

This chapter draws on a study in Scotland in 1998 which explored similarities and differences in the way district nurses and social workers assessed the needs of older people, with a view to identifying particular areas of expertise in this crucial area of practice (Worth 1999). A team of seven community care social workers and a sample of eight district nurses in the same geographical area were observed conducting eighteen assessments with people aged seventy-five years and over living in the community. The same two groups were also interviewed regarding their assessment practice. Four members of a multidisciplinary care management team in the same locality were also included in the study.

Observation was used to gain insights into what actually occurs during an assessment visit, while the interviews explored practitioners' views of the principles of assessment and the organisational influences on their practice. At interview, practitioners were also asked to describe assessments they had conducted where the boundaries between health and social needs and the responsibilities for meeting them were unclear. In this way, research methods were combined in order to explore both the 'ideal' and the 'real' in assessment practice, providing a more rounded understanding.

The process of assessment

Practitioners suggested that completing assessment documentation in front of the client forms a barrier between the client and practitioner and that clients are more 'open' if the assessment appears more like an informal conversation. They described using a 'mental guide' as a prompt to ask for information not covered in the course of conversation. After introductions, some practitioners, most commonly social workers, gave the client a strong lead in focusing the assessment. For example, one assessment began with the social worker saying to the client:

> *What I need is some sort of idea from you of what the problems are and what kind of help you need.*

Others, more commonly district nurses, began with a broad, open question such as 'How are you?', allowing the client more freedom to set the agenda. If the client responded at length, the practitioner tended to allow the assessment to flow naturally. Questioning became more focused as practitioners went through their mental checklists, or if time became short. Then a more closed questioning style was employed, which was also useful for gathering factual information.

In some cases, observed in both social work and district nursing assessments, it was the client who tried to focus the assessment, a comprehensive assessment strategy seeming to puzzle those clients who believed their needs were minimal. In one such case the clients, an elderly couple, said they needed a home help to do housework. This did not fit the eligibility criteria for home care and the social worker tried to identify another 'need' to allow a home help to be provided. Enquiries into their personal care abilities and social outlets appeared to worry the woman in particular, who found it hard to follow the assessment due to deafness. She tried to focus the assessment on getting help with the housework, seeming to find the social worker's comprehensive assessment strategy unnecessary and intrusive.

Social workers recognised that meeting health needs was central to quality of life. At interview, they generally claimed to understand such needs sufficiently to know when to refer a client to a health professional. They stressed the value of consultation with health professionals, often on an informal basis, if they were unsure whether a health need required further assessment. In observed assessments, social workers' questions about health needs were broad, such as 'How do you keep physically?' Often when clients responded by mentioning health needs such as pain and breathing problems, the social workers enquired no further. No social workers were observed to ask about continence, sleep or pain. The social workers' limited knowledge indicated that they experienced some difficulty in judging the significance of health information. One social worker said:

> *I always ask what medication they're on, not that it means anything to me, but at least it's there.*

District nurses, in contrast, were observed to ask detailed questions about health problems such as pain, continence, skin care and medication, and to enquire briefly into other health-related issues such as diet and sleep. Where problems such as pain existed, the district nurses followed this up with questions about the nature and site of pain, any treatment and its effectiveness and offered to ask the GP to call to assess further.

For both district nurses and social workers, a major component of assessment was functional ability. From observation, district nurses conducted more comprehensive assessments of this than social workers. District nurses' assessments encompassed detailed questioning about the client's ability in areas such as bathing and self-care, dressing, mobility and ability to prepare meals. They also examined the home to assess problems which might hinder mobility and, for bathing, they usually suggested a further visit to observe the client's ability. The social workers made only brief enquiries into functional ability, such as 'Are you able to get in and out of the bath?' and 'Can you cope with washing and dressing yourself?' Such questions were sometimes prefaced with statements such as 'Sorry if this is a personal question', indicating that such enquiries do not come naturally to social workers. If social workers thought a person might require a further functional assessment, they said they would make a referral to the occupational therapist.

District nurses' assessments of social needs were less comprehensive. The social workers asked more questions and offered more interventions, such as day care or voluntary sector support. Neither group enquired closely or routinely into mental health needs or potential abuse.

In observed assessments, only one district nurse, other than those acting as care managers, asked about the attendance allowance. In contrast, social workers were required to conduct extensive assessment of the client's financial circumstances. This caused some conflict for the social workers, who often prefaced their financial enquiries with disassociating remarks, for example:

> Sorry to ask all these questions, but I need to assess and also if you've got any savings as well I need to know. We should have been accountants not social workers.

In interviews and observed assessments, exploring options was identified as a vital part of determining need. When practitioners were under pressure to complete assessments quickly and where clients or carers were thought to be at risk, exploring options was necessarily time-limited. Social workers acknowledged that this was unsatisfactory, particularly where options included major life changes for clients, such as giving up their homes and moving into care.

The study revealed many similarities and differences in assessment practice amongst practitioners in the same group as well as between district nurses and social workers. District nurses in particular showed a wide variation, ranging from the health-care focused and service-led to a more comprehensive, needs-led approach. At interview, the social workers generally described a more unified, needs-led approach towards assessment. There was, however, a greater gap between social workers' descriptions of how assessment *should* be conducted and the reality identified through observation.

In observed assessments, the district nurses in the multidisciplinary care management team were the only practitioners possessing sufficient knowledge of health and social needs to conduct more holistic assessments. Their familiarity with health care enabled them to ask more detailed questions about health needs and functional ability, whilst the re-orientation of their work and close contact with social workers made them more aware of social needs. The district nurses and social workers in the care management team appeared to find that closer working relationships assisted their own decision-making and holistic assessment of clients' needs, and were particularly valuable where risks are high or conflicts arise between practitioner and client or carer views of need.

The skills of assessment

At interview, practitioners often described communication skills as being crucial. Observation revealed that practitioners displayed an impressive range of such skills, often with clients with whom establishing rapport could be difficult due to dementia, hearing loss or speech difficulties.

Another important skill was to go beyond what clients said explicitly: to consider what clients hinted at but might find difficulty expressing openly, and to gather cues from the environment. This was referred to in terms such as 'picking things up' and is developed, practitioners suggested, through knowledge and experience. Looking beyond the presenting problem appeared however, from observed assessments, to be a strategy applied more to the needs of the older person than to carers. Reasons given for not pursuing carers' needs were lack of resources to meet any needs uncovered and a suggestion that carers resist being viewed as clients.

Practitioners possessed considerable knowledge and expertise which they were observed to use to great effect to support clients and carers. Broadly speaking, the district nurses were best able to respond to health concerns and the social workers to financial problems. Clients and carers could resent questions about their finances but despite this, in the observed assessments, clients often expressed gratitude for the social workers' assistance in helping them with the complex financial assessment forms. Social workers were often able to correct misunderstandings about entitlements. The district nurse's role as judge of health needs and link with the GP were observed to be used effectively and were similarly appreciated by clients.

Anticipating the risks associated with a health state or a set of social circumstances was also perceived as a central assessment skill. The risks which practitioners focused on most were falling, deteriorating health, behaviour associated with dementia (such as wandering and dangerous use of electricity), carer stress, and inadequate understanding of medication regimes. From observation, risk assessment dominated some assessments, played a part in almost all, and was the most common source of disagreement about needs among clients, carers and practitioners. At times, carers' concerns about risk seemed, to practitioners, to be exaggerated; at other times, carers wanted to provide care at home when practitioners were sure they would be unable to manage. Between clients and practitioners, it was invariably the practitioner who perceived a risk which the client did not recognise. Risk of falling and dementia-related risks were particularly unlikely to be recognised by clients and they were reluctant to accept services designed to minimise such risks. Negotiating between clients, practitioners, carers and services in reaching agreements about risk is a sensitive and time-consuming business.

Although risk management was a strong feature of practitioners' assessment practice, they also recognised that they needed to allow clients the dignity of risk (Perske 1972). The uncertainty about making risk-related decisions was made clear by one social worker who, on leaving a house where an older woman had refused the extra home help the social worker believed she needed for safety reasons, said 'Oh dear, I hope I've done the right thing.' As accountable practitioners, district nurses and social workers face considerable pressure to prevent harm, but there can be a fundamental tension between needs-led assessment and risk management. A central assessment skill is therefore balancing clients' views of their needs with professional decision-making based on sound ethical principles.

Involving clients

Practitioners indicated that they understand the importance of gaining the client's view of their needs. One described client involvement as:

> *a fundamental principle, I would always try to involve the client as much as possible and as far as possible let them say what happens.*

Observation, however, suggested that practitioners had considerable difficulty in conducting client-led assessments. Clients are unaware of what is available, therefore practitioners have to suggest services, running through a list of those available such as meals on wheels, chiropody and home help.

One difficulty in incorporating the client's views was very apparent in many of the observed visits. Many clients were unable to define their needs due to mental impairment, and others wanted to pursue their expressed needs (for example not to have help at home) in circumstances which practitioners, family and neighbours felt would mean an unacceptable level of risk. Another factor for some clients was an inability to express their views due to severe hearing loss or speech problems following a stroke.

Observation and interview data suggest that assessment by a district nurse is viewed differently to an assessment by a social worker. Requiring help in meeting a health need appears to be more acceptable than help with more 'social' needs. Services such as home care and meals on wheels, and social interventions such as day care, were often strongly resisted by clients and carers as indicating 'failure to cope'. Comprehensive assessment, enquiring into areas where clients did not perceive themselves as having needs, could appear to be threatening to their self-image as capable people. In one assessment, a client with a serious vision impairment was persuaded by her family and the social worker to accept a home help and a community alarm which she made clear she did not want: 'I'm not the sort of person to have a home help' and 'I've been such an independent person and never needed any of this'. This suggests that, by accepting help, an older person has to face that they have become a different sort of person, the sort of person who needs help to manage. Such situations occurred in half of the observed assessments and were all associated with practitioners' perceptions of risks not being acknowledged by clients.

The ability of some practitioners to conduct needs-led assessment confirms, however, that it is possible. Although all practitioners enquired into the clients' views of their needs, only one, a district nurse, was observed to comprehensively establish need in detail before negotiating services. Throughout her assessments, the district nurse emphasised that the client may hold solutions, as well as the district nurse, treating needs as joint problems to be worked out together rather than the district nurse imposing a solution.

Constraints on assessment practice

Both social workers and district nurses said that resource constraints often did not allow the principles of needs-led assessment to be applied. Practitioners are required to set priorities, as resources are inadequate to meet all needs. In social work, the demand for assessment and home care services far outstripped resources of: social work and occupational therapy time, home care staff numbers and funding for care packages. Needs deemed least urgent included those for motivation or company, for help with housework and support for carers, such as sitter services. A number of mechanisms had been introduced to manage need, including the introduction of waiting lists for assessment and care provision and ever-tightening eligibility criteria. Social workers cited numerous cases where assessed needs could not be met due to resource constraints.

Due to pressure of work, social workers often complete assessments in one visit, giving little opportunity to explore client views in any detail and leading them to focus on 'the practicalities' or 'plugging the gaps'. For some practitioners, there is little point in conducting needs-led assessment as this raises client expectations. Resource constraints meant that assessment remained service-led, as one social worker described:

> I don't like to think in these terms, but in practice part of the assessment is influenced a bit by what you know you can provide . . . Now I don't ask questions about certain aspects of a person's support network because I know that the chances of giving them any help are zero.

Carers' needs are therefore rarely formally assessed, and unmet need is not formally acknowledged. The district nurses appear to have an advantage in aiding clients to discuss their views and address adjustment to increasing needs because they tend to conduct assessment over time, often while providing services and as part of a longer-term relationship with clients. The initial assessment visit can then focus on practical needs with on-going assessment giving opportunities for more detailed discussion of the client's views. Rationing of time was, however, increasingly necessary, as more people with acute, chronic and terminal illness and frail older people were cared for at home.

Conclusion

These findings suggest that district nurses and social workers have different and complementary areas of knowledge which together encompass the components of an holistic assessment of needs. They appear to cover similar areas of enquiry in their assessments, with some obvious exceptions, such as the detailed financial assessments which social workers are required to conduct. Assessment differed between the two groups in the degree of detail when enquiring into health and social needs and functional abilities. It appears that referral to either a social worker or district nurse results in a differently-focused assessment and, therefore, different outcomes for older people.

The study highlights the difficulty for practitioners in balancing needs-led assessment and the professional accountability which demands effective risk management. However, as some observed assessments showed, even with clients with dementia, listening to their views of their needs can be a means of establishing a relationship through which a degree of negotiation can take place regarding interventions.

For many older people, assessment seemed a marker of transition from independence to dependence, and thus was experienced with mixed emotions. Interventions might be welcomed as improving quality of life, but the recognition of becoming 'a person who needs help' has strongly negative connotations. Observation suggested that older people may not always understand the process and aims of comprehensive assessment, although understanding is essential to effective participation.

In many cases, resource availability drives the process of assessment. Practitioners experience a dilemma in being required to conduct needs-led assessment in a climate where needs are less likely to be met as resources are spread more thinly. In such circumstances, practitioners appear to find needs-led assessment a futile exercise and are unwilling to raise clients' hopes of receiving services they know they will not get.

Assessment is such a central part of everyday practice in community care that it often appears to be taken for granted. Evaluations of assessment practice often focus on criticisms, particularly regarding the gap between the policy rhetoric and the practice reality. Observation of practice reveals the reasons behind the gap, as well as the complex and highly skilled interpersonal and intellectual activities involved in the assessment of need.

The principles of community care are broadly welcomed by practitioners, but the lack of resources prevents them from being able to use their skills fully for the greatest benefit of clients. It appears that resource constraints and eligibility criteria for services drive assessment, rather than clients' views of their needs. Integrated working then becomes even more crucial, in order to pool expertise to meet the needs of clients most effectively.

REFERENCES

Caldock, K. (1994) 'Policy and practice: fundamental contradictions in the conceptualization of community care for elderly people?' *Health and Social Care in the Community*, 2, 133–141.

Ellis, K. (1993) *Squaring the Circle: User and Carer Participation in Needs Assessment*, Joseph Rowntree Foundation, York.

Perske, R. (1972) 'The dignity of risk and the mentally retarded', *Mental Retardation*, 10, 24–27.

Thompson, N. (1995) *Theory and Practice in Health and Social Welfare*, Open University Press, Buckingham.

Worth, A. (1999) *An Ethnographic Study of Assessment of the Needs of Older People by District Nurses and Social Workers*. Unpublished PhD thesis, Glasgow Caledonian University.

CHAPTER 37

THE IMPORTANCE OF HOUSING AND HOME

Christine Oldman

The importance of where vulnerable people live, and the suitability of that place, seems fairly self-evident. Despite this, housing is not central to national or local policies concerned with community care.

The words 'housing' and 'home' are distinct but closely related. Housing is a physical structure, for example a house or a flat, within which a self-selected household lives. It is a place in which the basic human activities of sleeping, eating, washing, storage of possessions, social contact, recreation and care take place (Harrison and Heywood 2000). The word may also incorporate the attributes of the structure: its location, size, design, condition, accessibility, warmth and comfort. The terms upon which housing is occupied (that is, its forms of tenure) will vary. They include owner occupation (freehold or leasehold, with or without a mortgage); renting from a council, private landlord or housing association (with varying degrees of security); and membership of a housing cooperative. 'Housing', thus, is a word imbued with technical meaning whereas 'home' denotes something much more intangible. Home is existential and experiential. It is where domestic lives are played out. Home is a myriad of things: a set of relationships with others, a statement about self-image and identity, a place of privacy, a set of memories, and a social and psychological space (Benjamin and Stea 1995).

Throughout the 1980s and 1990s, as the community care policies unfolded, anecdotes were told by various service providers of how housing and home mattered to vulnerable people. The following examples of the importance of both housing and home are derived from different reports which came out during that twenty-year period.

1   A person after three months in a psychiatric ward would be discharged straight back to the explosive family situation from which they came.

2   A seventy-five-year-old woman suffering from emphysema and with a history of severe bronchitic attacks, would be admitted to hospital with pneumonia from the poorly maintained and damp home she had lived in for the past forty years.

3   A sixteen-year-old would leave foster care and move to a supported housing project for young people, but would be unable to take a job because, without Housing Benefit, he would be unable to afford the rent.

4   A family with three children, one of whom suffered from complex physical and behavioural disabilities, would be moved to an adapted property on a poor estate some distance away from supportive networks.

Different issues emerge from these four vignettes. First, there is the issue of housing as home. Home is where much of our life is played out. The fairly confined space of most houses is the locus of complex social relationships. Second is the issue of supply. There are not enough homes of the right quality. Poor quality housing can adversely affect people's physical and mental health. Third, there is affordability, an issue which affects all tenures but in different ways. As the third vignette indicates, high rents can create work disincentives. Finally, there is the issue of accessibility. The majority of housing in Britain is not barrier-free. Domestic space is supposed to be designed for the majority but in reality it is designed for a minority, a super race of modal height, weight and age. Domestic environments can be disabling.

The aim of this chapter is to elaborate why housing and home are of importance in the lives of vulnerable people. It begins by reviewing the key elements of British housing policy and then goes on to plot the development of 'special needs' housing. It will be shown that the failure of social and housing policies to recognise the importance of housing and home adversely affects people's lives in many ways, as illustrated in the vignettes above. The chapter concludes by arguing that two fundamental issues remain, despite some welcome policy developments. First, the concept of need remains fragmented rather than holistic. Second, the need for community care will continue whilst investment in appropriate and adequate housing is woefully inadequate.

Issues and trends in housing policy

Fundamental to any analysis of housing in Britain is tenure. As far as this chapter is concerned it is of great importance since the tenure people occupy plays some part in determining both their housing and support

Table 37.1 Dwellings by tenure in England, Wales and Scotland (%).

	Owner occupied	Social rented*	Private rented
1950	29.0	18.0	53.0
1961	42.3	25.0	31.9
1971	50.5	30.6	18.9
1981	56.4	32.5	11.1
1991	66.3	24.4	9.6
1998	67.6	21.9	10.6

*Council, housing associations and other not-for-profit companies.
Source: Housing and Construction Statistics (various editions), Scottish Office, Welsh Office.

options and their life chances. The history of tenure change in the twentieth, as summarised in Table 37.1, is well known.

The table plots the rise in owner occupation over the last forty years. Before the Second World War the private rented sector was still the dominant tenure with less than a third of all dwellings in owner occupation (Hughes and Lowe 1995). It declined rapidly during the postwar period whilst the council house sector grew until around the mid-1970s but then went rapidly into reverse. Twenty years ago Britain had more than six million council houses. The total now stands at about 3.2 million (Perry 2000). The loss of council stock is accounted for by Right to Buy policies and, more latterly, by stock transfer to local not-for-profit housing companies and registered social landlords (housing associations). The latter sector has continued to grow modestly from a very small base in the 1970s, around two per cent of all dwellings, to around five per cent of all dwellings in 1998 (Wilcox 2000, Table 17d). Its role, however, has changed. Increasingly housing associations have been required to move away from their traditional task of catering for specialist need to being volume producers of general needs housing.

Tenure patterns and tenure changes are not uniform, however. Those people who form the focus of this book, those with support needs, are less likely to live in owner occupation and more likely to live in social housing (council or housing association properties) than the rest of the population. They are also more likely to live in private rented housing.

Owner occupation: a problematic tenure?

Surveys consistently show that owner occupation is the preferred tenure of most people. Much has been written about the symbolic significance of home ownership and, although discredited by some researchers, the thesis that ownership of a property confers 'ontological security' is still useful as an analytical construct (Saunders 1990). Young people, disabled people and others whose income is either low or insecure, however, are likely to have problems in both gaining access to, and maintaining, home ownership. The disability movement argues that disabled people should be able

to participate in the benefits of owner occupation such as equity appreciation. But housing policies and social security policies contribute to the disabling of people with impairments through practices which make it
difficult for people without the prospect of sustained employment to
obtain mortgages. Moreover, families (as in the fourth vignette) can have
difficulties finding or affording suitable properties in the private sector.

Despite its overwhelming popularity, events over the last ten to fifteen
years have highlighted the problematic nature of owner occupation. Its
recent growth is accounted for by large numbers of low-income households
entering the tenure through, in particular, the Right to Buy policies of the
1980s and 1990s and the ready availability of mortgage finance. Homeowner households now make up half of all poor households, but they
receive only eight per cent of the total support provided by the government
to assist low-income households with their housing costs (Wilcox and
Burrows 2000). Through the Income Support system, help is available to
home owners if they are unable to work through sickness or redundancy,
but this has eroded during the second half of the 1990s. During the down-
turn in the housing market at the end of 1980s, mortgage arrears and
repossessions increased steeply. Recently there has been some interest
among researchers in the impact of difficulties with the cost of owner occupation on mental and physical health. Problematic home ownership is now
a 'new' public health issue (Nettleton and Burrows 1998).

Home ownership then may work well for the majority but for some it
does not. The massive privatisation of housing since the 1970s, however,
underpinned by ideologies of personal responsibility and individualism,
has resulted in problems remaining out of sight and mind. Controlling for
health, studies have shown that tenants are more likely to be in receipt of
health and welfare services than older home owners (Evandrou 1997).
Older people living in social housing are more visible.

Housing disrepair

There is substantial under-investment, both private and public, in the
nation's housing stock. The very worst housing is to be found in the
private rented sector, but it is also much in evidence in both social housing
and in the owner occupied sector (Leather and Morrison 1997). Council
housing has attracted the jibe 'new slums for old' (Holmans 1999).
Increasingly, central government is showing less commitment to subsidise
repair costs and older home owners face considerable problems trying to
maintain their properties. Resources for home improvement grants have
been much reduced. At the time of writing, the government proposes to
reduce this help even further by abolishing the structure of the means
tested scheme and to devolve responsibilities to local authorities (DETR
2000). However, unfit homes are unhealthy homes (RICS 1997; Anchor
Trust 1998; Harrison and Heywood 2000). For example, despite the

evidence that older people's health can be exacerbated by the state of their homes, as the second vignette illustrated, local public health plans rarely link up to local housing strategies for home improvement (Harrison and Heywood 2000).

Housing and social exclusion

In recent years there has been some concern by academics that housing should be included in debates on social exclusion and that definitions of housing deprivation should be widened to include the impact of poor environments. Social exclusion is a fashionable, if contested, concept for describing the process of disempowerment and non-participation in mainstream economic and social life experienced by a sizeable minority in Britain today (Anderson and Sim 2000). The contribution of social housing to social exclusion has belatedly become a concern to politicians. Although always intended for those who would have difficulty competing in the market place, council housing, and to a lesser extent housing association accommodation, is now the tenure of 'last resort'. The processes of what many writers have dubbed 'residualisation' have left a rump sector. The housing sector has led the way in the massive process of welfare restructuring which began around the mid-1970s. All the best properties have been sold, leaving 'unbalanced' communities of (i) the original tenants, now old and possibly in poor health, (ii) high 'child-dense' populations, (iii) lone parents and (iv) 'community care cases': people with mental health problems and disabled people. These groups may have been moved by their local authority to properties on estates considered to be appropriate either through the provision of accessible features or the addition of support (as in the fourth vignette relating to the family with a disabled child). Local authority housing departments, persistently under-funded, are highly constrained in their task of trying to allocate suitable properties to vulnerable individuals who are unable to compete for housing in the market place. Estates are characterised by very high levels of benefit dependency, unacceptable levels of crime and, in some parts of the country, low demand: few people are willing to move to live there.

The housing dimension of social exclusion is not confined solely to council or housing association estates, although its more dispersed nature in the owner occupied and private rented sector makes it less visible. The latter is increasingly being asked to play a role in accommodating vulnerable people. Local authorities with less and less appropriate stock of their own are obliged to place those for whom they have a statutory responsibility – vulnerable homeless people – into what may be an insecure and, quite literally, unsafe tenure.

Issues relating to minority ethnic groups need separate attention. Although some minority ethnic groups are over-represented on the sorts of social housing estate described above, other minority ethnic groups are disproportionately likely to be owner occupiers. Regardless of tenure, however, there is evidence that high levels of vulnerability are to found (Law 1996; Mason 2000).

Housing affordability

Assisting low-income households with the high cost of housing has increasingly been the role, not of the housing system of the country, but of the social assistance system. Bricks and mortar subsidies have reduced significantly but subsidies to support the individual through the provision of Housing Benefit have risen dramatically. Governments for some time have looked for ways of reducing the Housing Benefit bill without, at the same time, going back to a policy of increasing capital subsidies. There is pressure on registered social landlords to narrow the differential between their rents and those of local authorities. There are particular problems in the private rented sector. As is so often the case, different policies conflict. The massive deregulation of the sector presided over by Conservative governments resulted in market rents which potentially increased the strain on the Housing Benefit bill but a number of social security measures in recent years have restricted the amount of benefit paid out. There are other problems. Private landlords need to guarantee their rental income and therefore look upon Housing Benefit tenants as 'unreliable'. They expect deposits which young and other vulnerable people cannot pay. Finally, mention must be made of the policy *Supporting People* (DETR 2001). One of the aims of this is to confine Housing Benefit to property or landlord costs. Rents of those who live in special needs or supported housing have typically been higher than equivalent rents in 'ordinary' housing, because Housing Benefit has been available to pay tenancy support costs (for example, the salary of a warden in a sheltered housing scheme for older people). From April 2003, these support costs will be taken out of the social security system and put into a cash-limited grant to be administered by multi-agency local authority commissioning panels. If – and it is a big if – this new pot of money is adequate, the work disincentive issue illustrated in the third vignette (about the care leaver needing supported accommodation but also needing to enter the world of work) will begin to be addressed.

It should now be clear that housing policies are at odds with health and social welfare policies. Inadequate levels of investment in housing have led to poor housing environments which contribute to poor outcomes for vulnerable people. Moreover, as the fourth vignette indicates, there is a shortage of resources for making housing more accessible for disabled people. Although there is some recognition that housing contributes to social exclusion, there has been a failure by policy makers to connect housing, social exclusion and community care. Where housing policy does butt on to welfare, is in the area of what has been called 'special needs' housing.

The development of 'special needs' housing

Accommodation provision ranges from ordinary housing at one end, through different types of special needs or supported housing, to institutional living arrangements such as residential care at the other. The argument has been that, beyond some level of need, people would benefit from a degree of communal living arrangement that offers care or support services in addition to accommodation services. Sometimes the decision to move someone to specialist provision coincides with what they themselves would choose, but it can also be seen simply as a more cost-effective option than supporting people with similar needs who are dispersed throughout a community.

The history of special needs housing goes back a long way, indeed to the Middle Ages and the provision of almshouses. From the 1960s, local authorities developed sheltered housing, the purpose of which was to offer older people with easy-to-manage housing and some minimal support – a warden, an alarm system and some communal facilities. The special needs housing movement started to grow fairly rapidly from the 1980s and its constituency is now very diverse. It includes those who are well outside the community care mainstream: people dependent on drugs and alcohol, and victims of domestic violence, as well as its priority groups such as older people, disabled people, people with mental health problems and learning difficulties. Special needs housing is seen as a preferred alternative to residential provision. It is also seen as preventing or delaying admission to the latter.

Its forms are quite varied and have changed as fashions change. The term 'supported housing' is now considered more acceptable than the label 'special needs'. Accommodation is now more likely to be self-contained with a minimum of communal facilities, and schemes are smaller. Built forms range from hostels to group homes, shared housing, 'core and cluster', and foyers for young people (that provide training opportunities as well as accommodation). Some schemes have 24-hour staffing; some have peripatetic support. Services offered vary, although past analysis has shown that resettlement, the teaching of independent living skills and tenancy support, accounted for a large part of the supported housing business (Watson and Cooper 1992).

The move away from special needs

There is now considerable criticism of special needs housing. It is increasingly seen as discriminatory and ageist. In order to attract any munificence, vulnerable people have had to be prepared to be labelled as 'in need'. Special needs housing highlights the special nature of people's housing need and is seen to reinforce negative stereotypes through segregation (Clapham and Smith 1990; Clapham 1997). A number of recent reports, policy guidance and pronouncements have reversed earlier policies, arguing that services should be brought to people rather than people having to move to schemes. Investment in sheltered housing and other special needs housing has been sharply reduced and encouragement given to housing related services which support people in their own homes, such as home improvement agencies called 'Care and Repair' or 'Staying Put'. Similarly 'floating support', provided for a specified period of time to people living in ordinary tenancies, has begun to be developed. Grants for adaptations to people's homes, principally the Disabled Facilities Grant, are seen as an alternative to moving a disabled person to a care home.

The most recent development in supported accommodation is *Supporting People*. Its title is significant, reflecting a desire to deliver services to people in ordinary housing settings rather than move them to supported accommodation. The aim of *Supporting People* is that there will be a more strategic approach in each local authority to the provision of housing-related support services than is currently the case. *Supporting People* is an important development to which all political parties appear committed. There does seem to be some recognition that the provision of low-level, housing-related support services is a key element of community care. However, although its philosophy is lauded by all involved in the provision of housing and community care, there is some scepticism that its actual implementation will be adequately funded. Critics see the initiative principally driven by a desire to reduce Housing Benefit expenditure by funding housing and support services from cash-limited monies administered by local authorities (Griffiths 2000).

Do developments like *Supporting People* represent a genuine conversion on the part of policy makers to the principles of independent living, empowerment and user choice? For these principles to become a reality there need to be adequate resources. Yet it has been shown above that there is a severe gap between need and the supply of services such as disabled facilities grants, which may provide alternatives to moving to specialist provision. I would argue, along with Allen (1997), that 'independent living' is a smokescreen behind which government investment in good quality housing can be reduced and the responsibility of care and support transferred back to families. Many vulnerable people will not want to move to a special needs scheme. However, some may want to live with others at some point in their lives, but without the 'special needs' baggage that has prevailed for so long. There is much evidence, for example, that some older people make a positive choice to live with other older people in a setting that is agreeable to them (Oldman 2000). What is important is being able to choose whether to move or not. Brenton, in a study of older Dutch people who had chosen co-housing, refers to one resident who said: 'It is important to move to a place you chose before other people move you to a place they choose' (1998: 1). The worry is whether *Supporting People* is going to increase the ability to choose between staying in existing accommodation or moving to an alternative.

Housing and welfare: divergence or convergence?

I now want to return to the vignettes in order to show that, despite some positive developments, housing and community care policies remain largely divergent. There are two aspects to this. The first relates to organisational, service delivery issues, and the second to more fundamental, structural themes.

Vulnerable people do not compartmentalise their lives into housing problems, social care problems or health problems. What is of fundamental importance to the middle-aged man recovering from a major psychiatric illness in the first vignette, or the abused young person in the third, is how to get their lives back in order. All too often, however, assessments are fragmented, one for social care, one for health care and one, if at all, for housing need. Where it is identified, housing need is very narrowly defined in terms of physical things such as stair lifts, hoists or ramps. The importance of housing as home does not come into the assessment (Allen *et al.* 1998). In the fourth vignette, the disability affected the lives of all the family members. They needed more space but were moved to a small and cramped, although allegedly adapted, property on a hostile estate. The adaptations met neither the child's nor the parents' needs, partly because issues about housing as home had not been addressed. Housing and community care continue to diverge because of the fundamental problems of joint working between different agencies in the housing, health and social care sectors (Audit Commission 1998). Professionals continue to argue about what each should do and what each should pay for.

As well as these organisational or tactical issues, the vignettes illustrate more fundamental or structural divergences between housing and community care. Adequate investment in the nation's housing stock, including adequate investment in accessible housing, would render the current 'fire-fighting' type of services obsolete. The necessity for moves to specialist schemes or for the provision of unwanted, expensive and unattractive adaptations would be reduced. There have been changes in the right direction. For example, from 1999, all new domestic dwellings in any tenure have had to comply with Part M of the building regulations, which require all properties to meet some, albeit basic, accessibility standards. In addition to problems of inadequate investment, the country's housing finance system also hinders the successful implementation of community care: in order to protect low income or vulnerable households and to minimise work disincentives, cutbacks in assistance with housing costs must be contained.

In this chapter, I have attempted to show that policies which acknowledge the importance of housing and home need to be part of welfare or community care programmes. If they are not, the effectiveness of the latter is undermined. Current developments are welcome but do not represent a fundamental 'sea change' in how housing and community care policies treat vulnerable people. 'Independent living' is a mantra rather than a reality, and housing and community care continue to diverge both for organisational and structural reasons. Joint working between housing, health and social care agencies works imperfectly. What is needed for housing and community policies to come together is recognition of the current inadequacy of investment in appropriate and affordable housing.

REFERENCES

Allen, C. (1997) The policy and implementation of the housing role of community care: a constructionist theoretical perspective, *Housing Studies*, 12(1): 85–110.

Allen, C., Clapham, D., Franklin, B. and Parker, J. (1998) *The Right Home? Assessing Housing Need in Community Care*. Cardiff: Centre for Housing Management and Development, Cardiff University.

Anchor Trust (1998) *Killer Homes: Facing up to Poor Housing as a Cause of Older People's Ill Health*. Oxford: Anchor Trust.

Anderson, I. and Sim, D. (eds) (2000) *Social Exclusion and Housing: Context and Challenges*. London: Chartered Institute of Housing.

Audit Commission (1998) *Home Alone: the Role of Housing in Community Care*. London: Audit Commission.

Benjamin, D. and Stea, D. (eds) (1995) *The Home: Words, Interpretations, Meanings and Environments*. Aldershot: Avebury.

Brenton, M. (1998) *Co-Housing Communities of Older People in the Netherlands: Lessons for Britain?* Bristol: The Policy Press.

Clapham, D. (1997) Problems and potential of sheltered housing, *Ageing and Society*, 17(2): 209–14.

Clapham, D. and Smith, S. (1990) Housing policy and special needs, *Policy and Politics*, 18(3): 193–206.

Department of the Environment, Transport and the Regions (2000) *Quality and Choice: a Decent Home for All*. London: DETR.

Department of the Environment, Transport and the Regions (2001) *Supporting People: Policy into Practice*. London: London: DETR.

Evandrou, M. (1997) *Baby Boomers: Ageing in the 21st Century*. London: Age Concern.

Griffiths, S. (2000) *Supporting People All the Way: an Overview of the Supporting People Programme*. York: York Publishing Services.

Harrison, L. and Heywood, F. (2000) *Health Begins at Home: Planning at the Health–Housing Interface for Older People*. Bristol: Policy Press.

Holmans, A. (1999) British housing in the twentieth century: an end of the century review, in Wilcox, S. (ed.) *Housing Finance Review 1999/2000*. London: Chartered Institute of Housing and Council of Mortgage Lenders.

Hughes, D. and Lowe, S. (1995) *Social Housing Law and Policy*. London: Butterworths.

Law, I. (1996) *Racism, Ethnicity and Social Policy*. London: Prentice Hall.

Leather, P. and Morrison, P. (1997) *The State of UK Housing*. Bristol: The Policy Press.

Mason, D. (2000) *Race and Ethnicity in Modern Britain.* 2nd edn. Oxford: OUP.

Nettleton, S. and Burrows, R. (1998) Mortgage debt, housing insecurity and health, in M. Bartley, D. Blane, and G. Davey Smith (eds) *The Sociology of Health Inequalities.* Oxford: Blackwells.

Oldman, C. (2000) *Blurring the Boundaries: a Fresh Look at Housing and Care Provision for Older People.* Brighton: Pavilion Press.

Perry, J. (2000) The end of council housing, *Housing Finance Review 2000/2001.* London: Chartered Institute of Housing and the Council of Mortgage Lenders.

Royal Institute of Chartered Surveyors (1997) *The Real Costs of Poor Housing.* Coventry: Royal Institute of Charted Surveyors.

Saunders, P. (1990) *A Nation of Home Owners.* London, Unwin and Hyman.

Watson, L. and Cooper, R. (1992) *Housing with Care: Supported Housing and Housing Associations.* York: Joseph Rowntree Foundation.

Wilcox, S. (2000) *Housing Finance Review 2000/2001.* London: Chartered Institute of Housing and the Council Mortgage Lenders.

Wilcox, S. and Burrows, R. (2000) *Half the Poor: Home Owners with Low Incomes.* London: Council of Mortgage Lenders.

CHAPTER 38

PARTNERSHIPS BETWEEN DISABLED PEOPLE AND SERVICE PROVIDERS

Frances Hasler

Background

Direct payments are a relatively new way of meeting social care needs. Although some pilot schemes date back to the mid-1980s, the Direct Payments Act did not come into effect until 1997. They offer new possibilities for partnership between disabled people and their local authorities, both on the individual level and collectively through their organisations.

The Community Care (Direct Payments) Act 1996 gives local authorities the power to offer disabled people a cash payment in lieu of a service. Direct payments allow disabled people independence: they can arrange support in ways that suit them. The disabled people's movement had campaigned for direct payments as a means to independent living. More recently, direct payments have been extended to carers, to parents of disabled children and to disabled sixteen and seventeen year olds.[1]

Partnership at the individual level

Direct payments alter the relationship between disabled people and their local authority. Government guidance on direct payments[2] suggests that they need to be introduced in a spirit of partnership and spells out how the partnership should work:

> *Local authorities should seek to leave as much choice as possible in the hands of the individual.*

This means the local authority has to ensure that information and support are available. They have to trust the user. The user has to contribute time, planning, and responsibility. In many local authorities it is being implemented. In some we are finding rules that seek to hedge the user's choice with conditions, rather than encouraging them to take full responsibility.

Guidance says that direct payments should:

> *allow people to address their own needs in innovative ways,*

but it does not allow local authorities to give up responsibility for a disabled person. They still have to satisfy themselves:

> *that the person's assessed needs are being met.*

How well these objectives are balanced is a good test of partnership:

> *The greater ownership the user has of the process by which his or her needs are assessed, and by which the decision is reached on the areas for which a direct payment will be made, the more likely it is that direct payments will be a success.*

All good in theory. How does it work in practice? The biggest problems in making this work in reality is the gap between disabled people's ideas on their needs and the local authority assessment of their needs. At the National Centre for Independent Living (NCIL) we have been told that 'care managers are reluctant to look holistically at need, for fear of raising expectations'.[3] Disabled people do not feel trusted to set their own priorities. Nor do they feel trusted about how they arrange their support:

> *The disempowering thing is that the system has to justify where the money is going and so we have to constantly account for our needs. It's as if they didn't quite trust you and give you something with a bad grace.*[4]

So partnership does not feel equal. One side has the power to decide what need is, to set the level at which need will be met and to operate the sanction of removing payments if they feel needs are being met inappropriately.

The other side has the power to use the local authority complaints process if they are unhappy with the process. Not a very equal start!

There is a problem with a rhetoric of partnership that does not recognise this huge imbalance. Although individual social workers may not feel they have a huge amount of power, they represent a large and powerful organisation, that literally can decide whether a person gets the resources to lead an independent life or not. Disabled people look to social workers to provide more and better information on what social services *can* provide, not just on what they must provide. To advocate for themselves, disabled people need true partnership, a generosity with information on behalf of social service staff.

Partnership at the organisational level

Direct payments often involve disabled people taking on responsibility for staff. To do this they need advice and sometimes training. So local authorities are encouraged to set up support schemes. Many of these schemes are run by disabled people's organisations.

> *Local authorities need to satisfy themselves that the scheme they develop serves all adult client groups equitably.*

It is a sad comment on some local authority practice that this part of the guidance was needed. Direct payments provide a huge potential for social inclusion. It is vital that all disabled people, whatever their ethnic origin or their impairment or their age, get a chance to explore this option. But prejudice and complacency were stopping this happening in some areas: prejudice against giving people with learning difficulties control over their lives; complacency that people from minority ethnic communities 'didn't want' independent living; lack of organisation to get information translated or put in new formats.

Partnership working is not easy. It requires creativity and tenacity. Disabled people need to learn huge amounts about the infrastructure of bureaucracies. Professionals need to learn new ways of communicating, that do not rely on a shared shorthand of jargon. At the most basic level, professionals have to learn to deal with the access barriers that disabled people face every day. For example this means ensuring that when meetings take place such things as wheelchair access, induction loops, sign language interpreters, support workers, audio taped and picture format information are all provided. In a few local authorities these things are now taken for granted. The fact that they are not readily supplied in *all* local authorities is a sign of how excluded disabled people have been in the past.

Disabled people bring so many different sorts of experience to the table. Finding a way to bring all sorts of people into your partnership means developing advanced communication skills, and ensuring that your practice does not inadvertently exclude. Getting the meetings right is just a start. Long experience of exclusion makes it hard for users to meet professionals on an equal basis. But, as in society at large, not all users are equal. Older people, users from minority ethnic communities, people without speech, can all find themselves excluded even within disability groups. Ensuring that partnership can be a reality for them involves targeted work, on a sustained basis.

Partnership fits within other policy objectives, such as best value. Authorities must ensure that:

> *public funds are being spent appropriately and with best value.*

However, guidance does not encourage a narrow view of value:

> *People with direct payments who have been involved with setting up their local scheme often act as advocates for and mentors of those who follow. This aids the rapid expansion of the scheme and ensures that an authority's investment in start-up costs provides good value for money.*

A real partnership between a local disabled people's organisation and the local authority can pay dividends. But we are still finding authorities that are reluctant to invest in this way, unable to make the culture shift involved in seeing disabled people as partners.

> *Partnership is a scary concept – it requires collaboration. In existing schemes disabled people do not actually have the lead. One lot of people (the local authority) have the authority and the power. For example – there is no budget for meetings for disabled people to get together. We need to talk about the power issue.*[5]

Even where the authority funds a scheme, it is often small scale and short term. The National Centre for Independent Living has been carrying out a research project on Centres for Independent Living. When we surveyed them recently an alarming number did not have sufficient funds for this financial year and had no idea where next year's money was coming from.

This is not partnership, if one party to the agreement is perpetually unable to plan, always living from hand to mouth.[6]

We also need partnership to achieve equity. Some local disability groups do not currently include people with mental health problems, for example. A local authority taking a partnership approach could help them to make the necessary contacts. Too often, authorities just dismiss a group for not being inclusive, rather than thinking how they can work together to promote inclusion.

[...]

Examples of good partnership

Partnership needs to involve mutual respect and trust, both at the level of individual assessments and in the relationships between organisations. An example is the Hampshire direct payments website, developed as a joint project by Hampshire Social Services in partnership with Southampton Centre for Independent Living (CIL) and Hampshire CIL. Technical know-how for the site came from the council, with content being devised by the CILs.[7]

Partnership needs to be nurtured and reinforced. At a joint direct payments conference in 2000 between Cheshire Social Services and Cheshire Disabilities Federation, the fact that the chair was a disabled person from the Federation, and the keynote speaker was the Director of Social Services underlined to all present that this was a real partnership. This was important, to help convince some frankly sceptical delegates, who had more fears than hopes about direct payments.

Partnership needs to be based on equity. For this reason the National Centre for Independent Living is working in partnership with REU (a race equality research organisation) to bring together disabled people's organisations and black community organisations, in order to learn from each other and thus to increase the opportunities available to black and minority ethnic disabled people. This recognises that, at present, black disabled people have unequal access to independent living options,[8] and seeks a mutually supportive way forward.

Partnership needs to be resourced. The partnership between West Sussex County Council and Scope to set up a direct payments support scheme includes a regular review of workload and a planned increase in staffing as user numbers increase. This scheme is now developing into a three-way partnership, as users are encouraged to take a greater part in running the scheme.

Partnership and power – examples from previous projects

More ambitious than the examples above was the Wiltshire Users' Forum scheme (pre-dating the Direct Payments Act) where the whole budget for independent living packages was devolved to a user-led group, and decisions on allocation were made by the group.[9]

A similar example in the voluntary sector was the Haringey On Call Support Scheme, where decisions on using local independent living funds from a research project were devolved to the user group. The project recruited a number of workers to act as 'on call' personal assistants, to supplement the usual support available to disabled people in the borough. Users were recruited to an advisory group that developed into a management group as the project progressed.

The open ended nature of the service was hard for some users to grasp at first. The fact that they could use their allocated hours of assistance for any activity they chose was a novelty for many. They were accustomed to local authority services, where staff could only carry out the tasks specified in the care plan.

The advisory group began with an idea that each person would have the same allocation of hours of assistance. But they quickly realised that different amounts were more equitable. Some had bigger support needs, such as night time assistance. A few could not 'budget' their hours as effectively as others. Some assessed their own needs as less than the suggested allocation. They decided that a 'pool' of spare hours should be available, to help those who ran out of their basic allocation. This turned out to be a good way of managing a shared resource. Users were able to make very mature decisions about relative need, free from the usual community care assessment framework.

Where the users had more difficulties was in negotiating a pay package for the on-call workers. The research team did not support the decisions to enhance the pay package, pointing out that this would make the unit cost of the service far higher than other comparable services. Users argued that other services suffered from the effects of paying low wages, with high turnover and poor motivation amongst staff. The users saw their ability to improve conditions for their workforce as proof that the project was a true partnership, with real control given to them. If the research team had insisted on maintaining control of rates of pay for on-call workers, the spirit of the project would have been lost. This was a testing time for the partnership between project team and users. It illustrates that partnership often involves one party giving up some power. In this case the project team, who held the purse strings, had to give up influence over wage rates, in the interests of empowering users to make management decisions.

This project, unlike the one in West Sussex, never became a three-way partnership, because the local authority never embraced the ethos of a user-led service. The overview report of the project notes that:

> *while the transition to a completely user-led service was experienced as a very positive and logical outcome by those closely involved, it did distance the project from local professional agencies, notably the Social Services Department.*[10]

Nonetheless, both it and the Wiltshire scheme are proof that users can rise to the challenge of a true partnership where it is offered.

Partnerships thwarted

The good experiences outlined above are not universal. In one London borough, a disabled people's organisation pioneered support for personal assistance users. They successfully provided a user-led service for ten years, developing a strong equalities ethos. But the introduction of tendering for the service (in the name of best value) led to them being undercut by an agency from another borough. No sense of partnership prevailed there.

There are also numerous examples of direct payments schemes that are still run from inside the local authority rather than being developed in disabled people's organisations.

> *An authority can be very politically correct about disabled people – yet still reluctant to hand over control.*[11]

Blocks to partnership

There are some fundamental blocks to partnership between disabled people and service providers. Each is linked. First is a social care system that is based on the notion that disabled people are vulnerable and incapable. Linked to this is a general (sometimes unspoken, occasionally explicit) consensus that people need social care because they are vulnerable and incapable. Finally, a social care and education system that schools disabled people into how to be good clients, rather than how to be active, assertive citizens, leaves them ill-equipped to take on real partnerships.[12]

The social care system is not conducive to independent living. It is based on an expert assessing your need and deciding how that need should be met. Recent guidance stresses the need to consult and involve the user, but this is not backed up with any guidance suggesting that users' own assessment of their needs should be given credence. The idea prevails that there is some 'objective' process of deciding on need. Straight away, users are being defined as the unequal partner. Their views are always less valid than that of the 'expert'.

More pernicious is the view that social care has to be decided and arranged for the user because he or she is incapable of doing this for her or himself. This view is particularly prevalent in mental health and learning disability services. Voluntary groups such as Values Into Action have been challenging this view, promoting models of assisted decision-making and the use of advocates to support independent living.[13]

The construction of disabled people as vulnerable and incapable underpins the entire charity approach to disability in this country (think, for example, of some advertising by charities) and also informs most social care. It is not surprising, therefore, that practitioners in social care have difficulty in seeing disabled people as true partners. The experience of disabled people working in social work departments and health authorities often bears this out. Crossing the line between client and colleague can make some of your colleagues very uncomfortable.

The traditional model of social care acts to ensure that disabled people cannot become true partners, by disempowering them at all turns. To get welfare benefits you have to emphasise your incapacity. To get services you have to emphasise your functional needs not your ambitions, hopes or strengths. Despite the growth of independent living schemes most social care is still provided in institutional ways – either in residential and day care or by home care workers 'doing to' disabled people. This all serves to reinforce feelings of dependency, and to de-skill disabled people.

Direct payments

Despite the problems outlined earlier, direct payments represent a very real move forward in the partnership between disabled people and service providers. At the individual level, they fundamentally alter the relationship. The disabled person is in control of the 'service' because she or he is hiring (and if need be, firing) the workers who provide it. She can set the job tasks, the times and manner in which they are carried out. Disabled people need their personal assistants, so there are limits to the power they exercise in the 'partnership', but they are the stronger partner in many respects, because they are the purchaser.

At a more general level, direct payments enable disabled people to use their social care to do different things. Going out with your personal assistant, to a meeting, to a shop, to your friend's house or your child's school, is a long way removed from going to the day centre. All are 'day time activity' in care plan terms. But in using direct payments the disabled person has changed the role of social services from a provider to an enabler and thus changed the relationship too.

Conclusion

Relationships between disabled people and the local state are never going to be fully equal. The notion of partnership is an expression of an ideal, influencing the style of the relationship. But some smaller scale experiments in allowing disabled people to manage general, as well as personal budgets (for example Wiltshire and Haringey) have shown that partnership can be more than a buzz word.

Direct payments in the UK came about because some disabled people had a good idea: they thought they could make better use of the money that was being spent on keeping them in residential care, if they were allowed to use it to hire their own assistants in the community. Some local authority staff were prepared to take a leap of faith and back the idea.[14] At that stage, the partnerships were very informal, based on personal contact. As direct payments have developed to the point where they are a mainstream community care option (local authorities are required to provide them), the partnerships have become more formalised. Service level agreements, 'contracts' between authority and user and close monitoring of spending, have all arrived. The partnership is, in effect, controlled by the local authority. Perhaps the future challenge is rediscovering the simple partnerships of the early days of direct payments.

One of the pioneers of direct payments in the UK sums it up thus:

> We dreamed a dream ... Our dream was that disabled people would be enabled to fulfil their roles in terms of taking the opportunities society offers and meeting the responsibilities society requires ... The dream was to do with being enabled to be an active citizen at work, rest and play. The fact of the matter is this is not available because nobody else is enabled to achieve these ends through social welfare provision.[15]

Disabled people are interested in partnerships because we are still dreaming that dream.

NOTES

1. Carers and Disabled Children Act, 2000 (HMSO). Also see www.carers.gov.uk.
2. *The Community Care (Direct Payments) Act Policy Guidance and Practice Guidance*, Department of Health, 1999.

3. Contributor to focus group, April 1998, part of the Implementation of Direct Payments project. Outcomes published as *Direct Routes to Independence*, Hasler, Campbell and Zarb, PSI, 1999.
4. Quote from *Cashing in on Independence*, Zarb and Nadash, BCODP, 1993.
5. Contributor to focus group (as note 3).
6. *Creating Independent Futures*, Stage One report, University of Leeds, 2000.
7. www.hampshire.gov.uk/socservs/directpayments.
8. *Double Invisibility*, Banton and Hirsch, Council of Disabled People Warwickshire 2000.
9. Evans, C. Disability, discrimination and local authority social services: the user perspective, in *Community Care: A Reader*, 2nd edition, J. Bornat, J.S. Johnson, C. Pereira, D. Pilgrim and F. Williams (eds), London: Macmillan, 1997.
10. *Community Care Projects*, Report to the King's Fund, Judith Unell, 1994.
11. Contributor to focus group, April 1998 (as note 3).
12. 'The Crafting of Good Clients', Ken Davis in *Disabling Barriers: Enabling Environments*, Swain, Finkelstein, French and Oliver (eds), Sage/OU, 1993.
13. *Choice and Control – decision making and people with learning difficulties*, Bewley, Values into Action, 1998.
14. Philip Mason, quoted in *Shaping Our Futures* report, NCIL/HCIL, 1998.
15. As note 14.

CHAPTER 39

CARE AS A COMMODITY

Clare Ungerson

Since the nineteenth century and well into the second half of the twentieth century, there has been a clear distinction in industrialised societies between 'unpaid' and 'paid' work. Similarly there have been well-laid boundaries between public and private domains of life. Despite this there have always been strong similarities between 'unpaid' and 'paid' work and the feminist literature on care has been extremely important in delineating this (Thomas 1993). It has also outlined the way in which the demands and exigencies of unpaid work impact on opportunities for (and status within) paid work, particularly for women (Joshi 1992).

In this chapter, I argue that the dualism of 'paid' and 'unpaid' work is dissolving, and that we are moving into a period where the boundaries between public and private domains are beginning to crumble. Nowhere is this more obvious than in the policy area of care for people with disabilities. To date, much of this has been delivered by kin, neighbours and friends. Usually it has been named 'informal' care and assumed to be provided without payment. There is evidence now, however, from both Europe and North America, of a search within the welfare state for ways of *underwriting* the provision of care within households and kin networks. Many of these ideas entail cash subvention both to carers and to care-recipients and one consequence of this, I argue, is the *commodification* of care. By this I mean that the type of care which is delivered is increasingly being paid for, either directly or indirectly by the state, and/or by the care user. Anything that is delivered and paid for is a commodity. This is what care is becoming. In this chapter, I draw on literature and research that has been reviewed in more detail in Ungerson (1997).

This development raises issues of explanation and of evaluation. Why is informal care increasingly commodified? Is it likely to increase the supply of carers? Will it improve the care relationship? And is this commodification in the interests of carers, particularly women carers?

A typology of payments for care

Cross-nationally, the ways in which care is being commodified are manifold. It is important to devise a typology that makes some generalisable sense of the policies that are in place. There are five types of payment:

1. *Carer allowances*, paid through social security and tax systems
2. *'Proper' wages*, paid by the state or state agencies
3. *Routed wages*, paid directly to care users (e.g. 'direct payments')
4. *Symbolic payments*, paid by care users to kin, neighbours and friends
5. *Paid volunteering*, paid by voluntary organisations and local authorities to volunteers.

This typology is a route to understanding the way in which cash impinges on and structures the care relationship. Clearly each one of these types of payment, when it enters the caring household or caring relationship, gives rise to different kinds of working conditions. Moreover, these are not discrete categories – within particular countries, they can and do overlap.

Carer allowances

These are benefits for carers that are paid through either tax or social security systems. They are often construed as recompensing carers of working age for not being able to take up paid work as a result of the exigencies of the unpaid work of care. The British Invalid Care Allowance (ICA) dating from 1977 and extended to married women in 1988, is an example. It is a non-contributory benefit within the National Insurance Scheme, that is payable only to carers of 'working age'. In the United States, the Federal Dependent Tax Care Credit (a rather small amount) is similarly available to taxpayers who are normally in paid work. Since the 1980s, carers of severely disabled and chronically ill children in Denmark have been able to claim, under the Social Assistance Act, a care allowance equivalent to the 'normal earnings' that have been foregone by the carer. Further financial provision for Danish carers of seriously ill children and of terminally ill adults was made in 1990. The payments to carers who care for the terminally ill are the same as are paid to conventionally employed home helps. In Ireland, the means-tested Carers Allowance (introduced in 1990 and replacing a previous, very restricted 'Prescribed Relatives Allowance') is somewhat different. Barely covering subsistence costs, it is seen primarily as a way of encouraging the long-term replacement of residential care by informal and family care, rather than as a compensation to carers for giving up paid work (McLaughlin 1994).

What is so fascinating about these social security and tax-related carer allowances is that they are payable to 'carers' who do not have to demonstrate that they are actually caring. It is normally sufficient to demonstrate a relationship (relational or geographical proximity) to someone who is able to produce documentary evidence of a need for care, something that is usually assessed on a medical basis. These carer allowances are, essentially, citizenship-based rights to income for carers: they are funded on the basis that the risks of becoming a carer should be pooled, and that there is a collective responsibility to alleviate at least some of the income needs of carers.

'Proper' wages

There are nations such as Denmark which pay 'carer allowances' which are equivalent to the wages that carers could otherwise earn. But there are also systems of payments for care which are based on the direct employment of carers by the state. Such arrangements, commonly available to relatives, exist, and have done for sometime, in Sweden and Norway. Such wages are usually set at the prevailing wage for home helps paid by the municipalities. Thus, in these situations it is possible for carers to become state employees, often with similar contractual employment and social security rights to those of more 'formal' carers who work within the collectivised personal social services. In this case, however, the care work actually takes place within a one-to-one setting of intimacy and an established biography between carer and care-recipient. Related as these systems are to prevailing wage rates for care work, and in countries where there is minimum wage legislation which applies, such 'proper wage' systems are very expensive. After all, they constitute a full-blown version of 'wages for housework'. There is some evidence that these systems are in decline, particularly in Sweden (Ungerson 1995), but it is noticeable that the 1998 Danish Social Services Act has recently introduced similar provision in 'exceptional circumstances' (Glendinning, Chapter 34 in this volume).

Routed wages

These are the systems where care users are given the means to employ care-givers directly in an employer/employee relationship. Many of these schemes seem to take their cue from early direct payment schemes developed in the United States for disabled veterans of the Second World War. As Keigher and Stone (1994) state, 'veterans are free to purchase necessary services from professional providers, pay a relative or friend for help, use the money for living expenses, or anything else they choose'.

These patterns of consumer autonomy which allow care users to purchase their own services, including the direct employment of care assistants, are now being widely copied in Europe. Italy has had 'Companion Payments' at least since the 1980s, payable to the care-recipient but expected to be spent on the purchase of care, and the level of it (about £75 a week) is high enough to do so. In 1990 there were 1.1 million recipients of this benefit (Glendinning and Millar 1992). Also in the 1980s, Denmark introduced allowances to care-recipients to pay for 24-hour assistance which they can use to pay relatives. These allowances can reach the astonishing figure of £50,000 per year per person. In France, 'decarceration' policies were introduced in 1975, and these included two benefits, one for those aged sixty-five or more and one for those aged less. Although payable to care-recipients, these were expected to be handed over to care-givers. In 1996, France developed a voucher scheme and tax breaks to care-recipients which they have to spend on the employment of personal assistants recruited from neighbourhood and kin networks (so-called *emplois de proximite*). This is a policy not so much to resolve a problem of care, but rather designed, at one and the same time, to increase the absolute number of jobs during a period of high unemployment, and also to formalise and regulate paid work previously located in the invisible grey economy. Austria has converted its entire care system to high cash payments to care recipients in the expectation that they will purchase their own care. In Britain, the Community Care (Direct Payments) Act, 1996, introduced the option for disabled people under sixty-five to go for cash rather than services, and the expectation is that they will use the cash to purchase personal assistance. Since 2000, this has been extended to older age groups and to carers and young disabled people under the Carers and Disabled Children Act, 2000.

These developments constitute the sharp end of commodified care and marketised intimacy. The state, in effect, has underwritten a employer/employee relationship within the care dyad. This is, at least for European welfare states, a radical innovation in care delivery, apparently reversing the professional and bureaucratic control of health and social care that has developed since the Second World War.

Symbolic payments

These kinds of payment are the least visible of all payments for care and, hence, there is the least documentation of them. However, in an empirical and longitudinal study of stroke patients and their carers (Baldock and Ungerson 1994), many households containing a disabled person mistakenly understood the benefits they received to be a form of 'direct payment'.

In Britain, well over a million disabled people receive such benefits and if only a substantial minority use them to pay their carers, then this benefit still constitutes an important flow of money. These cash transfers are unregulated and informal and they fudge the boundaries between the two rationalities of gift and market. They therefore constitute arrangements that are not strictly contractual, although they can be brought to an end – with difficulty and embarrassment – if the participants are unhappy with caring aspects of their extant relationship.

Paid volunteering

This form of paid care-work is probably unique to Britain. 'Paid volunteering' involves contracting caring labour from strangers to work in the private domain, and paying them symbolic payments rather than 'proper wages'. In Britain there are now numerous schemes, organised by voluntary organisations and local authorities, which recruit 'volunteers' to undertake care-work for someone in their neighbourhood and which then 'cement' the contract through symbolic payments. The payments can range from £1.00 a visit (and there may be as many as four visits contracted per day) to a limited amount of money per week. Many of these schemes seem to be deliberately targeted at the recruitment of women 'volunteers', women who are seeking small additional incomes which neither push them into compulsory social security contribution bands nor take them above social security benefit earnings disregards (Baldock and Ungerson 1991). Although these paid volunteering schemes are sometimes said to cover expenses rather than represent any emolument for the actual work undertaken, they tend to pay standard amounts and over the odds.

It is likely that such schemes will expand, particularly in countries with high unemployment: 'workfare' schemes, which make social assistance for the unemployed contingent on taking up paid work, may well spread from the United States and be used, in conjunction with voluntary organisations, to provide a reliable supply of symbolically paid 'voluntary' care-workers. Whether these schemes remain as gendered as 'paid volunteering' currently is remains to be seen.

Reasons for these developments

It should be clear by now that arrangements for paying carers vary from nation to nation. The research into why developments have taken a particular turn in any particular nation has not yet been undertaken, so explanations of these variations in emphasis are somewhat speculative. In the discussion that follows, I identify the basic parameters of their political contexts.

'Carer allowances' and 'proper wages' appear to be a feature of the countries of Northern Europe. The Scandinavian arrangements arguably follow from a long-standing view of the welfare state as the 'people's home' where care has become more integrated into concepts of citizenship. It is also possible to argue, however, that payments to carers reflect a concern of policy makers with a growing 'care deficit' and that this feature applies to all the developed nations in the 1990s. Certainly policies of decarceration are converging (Baldock and Evers 1992) while, at the same time, features of marriage breakdown, geographical mobility and women's participation in the labour market, mean that traditional concepts of gendered kinship obligation are likely to loosen considerably. In this situation, in order to maintain an adequate supply of care, the temptation for governments to reinforce care responsibilities through payments to informal carers is likely to be great.

Carers themselves are acquiring political leverage. In Britain, associations of carers act directly on the political agenda, driving the point home that carers should be supported by recognition, services and income. In addition, there is a feminist politics that argues that citizenship is an essentially masculinised concept of the public domain and that, in order to underwrite women's citizenship, it is vital that welfare states recognise unpaid work that takes place within the household (Fraser 1994).

Concerns about the supply of informal care also feed the development of symbolic payments and paid volunteering. A particular feature of these types of payment is that, through implicit and explicit contract, they are designed to maintain the continuity and reliability of care (Ungerson 1994). Symbolic payments, particularly where they occur between kin and neighbours, also have reciprocity at their heart. The wider political context of this is the cross-national development of service delivery based on the 'mixed economy of welfare'. Here, the idea is that multiple welfare partners, including the voluntary and informal sectors of care delivery are managed by public sector brokers of care (Baldock 1993). These are often part and parcel of a withdrawal of public provision and the development of charged-for and for-profit systems of delivering care. Where prices for care are highly visible and informal care is part of the care delivery system, users of care become increasingly aware that the services they receive from their kin and neighbours have a value attached to them. Hence one can expect both these types of payment to develop further within a marketising and commodifying system of care delivery.

Payments to care users that lead to 'routed wages' have another set of politics and political actors. To date the major actors have been disabled people making claims for payments to underwrite 'independent living'. Their voices have been echoed and supported by the new right, who argue that direct payments to care users promote the key objectives of choice and efficiency which, it argues, are uniquely available through the operation of free markets. Clearly the power of these political actors is variable: in

2001, the new right appears to be in decline in Europe (although their legacy of marketised services holds firm) while the views of disabled people have only recently moved centre stage. 'Routed wages' may also have a political context which has less to do with the management of care and more to do with the control of unemployment. In France *emplois de proximite*, a system of local domestic and care services funded through managed vouchers given to care users, has been put in place. This may be adopted by other European countries seeking to shift the unregulated, cash-based, informal economy into formal recognition and control.

Predicting the impact of payments

There are four streams of literature that predict that payments for care may transform important aspects of post-industrial society. The first two streams come from the new right arguing for cash rather than services for users in order to develop more efficient markets for care, and from the disability lobbies arguing for the same policy but specifically to empower an oppressed minority (Morris 1993). Both have been discussed above as part of a politics of payments for care that is already 'in place'. Both these streams of thought make large claims for the impact of redirected cash flows, suggesting that cash has enough potential power to chip away at, if not topple, economic and cultural oppressions, and the professionalisation, medicalisation and bureaucratisation of social and personal life.

The third stream is a feminist analysis of social policy in which the discussion of payments for care takes place within the context of a larger debate about how to establish women's rights to citizenship. Nancy Fraser, the American feminist political theorist, has suggested that a new world of economic production and social reproduction is emerging where we should ask what new, postindustrial gender order should replace the family wage. She suggests that two models qualify as feminist: the 'Universal Breadwinner' model fosters gender equity by promoting women's employment in paid work. The 'Caregiver Parity' model aims to promote gender equity by supporting informal care, largely through state provision of carer allowances (Fraser 1994). However, other feminists have been quick to point up the difficulties of developing the latter model:

> *we are torn between wanting to validate and support, through some form of income maintenance provision, the caring work for which women still take the main responsibility in the 'private' sphere and to liberate them from this responsibility so that they can achieve economic and political autonomy in the 'public' sphere.*
>
> *(Lister 1994: 19)*

It is perhaps because of this conundrum that so many feminists write articles with 'dilemma' in the title. Be that as it may, in considering the delivery of care, any policy discussion as to whether or not carers should be
paid has to take on board this wider debate about the appropriate route to
women's full citizenship and whether women, as a category, should be
treated as different from men because they have caring responsibilities.

The fourth stream of thought, like the first and second, is far less
equivocal about the merits of payments for care. This is the 'welfare plu-
ralist' argument of, in particular, the German policy analyst, Adelbert
Evers. He suggests that a policy of 'payments for care', paid primarily to
care users but also to care givers, leads towards a new middle ground, that
stands between the polarities of state, family, and market. Lying between
the land of consumerist individualism on the one hand, and service-orien-
tated collectivism on the other, there is this middle ground of solidarity
and community which can be rediscovered through the commodification
of the care relationship. Thus Evers argues that payments to care users:

> strengthen those economies of care which are easily overlooked in the
> consumerist model ... these care services work through trust and
> unwritten rules quite different from the 'easy in / easy out' norms and
> values of larger commercial suppliers.
>
> (Evers 1994)

Such arguments are concerned neither with questions of power nor with
issues of citizenship, but rather with issues of cooperation and social cohe-
sion. As with the other three streams of thought, the argument makes
major claims for the transformative powers of payments for care.

Arguments such as these are pitched at a very high level of generality. In
my view, they lead to oversimplified claims for the power of cash to transform social relationships in a single and particular direction. It seems to
me that the social, political and economic contexts in which payments for
care operate, and the way in which payments for care are themselves
organised, are just as likely to transform relationships as the existence of
the payments themselves. One of the particularities left undiscussed in
these streams of thought is the level of payment, whether to user or carer:
whether they are talking about symbolic amounts, or amounts high
enough to guarantee financial independence for the care recipient and care
giver. The actual amounts of money involved will radically affect the
labour market behaviour of potential carers, their relationship to the state
and the household and, last but not least, they may have real impact on
the prevailing sexual division of caring. It will also affect the types of care
relationships that both users and carers can afford to enter, and the mixes
of time, personnel, sources of income and location of care, that carers and

care-recipients would have to put together. Similarly, with the exception of the disability lobby, no thought has been given to how such payments would flow, and whether and how the way in which the flow is organised would affect the location of power and decision-making within and beyond the caring relationship.

In my view, these kinds of detailed empirical questions have to be asked and answered before we can come to any conclusions as to whether or not commodified care will benefit women carers and care recipients, and whether it will ameliorate problems resulting from the 'care deficit'.

REFERENCES

Baldock, J. 1993. 'Patterns of change in the delivery of welfare in Europe', in *Markets and Managers: New Issues in the Delivery of Welfare*, P. Taylor Gooby and R. Lawson (eds). Buckingham: Open University Press, 24–37.

Baldock, J. and Evers, A. 1992. 'Innovations and care of the elderly: the cutting edge of change for social welfare systems. Examples from Sweden, the Netherlands and the United Kingdom'. *Ageing and Society*, 12, 3, 289–312.

Baldock, J. and Ungerson, C. 1991. 'What d'ya want if you don't want money?', – a feminist critique of paid volunteering, in *Women's Issues in Social Policy*, M. Maclean and D. Groves (eds). London: Routledge.

Baldock, J. and Ungerson, C. 1994. *Becoming Consumers of Community Care*. York: Joseph Rowntree Foundation.

Evers, A. 1994. 'Payments for care: a small but significant part of a wider debate', pp. 19–41 in *Payments for Care: A Comparative Overview*, A. Evers, M. Pijl and C. Ungerson, (eds). Aldershot: Avebury.

Fraser, N. 1994. 'After the Family Wage: Gender Equity and the Welfare State'. *Political Theory* 22, 4, 591–618.

Glendinning, C. and Millar, J. (eds) 1992. *Women and Poverty in Britain: the 1990s*. Hemel Hempstead: Harvester Wheatsheaf.

Joshi, H. 1992. 'The Cost of Caring'. In *Women and Poverty in Britain: the 1990s*, C. Glendinning and J. Millar, eds. Hemel Hempstead: Harvester Wheatsheaf.

Keigher, S. and R. Stone. 1994. 'United States of America', pp. 321–45 in *Payments for Care: A Comparative Overview*, A. Evers, M. Pijl and C. Ungerson, eds. Aldershot: Avebury.

Lister, R. 1994. 'Dilemmas in Engendering Citizenship', paper presented at Crossing Borders Conference, University of Stockholm, Stockholm, May.

McLaughlin, E. 1994. 'Ireland', pp. 275–94 in *Payments for Care: A Comparative Overview*, A. Evers, M. Pijl and C. Ungerson, eds. Aldershot: Avebury.

Morris, J. 1993. *Independent Lives? Community Care and Disabled People*. London: Macmillan.

Thomas, C. 1993. 'De-constructing Concepts of Care'. *Sociology* 27, 3, 649–69.

Ungerson, C. 1995. 'Gender, Cash and Informal Care: European Perspectives and Dilemmas'. *Journal of Social Policy* 24, 1, 31–52.

Ungerson, C. 1997. 'Give Them the Money: Is Cash a Route to Empowerment?'. *Social Policy and Administration* 31, 1, 45–53.

■■■■■■■■

CHAPTER 40

GOOD COMPANIONS

40.1 WORKING AS A 'COUNTRY COUSIN'

Alice Kadel

A typical day with Odette

7.30 Arise and breakfast. Feed the dog Sara and let her out into the garden, then let her in and lock up again. Vacate the kitchen by 8.00 so Odette can breakfast quietly by herself. Make Odette's bed and wash through her overnight catheter bag. Shower and dress.

9.00 Take dog for a walk for about half an hour. The village is beautiful so this is usually a pleasure. Clean bathroom, kitchen, toilet as appropriate. (A cleaner comes once a week for more general cleaning.) Wash up and prepare lunch, usually soup or something quite simple. Odette has strong views on food and everything is usually strictly prescribed, except sometimes when she wants to be surprised! Dictatorial ways and boredom are evidently related. Fortunately what I do naturally she generally likes. Hand washing and machine washing clothes as required. At odd moments during the day I am knitting a cardigan for Odette in the colours she likes. Hopefully it will give some variation from the catalogue clothes she relies on.

11.00 Walk with Odette and dog around the village. These walks are crucial to Odette. She does not encourage visitors so the people she meets along the way are her social life. She used to go out alone but now does not feel safe, as she has pain in one leg from arthritis as well as general instability due to Parkinson's. She does not like her physical difficulties to be ignored, so quite a lot of our talk revolves around them.

12.00 Eat lunch, chat and wash up.

1.00 Usually I have free time now, walking on the downs with cattle, sheep, birds and butterflies. The sea sparkles in the distance, but it is too far to walk or bus there in the time available. Once or twice a week I walk into Lewes and run errands for Odette.

3.30 (later in summer) I walk with Odette and dog again. The talk at this time, and sometimes over tea, I find the hardest part of the day. I think it is because she wants to me to talk about what I have seen, while I am rather tired, and would rather keep my impressions to myself.

5.00 Make supper, again generally something fairly simple, but it can get complicated.

6.30–7.00 Wash up, and lay out breakfast things. Then free time: reading, knitting, phoning, watching television.

This is a very simple routine which I like. However, it can always be interrupted by Odette's health and state of mind, which can result in quite difficult negotiations with doctors, consultants and nurses, or with a variety of suppliers and services.

A short biography

Odette was born in 1920 in Paris. She is generally very well, and a good advertisement for all the health foods and supplements that she eats. She has plenty of money. She is divorced now, but was married three times. She gets some emotional support from the second of her husbands who lives not far away, and their son Andrew who is her only child. Andrew visits her about six times a year, always with his wife and children. She longs to see him on his own. Most clients have more substantial family links. It is perhaps partly because she is so good at looking after her own interests that she has cut down on these. She is highly manipulative, but often perceptive and amusing, even empathetic.

After a traumatic time as a young woman in occupied Paris, she has had a romantic and perhaps romanticised life story, which she un-fortunately stopped telling me since, she complains, I began to put on a little smile which she interprets as disbelief. I try not to do this, except perhaps in relation to her ideas on aliens. She belongs to a group convinced that aliens are walking around with us all the time, and she prays for them to come and take her with her little dog up to heaven in a spaceship. She also has more conventional religious ideas learnt from an English guru. The thing about Odette that I find most worrying is the way she treats her dog. Sara weighs two thirds more than she should, but Odette continues to feed her from the table four or five times a day. She is actively destroying what she says she loves and I wonder why this should be.

The agency

Odette is one of ten or more clients I have lived with since working for Country Cousins. This is an agency set up by a woman who came back to England from India around 1950, after Independence. She complained of boredom so her husband gave her £100. She set up an office to put nannies left stranded in postwar Britain in touch with onetime ladies of the Raj who found themselves suddenly servantless. It has outgrown these beginnings now, and is one of the larger agencies in the UK that supply freelance carers to clients 'unable to cope alone'.

The work involves going to live with someone two or three weeks at a time, doing whatever needs doing to keep things ticking over – shopping, cooking, cleaning, washing, ironing, visits, walks, care of pets and so on. There is usually a write-up of a typical day left by a previous carer to start things off. My category of work is known as Emergency Help (paid at £40 a day). It means that personal care is usually fairly minimal, but it can reach quite substantial proportions. Some clients want and demand a lot of companionship, others very little. Some encourage you to take time off in the afternoons, others hate it.

Clients' personalities, mental states, homes and families are infinitely various. It is the great strength of this work, and I imagine the client remaining in their own home fosters it. Almost always there is substantial family support which means, among many other things, that clients can call on help to get rid of 'the carer from hell' that most have experienced at some time. Generally clients invite carers they like to return again and again.

I began doing this work in 1997, aged fifty-seven, mostly because I wanted to get away from home for some time. A lot of the time I have enjoyed it, and have met a lot of other carers – who are almost as various as clients – who enjoy it too. The Agency will continue to supply work up to your 70th year, so I may continue with it for some time!

40.2 'BEING A THING CALLED A COMPANION'

Daphne du Maurier

Source: From *Rebecca*, Daphne du Maurier, du Maurier, Gollancz, London, 1938, pp. 19–22.

The morning after the bridge party Mrs Van Hopper woke with a sore throat and a temperature of a hundred and two. I rang up her doctor, who came round at once and diagnosed the usual influenza. 'You are to stay in bed until I allow you to get up,' he told her; 'I don't like the sound of that heart of yours, and it won't get better unless you keep perfectly quiet and still. I should prefer,' he went on, turning to me, 'that Mrs Van Hopper had a trained nurse. You can't possibly lift her. It will only be for a fortnight or so.'

I thought this rather absurd, and protested, but to my surprise she agreed with him. I think she enjoyed the fuss it would create, the sympathy of people, the visits and messages from friends, and the arrival of flowers. Monte Carlo had begun to bore her, and this little illness would make a distraction.

The nurse would give her injections, and a light massage, and she would have a diet. I left her quite happy after the arrival of the nurse, propped up on pillows with a falling temperature, her best bed-jacket round her shoulders and be-ribboned boudoir cap upon her head. Rather ashamed of my light heart, I telephoned her friends, putting off the small party she had arranged for the evening, and went down to the restaurant for lunch, a good half hour before our usual time. I expected the room to be empty – nobody lunched generally before one o'clock. It was empty, except for the table next to ours. This was a contingency for which I was unprepared. I thought he had gone to Sospel. No doubt he was lunching early because he hoped to avoid us at one o'clock. I was already half-way across the room and could not go back. I had not seen him since we disappeared in the lift the day before, for wisely he had avoided dinner in the restaurant, possibly for the same reason that he lunched early now.

It was a situation for which I was ill-trained. I wished I was older, different. I went to our table, looking straight before me, and immediately paid the penalty of gaucherie by knocking over the vase of stiff anemones as I unfolded my napkin. The water soaked the cloth, and ran down on to my lap. The waiter was at the other end of the room, nor had he seen. In a second though my neighbour was by my side, dry napkin in hand.

'You can't sit at a wet tablecloth,' he said brusquely; 'it will put you off your food. Get out of the way.'

He began to mop the cloth, while the waiter, seeing the disturbance, came swiftly to the rescue.

'I don't mind,' I said, 'it doesn't matter a bit. I'm all alone.'

[. . .]

'Your friend,' he began, 'she is very much older than you. Is she a relation? Have you known her long?' I saw he was still puzzled by us.

'She's not really a friend,' I told him, 'she's an employer. She's training me to be a thing called a companion, and she pays me ninety pounds a year.'

'I did not know one could buy companionship,' he said; 'it sounds a primitive idea. Rather like the Eastern slave market.'

'I looked up the word companion once in the dictionary,' I admitted, 'and it said "a companion is a friend of the bosom".'

'You haven't much in common with her,' he said.

He laughed, looking quite different, younger somehow and less detached. 'What do you do it for?' he asked me.

'Ninety pounds is a lot of money to me,' I said.

'Haven't you any family?'

'No – they're dead.'

40.3 IT'S MY PARTY: PERSONAL ASSISTANTS AND YOUR SOCIAL LIFE

Ruth Bailey

Source: S. Vasey, *The Rough Guide to Managing Personal Assistants*, National Centre for Independent Living, London, 1998, pp. 69–76.

I've been using PAs for the last ten years, but it is only in the last year that I have needed, and, crucially, had the funding, to enable me to have PA support when I go out. Yes, this is liberating; less stress about access, as I know, for example, that if there is a step at the front entrance I can send a PA inside to find the side entrance. I do not have to restrict my menu choices to what I can manage to carry or cut up, or have to metaphorically cross my leg for hours on end. Yet liberation, of this sort at least, brings its own headaches...

The question I constantly grapple with now is how to manage my relationship with my PAs, so that, on the one hand I get the help I need and on the other get the space to be alone with my friends. Or simply to be 'alone', in the sense of not having to talk! If only this were an academic question! In fact, daily it sometimes seems to stressed old me, I have to deal with its practical manifestations. Here's a taste of some of them...

Being a keen cinema/theatre goer, should I get my PA a ticket or, given that I don't need assistance once settled in the auditorium, tell them to come back at the end? At first I did the former, but I soon realised that this was expensive – and didn't feel right in terms of my relationship with my PA. If I'd shelled out £20 for a ticket and they didn't seem interested or wouldn't discuss it with me afterwards, I felt pissed off. I knew that was unreasonable on my part, because their job was to assist me, not be my companion. It also made me lazy. I'd think, oh I won't ring so and so and see if she wants to come to the pictures, I'll go with my PA. So now I don't get my PA a ticket, but tell them to bring a book and come back for me at the end of the performance. True, this does lead to some raised eyebrows – 'isn't you're friend coming with you?' ask the trying-to-be-friendly and actually being-patronising box office staff. 'No' I reply, without explanation, which isn't helpful I know but a girl's gotta have a rest...

I do have exceptions to my no ticket policy – or perhaps, more honestly, I should say my policy is inconsistent. Some of my PAs are also good mates, and if there is a particular film we both want to see, I arrange to go and see it when they are working – and pay for their ticket. This can lead me into tricky situations, such as feeling under pressure to go out with my PA, because from her point of view, a night out at the cinema is preferable to doing my ironing. At one stage, I did think that I'd give my PAs a choice. I'd say if she was interested in the play she could come if she wants, provided she buys her own ticket. But I'm beginning to realise that even that only feels OK if I'm fairly friendly with the PA and she knows the friend I'm with. Why? Well on a precious night out with a friend, to share her or him with a PA who I have little in common with – and who I spend more time with than my friends anyway – just isn't what I want.

It has taken me a while to find the confidence to say this, and will probably take even longer to feel OK about it!

More complicated than the ticket question is that of my handling of the role of PAs when I am with other people, say going out for a meal or at a party. When I first started using PAs, I tried to include them in the conversation, 'putting them in the picture' as it were, about whatever it was my friends were talking about. But this was very tiring for me, and it felt the PA was getting to know too much about me and my friends – either that or the conversation never ceased to flow beyond the superficial and, for me, that isn't satisfying. I can remember feeling full of despair that I would never again experience intimate dinners with friends where we talked and talked about really personal stuff. I felt I would lose my sense of being an individual, that I was becoming one of a couple, yet my partner was a PA whom I had no particular knowledge of, or feelings for, and vice versa. (Interestingly, when I am in a relationship, it has always been important to maintain my other friendships, to see friends alone as well as with my partner.)

My next strategy was to try to ignore my PA when I was in social situations, talking with her only so far as was necessary for her to assist me. After all, that is the theory, that a PA's role is to facilitate, and therefore in any social situation, such as when I go out for a meal with friends, they should ideally remain stumm unless talking with me about my needs. This does work ... up to a point, although I am still at that stage of feeling quite uneasy about chatting away to a friend and ignoring the person sitting next to me, cutting up my food, holding my drink, or whatever. And, of course, it is not easy for the friend – still less the stranger, who may never have come across the concept of facilitation. I have yet to come up with a formula of words to explain to those friends and strangers why I am ignoring the person helping me. My fantasy, my fear, is that people think I'm rude, and an ungrateful crip, but hopefully in time I'll get over that, as I convince myself that what I'm doing is OK and I'd quite like them to do the same!

I do try and talk openly with my PAs about all this. Recently, when discussing the role of a PA with an interviewee, she said 'I can be a very good broomstick'. My liberal instinct nearly made me say 'Oh you're a human being, not an inanimate object', but then I realised that actually, this was a pretty good way of describing how I wanted her to be in a particular situation, and I needed to have the confidence to acknowledge this. As an aside, I offered this person the job – but her broomstick skills (and I do think being a 'broomstick', that is being self-effacing, without appearing to be bored or sullen, is a skill, and one which doesn't come easily to a lot of people) do sometimes slip. Once when this happened, I sat there in quite a stew, trying to decide if she was being patronising and intrusive or if it was just me being over-sensitive. Then the friend I was with, a non-disabled woman with no knowledge of PA issues, commented that my PA was a bit OTT motherly. Time to act!

Another problem area for me is my tendency to worry too much about whether my PAs are bored. This has led me into some sticky situations. For example, I swim regularly, and while in the pool I tell my PA to go up to the café and come back to the poolside in twenty minutes. However, some people just don't have a sense of time. On one dramatic occasion, after thirty minutes there was no sign of my PA and I was freezing and seizing up, so I commandeered the help of my friend to get me out and stick me under the shower. Now, my friend has epilepsy, and if he's swim-ming, he gets sufficient warning of a fit to jump out. Unfortunately, while he was being an emergency PA and pulling me up the ramp, he got a warning, but he just tried to keep going, hoping he'd get to the top before passing out. He didn't, and things got a bit hairy for both of us ... When my PA came back, I was pretty angry. It took a friend of mine to point out, that to send my PA off for a coffee was for their convenience, not mine, and I was not really taking due care of myself. It would be perfectly OK for my PA to sit by the pool and read a book, which would then give me the freedom to get out whenever I chose.

As I become a more experienced PA employer/user, I hope that perhaps I can 'let go' a bit and not worry so much about what my PA might or might not say in any given situation. I need to recognise that I can't control a PA – and, more importantly, don't have to – but what I can do is give a clear instruction as to my expectations and my needs, and then trust them to get on with it. Then I will be able to enjoy myself even more, and probably have a much better, more professional, relationship with my PA. Certainly in the early days I craved for somebody to be by my side, teaching me how to be a PA user. That would be good, but in a way one has to learn by doing, by testing things out yourself. After all, we are talking about relationships here, and these have to be shaped by one's own needs and personality – and that of the PA. What feels 'right' with one PA, may not feel so good with another. *The Rough Guide to Managing Per-sonal Assistants* is invaluable, giving reassurance that 'it's not just socially inept me' who struggles with these questions and also a framework for considering them.

INDEX

abuse 56, 125, 139, 181, 185, 197–201
  in care homes 232–239
  of children 9, 52, 205
  of disabled people 250
  of older people 192–193, 197–201,
    227, 245
access 33, 35, 247–248, 338
  for disabled people 278–279, 331,
    364
accommodation 3–4, 14, 127, 201,
    222, 276, 304
  shared 274–275
  see also housing
adult training centres 256, 282
advocacy 245, 248, 253
  see also self-advocacy
African-Caribbean community *see*
    black and minority ethnic groups
age 13, 45, 48, 94, 168, 172, 275
Age Concern 71–73, 75, 124, 249
ageing 47, 49, 122–124, 151–157, 210,
    300
  ageing in place 300
ageism 153–157, 197, 230, 336
almshouses 336
Alzheimer's disease 174–180, 181, 211,
    222, 225–231, 325
animals (pets) 15, 99, 170, 218,
    360–361
assessment
  'care dependency' 6, 306, 308
  disabled people 346–347
  home care 304, 309
  nursing home care 84, 302
  older people 175–177, 178–179,
    192–193, 221, 227, 301–304, 310,
    321–329

  see also risk assessment
Association of Directors of Social
    Services 33
Attendance allowance 324
autonomy 192, 195–197, 200,
    217–223, 268, 296

Barclay Report 47, 104
bathing 4, 9, 205–206, 219, 221, 223,
    227, 233, 291, 323
Benefit Agency 18, 30, 31
benefits 6–7, 24, 33, 35, 42, 171, 201,
    252, 281, 306
Beveridge Plan 30–32, 249
black and minority ethnic groups 105,
    156, 334, 343, 345
  African-Caribbean community
    122–123, 124–126, 127–128
  Bangladeshi community 118,
    122–124, 125, 127–128
  black community 64–65, 121–123,
    127, 128
  Indian 123–124, 126, 128
  Pakistani 122–124, 125, 127–128
  South Asian 121–123, 125, 126, 128,
    129
Blair, Tony 41, 265
blindness *see* visual impairment
bodies 11, 50, 130, 135–136, 143–144,
    163, 168, 226, 292–296
boundaries xii, 5, 12, 263, 285, 296,
    351
  administrative 58, 311, 338
  professional/occupational 5, 313–320
bureaucracies 166, 187, 267, 270, 343
  bureaucratisation 357
  record-keeping 171, 242–245, 280

campaigning 65–67, 69–70, 71, 73–75
care xi, 12, 57, 61–62, 81, 122,
 130–137, 147, 220, 285–298
 care deficit 356
 care dependency *see* assessment
 care homes *see* nursing homes;
  residential homes
 care insurance 306–307, 311
 care managers 6, 268, 301, 342
 care settings 230–231, 240, 263
 commodification 351–361
 contracts 32, 304, 333
 custodial care 54, 146, 216
 intimidation 198, 230
 private sector care 217, 218, 219,
  221, 222, 301
 see also long-term care
Care Orders 281
Care Standards Act 2000 245
Care Trusts 319
care workers 290
carer allowances 352–353, 356–357
carers *see* informal care
Carers and Disabled Children Act 2000
 354
careworkers 153–154, 210, 232, 241,
 285–297, 300, 328, 352, 360–362
Caring for People 34, 317
cash 16–17, 21, 25–27, 30, 35, 41, 45,
 47, 127, 232, 245, 275, 357
 cash benefit option 307–308
 see also direct payments
Castle, Barbara 70
Centres for Independent Living (CILs)
 344, 345
charges 33, 35, 61, 83–86, 174, 216,
 301, 309, 319
charities 17, 91, 238, 241, 259, 276
Child Poverty Action Group 1
childcare 107, 200, 280–284
 adoption 281
children 15, 22–23, 25–27, 36, 96, 99,
 130–137, 206, 250, 277, 281
choice 14–15, 22, 25–26, 41, 76, 85,
 156, 161–162, 192, 195–198, 202,
 216–223, 255–256, 277, 311, 341
CILs *see* Centres for Independent Living
Civil Procedure Rules 248
client involvement *see* user-led groups
clothing 11, 27, 50–51, 93–94, 133,
 136, 141, 148, 176–177, 256, 280,
 291, 295, 360, 363
CMHT *see* Community Mental Health
 Team

coercion 147, 196, 197
commitments *see* responsibilities
common law 198, 248
common sense 183–187
communication 9, 117, 188, 206, 254,
 256, 263, 269, 274, 325, 343–344
communitarianism 100–102, 104–105
communities 87, 89–99, 121–129
 regeneration 103–111
Communities First 108–109
community xi, 87, 100–102, 130–137,
 148–150
community care 32, 53–63, 229,
 265–273, 311, 317, 328–329,
 330–340
 agencies 8
 law 247–254
 virtual 269–270
Community Care Act 1990 249
Community Care (Direct Payments) Act
 1996 264, 341, 354
community development 105–108
Community Health Councils 74
Community Mental Health Team
 (CMHT) 6, 275
companions 212, 264, 327, 360–366
complaints procedures 85, 218, 227,
 343
concealment 11, 248, 296–297
confidence 20, 228, 256, 277
 see also self-esteem
control 5, 54–55, 57, 59–60, 62, 107,
 147, 172, 184, 188, 198, 201, 218,
 220, 260–261, 288, 289
Cooper, David 94–95, 145–146
coping 22, 169, 176, 293–296, 326,
 362
counselling 19
Court of Protection 178
crime 28, 39–40, 53, 100, 199, 334
criminal justice services 183
critical psychiatry 146–148
cultural competence 159–161
Cyrenians 18

dangerously severe personality
 disorders (DSPD) 146
dangerousness 39, 52, 56, 62, 144,
 181, 183–191, 325
Data Protection Act 1998 249
day care 240, 282
 day centres 155, 227, 228, 258–259
death 17, 41, 51, 161, 163, 187, 206,
 228, 237

suicide 7, 144
decarceration 354, 356
decision-making 187, 198, 199, 200, 201, 348
deinstitutionalisation 142
dementia *see* Alzheimer's disease
Denmark 303–306, 311, 352–354
Department of Social Security (DSS) 266
dependence 152–155, 197, 275, 288, 306, 308
depersonalisation 288
depression 5–8, 16, 18, 22, 171, 275
deviancy 24, 27, 138, 139
difference xii, 21, 65–67, 89–102, 144, 161, 173
dignity 21, 139, 221, 222, 326
direct payments 264, 341, 347, 348–349, 352–354
Direct Payments Act 1996 264, 341, 354
disability 11–12, 64–67, 168–173, 250, 301, 302
    barriers 169, 248, 278–279
    beg confinement 289–290
    disabled people's movement 45, 64–68, 173, 341, 359
    employment 45–47
    housing 332–333
    poverty 34
    rights 251, 259
    social model of 64, 67, 278
    support 276, 282
Disability Equality Training 171
Disability Living Allowance 45
Disabled Facilities Grant 337
Disabled Persons (Services, Consultation and Representation) Act 1986 248
discrimination 1, 46, 67, 248, 276
disempowerment 230, 342
domestic help 60, 286, 305
domiciliary care *see* home care
drugs 98, 146, 178–179, 227, 336
    drug abuse 39, 100
    pharmaceutical industry 147
DSPD *see* dangerously severe personality disorders
DSS *see* Department of Social Security

economic policy 31, 107, 265–266
elderly people *see* older people
eligibility criteria 217, 301, 303, 322, 327–329

emergency accommodation 16, 282
Emergency Housing Officer 14
emotions 3, 153, 158–167, 234
    emotional capacity 115, 200
    emotional labour 29, 164–165, 212, 293–294, 361
employment 19, 45–47, 60, 98, 126–127, 159, 169, 266
empowerment 8, 163, 172, 185, 200, 230, 346
entitlements 7, 51–52, 311, 325
environment
    of kin 112, 115
    locks 9, 94, 146, 206, 223, 226, 229
    protected 6, 95
ethnicity *see* black and minority ethnic groups; race
Europe 229, 299–312
Exceptional Hardship payments 30
exile 3–4
experts 11, 147–148, 186, 188, 190, 221, 223, 260, 270, 325, 348
Expert Patients Task Force 148

familiarity 78
families 14, 32, 36–37, 43, 50, 87, 228–229
    community care 32, 36–37, 55–57, 61, 303
    extended 79, 92, 112, 118, 170
    family life 97–98, 112–120, 251
    family support 6, 83–86, 168, 174–180, 361
    older people 194, 219, 300, 303
    social change 112–120
    ties 113, 115, 124–126, 226
    see also informal care
Family Law Act 1996 200
feminism 61, 64–66, 357
festivals 97, 98
    Christmas 18, 22, 26, 72
food 16, 18, 21–22, 26, 51–52, 132–133, 176, 187–188, 218, 242–243, 360–361, 365
    malnourishment 21–22, 194, 200, 227–228, 233, 275
football 89–91
foster care 8–9, 281, 331
    adult foster care 240
Foucault, Michel 188–189
freedom 42, 55, 76, 97, 124, 198, 207, 366
    see also autonomy; choice

freedom of expression 145–146, 251–252
friends 6–7, 14, 29, 46, 55, 79, 96, 117, 161, 172–173, 206, 365

gender 11–12, 34, 40–41, 229, 287, 358
general practitioners (GPs) 7, 19, 95, 178, 194, 200, 226, 233, 283, 323
genetic screening 61
Germany 306–308, 311
Griffiths Report 1988 268–269, 317–318
groups 20, 160, 169, 212, 214, 260, 269–270, 345
guardianship 54, 57–58
Guardianship Society, Brighton 59

health care 147, 313–320, 321–329
  see also National Health Service
Health and Safety legislation 185, 242
health services 107, 278, 306
  see also National Health Service
Health and Social Services and Social Security Adjudications Act 1983 34
helplessness 196
Herefordshire Lifestyles 276–279
holidays 26, 92, 127, 282
home 43, 57, 81, 97–98, 207, 277, 285–289, 300, 330–340
home care 34, 194, 240, 263, 299–313, 315
home help 174, 194, 282, 283, 300, 304–305, 309, 314, 322
homelessness 14–19, 275, 282
hospitalisation 5–11, 46, 51, 174–175, 274–275, 288–289, 300, 302, 315
hospitals 11, 205–208, 220
  admission 9, 17, 168, 174, 206, 315, 331
  bed blocking 175, 314
  bed closures 74, 149, 301
  day hospital 7
  discharge 5–8, 300, 331
  doctors 11, 83–84, 174, 206, 314
  geriatric beds 84, 314–316
hostels 4, 13, 14, 55, 206–207, 275
hotels 174, 216–217, 222
house calls 274–275
households 269
  expenditure 42
  low income 42, 335, 338
  structure 114, 124–126

housing 34, 126–128, 149–150, 281, 304, 310, 330–340
  affordability 43, 331, 335
  benefits 6, 32, 335
  services 14, 18
human error 184
Human Rights Act 1998 181, 182, 247–254
human services 140, 141, 185–186, 190, 267
hygiene 4, 218, 242
  dirt 14, 24, 39, 42, 56, 176, 200, 232, 286, 292–297

ICA see Invalid Care Allowance
ICTs see information and communication technologies
identity xii, 12, 13, 21, 65, 87–89, 143–144, 160, 162, 165–166, 168, 171–172, 177, 213, 285, 288–289, 330
illness 5, 44, 46, 122–124, 171, 174, 227, 270, 287, 306, 317, 331, 360
  diabetes 168, 206
  sickle cell anaemia 90–91
immigrants see migration
impairment 11–12, 64, 66, 84, 192, 210, 252, 279
Incapacity benefit 7, 45, 46
inclusion 31, 37, 105–106, 109, 146
  see also social exclusion
income 6, 42, 99, 306
Income Support 16, 31, 333
independence 61, 151–157, 168, 181, 216–224, 275, 341
  see also autonomy
independent living 181, 339, 345, 347–348, 356
inequality xii, 1, 31, 35, 67, 128–129, 147, 345
infantilisation 230, 293
informal care 29, 130–137, 153, 175, 300, 328, 351–353, 356
information and communication technologies (ICTs) 265–271
Inspection Units see Registration and Inspection Units
institutional care 53–54, 56, 169
institutionalisation 210, 212
institutions 8–11, 148–150, 311
insurance 31, 43, 306, 308, 311
inter-agency cooperation 8, 107–108, 193, 198, 263, 342
  see also team work

Internet 263, 269, 270
Invalid Care Allowance (ICA) 352
Invalidity Benefit 32
Ireland 13, 40, 43, 92–93
isolation 3, 14, 23, 47, 115, 122–123, 125, 147, 156, 170, 173, 214, 229, 236

Jones, Jack 70–71

labelling 27–28, 38–41, 139, 230, 258–259, 261, 336
labour market 42, 303, 356
Laing, R.D. 94, 145
learning difficulties 53–62, 88, 185, 241, 250–251, 281, 282
    Down's syndrome 58
    older people 151–157
    self-advocacy 182, 255–262
legal representation 247
legislation 181, 247–253, 261
liberation 145–146, 149, 364
life cycle 42
Lister, Ruth 31, 357
litigation friend 248
local authorities 33, 34–35
    community development 107
    councils 238, 303–304
    direct payments 341–345, 349
    guardianship 54, 281
    home care 300–311
    housing 332, 334
    local democracy 303
    municipalities 304
    nursing home care 84
    residential homes 216, 219–222, 240
    service provision 252, 313–317, 341–350
    unitary authorities 317
Local Authority Social Services Act 1970 282
Local Government Anti-Poverty Unit 33
London 43–45, 95–96, 112, 184
lone parents 24–25, 39, 42, 101, 269, 334
long-term care 61, 75, 148, 196, 317–318

marriage 6, 13–19, 43, 50, 56, 87, 177, 207, 212, 356
means-testing 33, 35, 313
media 24, 27–28, 70, 72, 74, 94, 184
medication 4, 46, 94, 147, 175, 179, 226–228, 242, 245, 274–275, 295, 323
    see also drugs
memory 51, 92–93, 179, 208, 274
mental capacity 198, 199, 200, 248
Mental Deficiency Act 1913 53–54, 61
Mental Deficiency Act 1927 54
mental health 5, 9, 45, 94, 146–147, 184, 241, 249, 275
Mental Health Act 1959 283
Mental Health Act 1983 146, 200, 247
Mr Micawber 41
migration 40, 125–126
    see also refugees
MIND 249
models 147, 172, 211, 223, 230, 291, 314, 348, 357
    see also disability
Modernising Government 317
Modernising Social Services 187, 240
moral panic 184
multi-agency see inter-agency
multicultural society 87, 119, 159

National Assistance Act 1948 200, 314
National Centre for Independent Living (NCIL) 264, 342
National Health Service Act 1946 314
National Health Service and Community Care Act 1990 317, 318
National Health Service (NHS) 266, 268, 301, 311, 314, 318–319
national insurance see insurance
National Lottery Charities Board 278
National Schizophrenia Fellowship 46–47
National Service Frameworks 146
NCIL see National Centre for Independent Living
needs 48–49, 50–52, 87, 104, 121–129, 216, 270, 323–324, 327–328, 365
negative freedom 196, 198
neglect 57–58, 61, 175
neighbours 29, 50, 101, 283, 356
The Netherlands 308–311
networks see social networks
New Age travellers 96–99
New Deal 36, 46
New Labour 36–37, 41, 45, 70, 103–104, 146, 319
NHS see National Health Service

normalisation 46, 87–88, 138–143, 152, 156–157
 normality 12, 27, 57, 145, 151, 169, 172, 189, 221
North Staffs Pensioners Convention 69–75
NSPCC 281
nurses 89, 226, 241, 297, 361, 363
 community nurses 302, 309
 community psychiatric nurses 283
 district 58, 227, 283, 321–329
 health visitors 54, 281, 283
 home nursing 300–311, 314
 hospital nurses 17, 45–46, 51, 94–95, 174, 206, 281
 nursing 292, 315
nursing home care 76–82, 83–86, 155, 212, 241, 310, 311

objectivity 188
occupational therapists 283, 323
older people 31, 48, 50
 abuse 232–239
 assessment 321–329
 care 263, 299–312, 313–320
 caring for 174–180
 citizenship 311
 disabilities 66, 302
 families 112–120, 300
 learning difficulties 151–157
 minority communities 121–129
 poverty 25, 37
 residential care 76–82, 209–214, 216–223, 232–239, 240–246, 250, 282
 self-determination 192, 197–201
 see also pensioners
on-line help 269–270
one-to-one assistance 276
oppression 64–68, 163–164, 169, 173, 196, 262
oral history 57, 60
owner occupation 332–333

paid volunteering 355, 356
panic attacks 45
PASS see Program Analysis of Service Systems
paternalism 42, 192, 197, 221, 270
patronising behaviour 155, 230, 366
pensioners 69–75
pensions 31, 32, 43, 216
pensions-earnings link 69–70
People First 255

personal assistance 264, 300
Personal Assistants 346, 348–349, 364–366
personal budgets 310
personal care 302, 304, 311
personal competence 139, 141
personal development 171
personhood 181, 216, 229
police 48, 50, 94, 100, 193, 194, 200, 226, 234, 237
Poor Law 38, 58, 216, 249, 315
1991 Population Census 123, 125
positive freedom 196
poverty 1, 13–19, 20–28, 29–37, 38–41, 42, 50–51, 58, 127, 147
 effects of 21–27, 99
 labelling 27–28, 38–41
 social services 29–37
power xii, 1, 21, 26, 33, 64, 106, 220, 285, 289
 power relations 158, 264
power of attorney 178
pregnancy 14–17, 23, 96
prisons 27, 144, 176, 178, 188, 206, 281
privacy 181, 182, 216–224, 251, 285, 287, 291, 292–296, 307, 330
private rented housing 332
probation officers 184, 281, 283
Program Analysis of Service Systems (PASS) 140
protection 183–186, 192, 193, 206
psychiatry 22, 93–95, 146–148
psychological care 139, 225–231
Psychology Service 6, 7
psychotherapy 6
Public Assistance Act 1948 288
Public Assistance Institutions 216
public authorities 249
public protection see protection

R&I see Registration and Inspection Units
Race Awareness Training 163
race equality 158–167, 345
racialisation 159, 291, 295
racism 15, 44, 65, 67, 90, 125, 128, 144, 164–165
 institutional racism 166
referrals 6, 34, 301, 304
The Reform of Social Security: Programme for Action 31
Refugee Council 3–4
refugees 4, 93–94

Registered Homes (Amendment) Act 1991 240
Registration and Inspection (R&I) Units 234–237, 240–246, 301
rehabilitation 5–8, 168–169, 300, 315
reinstitutionalisation 156, 249
relationships 1, 79
    caring 29, 281
    older people 113–119
    poverty 23–25
religion 10, 17, 93, 142, 144, 161–162, 259, 361
    the church 38, 71
    churches 4, 11, 24, 206
research methods 20, 77, 114, 160, 218, 230, 241, 321–322
residential care 32, 205–208, 232–239
    adjustment to 76–82, 209–215
    older people 76–82, 155, 177, 209–214, 216–223, 227, 250, 282
    small homes 240–246
    trends 304, 307, 310–311
residualisation 35–36, 334
resources 8, 33, 105, 252–253, 310, 313, 327
responsibility 181, 209, 263, 358
    collective 84, 229, 281, 311, 316
    personal 42–43, 51, 100, 113, 169, 172, 255, 333, 342
revolving door syndrome 275
Right to Buy 333
rights xii, 35, 41–43, 51, 65, 67, 87, 181–182, 221, 247, 311
    disabled people 251, 252, 259, 279
    individual 162
    older people 192
    parental 52, 58, 281
    to life 249–250
risk xii, 165, 181–182, 183–191, 192, 197–198, 216–224, 252, 326
risk assessment 186, 188, 190, 325
risk management 184, 189–190, 219, 220–222
RNIB 169, 171
roles 61, 113, 138–139, 170, 263
rural communities 11, 92–93, 98, 105, 360–361

safety 45, 55–56, 187, 197
SCAR see Sickle Cell Anaemia Relief
schizophrenia 45–46, 145–146, 275
Scope 34, 345
Scotland 33, 181, 321
security 3, 15, 115, 222, 334

Seebohm 32, 282
self-advocacy 8, 20, 182, 247, 252, 255–262
self-determination 181, 192–204, 291
self-esteem 61, 91, 139, 277
self-fulfilling prophecy 27, 153
self-help groups 269–270
sexism 65, 67, 127
sexual activity 9–10, 56, 59, 189, 248, 251, 259
Sexual Offences Act 1956 251
sexuality 65–67, 189, 251, 291–292, 294
sheltered housing 310, 337
    extra-care 240
shopping 15, 21, 23, 24, 51, 96, 142, 148, 174, 225–226, 276, 304–305
sick leave 42, 170
sick role 139
Sickle Cell Anaemia Relief (SCAR) 90–91
smoking 10, 15, 148, 169, 220–221
social care 158–167, 220–222, 263–264, 266, 313–320, 321–329, 341–349
    needs 121–129
social class 13, 39, 40, 45, 48–49, 59, 66–67
    middle class 49, 90, 118–119, 286
    working class 49, 89
    see also underclass
social exclusion 31, 107, 147, 152, 231, 334–335, 344
Social Fund 30, 31, 34
social images 139, 141
social life 290
social movements 12, 20, 64–65, 69–75, 189
    see also disabled people's movement
social networks 5, 77, 79, 112–120, 125, 156, 212–213, 310
social psychology 230–231
social security 17, 24, 30–32, 99, 252, 281, 301
social services 29–37, 47–50, 61, 85, 159, 266–269, 278, 299, 312
    older people 176, 220, 226–227
    poverty 29–37
    risk assessment 187–188
    see also human services
Social Services Inspectorate (SSI) 192, 266
social settings 144
social systems 140

social work 29–37, 47, 162, 192–204, 280–284
  codes of ethics 184–185
  values 194–195, 218, 222, 267
social workers 6, 51–52, 200, 208, 227
  hospice social workers 159–162
  ICTs 267
  intuition 194
  medical social workers 282
  and older people 83–84, 193, 194, 227, 321, 322–328
  poverty 30, 32, 33
societal integration 142
special needs housing 331, 335, 336–337
SSI see Social Services Inspectorate
stereotypes 5, 98, 121, 142, 144, 151–152, 154, 156, 194, 269, 336
sterilisation 61
stigma 14, 50, 66, 139, 141, 143–145, 147, 216
  dementia 230
  homelessness 19
  learning difficulties 88, 152
  poverty 23–24, 27, 29, 32, 37, 38
  single pregnant women 14
Stoke-on-Trent 69–75, 89–92
strangers 50–52, 144, 220, 286–287, 291, 365
stress 4, 21–22, 46, 125, 175, 229–230
support 1, 6, 19, 274–284
support networks 8, 214
support schemes 343
supported housing 336
Supporting People 337
Sure Start 36
surveillance 37, 54, 62, 223
survival 42, 51–52, 147

taxation 303, 311
team work 5, 81, 283–284
telephones 117–118, 177, 227, 361
television 22, 73, 132, 134–135, 176, 222, 226, 269, 271, 361
tenure 331–332
territories xii, 263, 290
Thatcher, Margaret 104, 249
Titmus, Richard 35
Townsend, Peter 114, 216
training 54, 59, 171, 231, 245, 284
  self-advocacy 256–257

transport 14–17, 26, 44, 70, 92, 95–96, 99, 115, 127, 187
  disabled people 45, 67, 169, 258

underclass 27–28, 40, 104–105
unemployment 32, 42, 43–45, 127, 147, 169
Unemployment Assistance Board 43–45
United Response 275
United States 38–41, 100–102, 104, 138, 353
universalism 32, 308
user-led groups 346–347
  user involvement 140, 147, 326–327
users 152, 161, 185

values 104, 195, 198, 218, 286, 311, 344
Values Into Action 348
victims 42, 196, 200, 201, 210
violence 44, 53, 90, 93, 235
visual impairment 88, 168–173, 326
voluntary organisations 58–59, 65, 72, 105, 241, 268, 355
  non-profit foundations 309
voluntary support 126, 276–280, 324
voluntary work 46, 51, 56, 74

wages 60, 353
  routed wages 353–354, 356–357
Wales 13–19, 103–111
welfare xi, 29, 32, 38–52, 58, 221, 349
  agencies 185, 282
  recipients 47
  rights 41–43, 84–85
  services 299–311
  welfare state 30, 32, 42, 51–52, 61, 84, 104, 189, 249, 299, 311, 351, 354, 356
  see also benefits
Welfare Rights Office 7
welfare-to-work 45, 61
whiteness 159, 165
Winter Fuel Allowance 73
Wolverhampton 112, 171
work 18–19, 165
  disincentives 45–47
  learning difficulties 57, 59–60, 61
  unpaid 351
working class see social class
Working Families Tax Credit 36
WRVS 282